SOCIAL DETERMINANTS OF HEALTH

An interdisciplinary approach to social inequality and well-being

Edited by Adrian Bonner

GW00496777

P

First published in Great Britain in 2018 by

Policy Press   North America office:
University of Bristol   Policy Press
1-9 Old Park Hill   c/o The University of Chicago Press
Bristol   1427 East 60th Street
BS2 8BB   Chicago, IL 60637, USA
UK   t: +1 773 702 7700
t: +44 (0)117 954 5940   f: +1 773-702-9756
pp-info@bristol.ac.uk   sales@press.uchicago.edu
www.policypress.co.uk   www.press.uchicago.edu

© Policy Press 2018

British Library Cataloguing in Publication Data
A catalogue record for this book is available from the British Library

Library of Congress Cataloging-in-Publication Data
A catalog record for this book has been requested

ISBN 978-1-4473-3685-3 paperback
ISBN 978-1-4473-3684-6 hardcover
ISBN 978-1-4473-3687-7 ePub
ISBN 978-1-4473-3688-4 Mobi
ISBN 978-1-4473-3686-0 epdf

For Gill, Adam, Kirsten, Gemma, Jake, Hope,

Thea, Cassian and Freya.

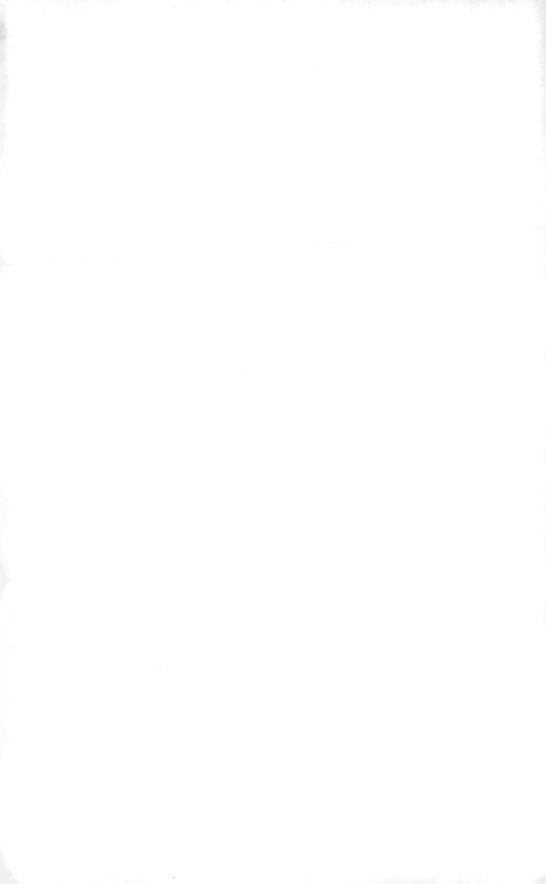

Contents

List of tables and figures

Tables

Figures

Notes on contributors

Editor

Adrian Bonner

Addictive behaviour: Molecules to mankind (Bonner and Waterhouse, 1996) is the title of the book that symbolises the trajectory of Adrian's academic career. His early research was concerned with neurobiological aspects of alcohol, as reflected in publications and teaching activities in the 1990s at the Universities of Surrey and Kent (UK). At this time, he became Chairman of the Congress of the European Society for Biomedical Research into Alcohol (Bonner, 2005). *Social exclusion and the way out: An individual and community response to human social dysfunction* (Bonner, 2006) provided the basis for research into *The seeds of exclusion* (Bonner, Luscombe et al, 2008), a major report that continues to influence Salvation Army strategic planning. These activities were undertaken while he was a Reader in the Centre for Health Service Studies, University of Kent, and was Director of the Addictive Behaviour Group, which facilitated the development of undergraduate and postgraduate teaching and research activities.

From 2010 to 2012, he was seconded from the University of Kent to become the Director of the Institute of Alcohol Studies. This involved participating in the UK government's Responsibility Deal (Bonner and Gilmore, 2012) and membership of the European Alcohol Health Forum, an advisory group supporting the work of the European Commission. These insights into UK and European policy development have influenced his current activities, which include interdisciplinary research into health inequalities and local political action working with the London Borough of Sutton. Current research, as Honorary Professor in the Faculty of Social Science at the University of Stirling, focuses on the impact of economic austerity policies on health, social care and housing strategies.

References
Bonner, A.B. (ed) (2005) *10th Congress of the European Society for Biomedical Research into Alcohol, Canterbury, 4–7 September*, Oxford: Oxford University Press.

Bonner, A.B. (2006) *Social exclusion and the way out: An individual and community response to human social dysfunction*, Chichester: John Wiley & Sons.

Bonner, A.B. and Gilmore, I. (2012) 'The UK Responsibility Deal and its implications for effective alcohol policy in the UK and internationally' (Invited Editorial), *Addiction*, 107: 2063–5.

Bonner, A.B. and Waterhouse, J. (eds) (1996) *Addictive behaviour: Molecules to mankind*, Macmillan Press.

Bonner, A.B., Luscombe, C., Van den Bree, M. and Taylor, P.J. (2008) *The seeds of exclusion*, London: The Salvation Army.

Contributors

Anne-Marie Bagnall

Dr Anne-Marie Bagnall is a Reader in Evidence Synthesis (Health Inequalities) in the Centre for Health Promotion Research at Leeds Beckett University. She is also an Associate Lecturer for the UK Cochrane Centre Learn and Teach Faculty, and a member of the What Works for Wellbeing Centre's Communities Evidence Programme and National Methods Advisory Group.

Clare Bambra

Clare Bambra is Professor of Public Health at Newcastle University. Her research examines the political, social and economic determinants of health; and how public policies and interventions can reduce health inequalities. She is the Associate Director for Health Inequalities in Fuse: Centre for Translational Research in Public Health and an Executive Member of the National Institute for Health Research School for Public Health Research where she is a Senior Investigator on the Communities in Control Project. She holds a Leverhulme Research Leadership Award which examines Local Health Inequalities in an Age of Austerity and she is the Principal Investigator on the Norface-funded grant 'HiNEWS' which examines health inequalities in Europe with partners in Norway, the US and Germany. She is also a collaborator on the ESRC Rethinking Incapacity project. She works closely with public health policy and practice and is currently the co-Director of the Equal North: Research and Practice Network in partnership with Public Health England.

Claire Bonham

Claire Bonham currently works as the Volunteer Development Manager at The Salvation Army, where she is responsible for volunteering across the UK and Ireland. Claire has over 15 years' experience of working with volunteers in a variety of sectors, including International Development and Criminal Justice. Claire has a PhD in International Relations from the University of Exeter, focussing on international social movements.

Naomi Brooks

Dr Naomi Brooks is a Lecturer in Sport, Health and Exercise Science at the University of Stirling. She has a PhD from Ohio University, and has been a Post-Doctoral Fellow in Human Nutrition at Tufts University (Boston) and Post-Doctoral Associate at Stellenbosch University (South Africa).

Katherine Brown

Katherine Brown is Director of the Institute of Alcohol Studies, an independent research institute that brings together evidence, policy and practice from home and abroad to promote an informed debate on alcohol's impact on society.

Paul Burstow

Professor Paul Burstow is a social policy entrepreneur and thought leader. He chairs the Tavistock and Portman NHS Foundation Trust, is Professor of Mental Health Public Policy at the University of Birmingham and Chair of the National Advisory Board of Design Council project Transform Ageing. He was a Liberal Democrat MP for Sutton and Cheam between 1997 and 2015. He served as the Minister for State for Care Services between 2010 and 2012. In that role, he covered a range of social policy issues, including mental health, adult social care, carers, personal health budgets, safeguarding vulnerable adults, end-of-life care and long-term conditions. He is a member of the Privy Council.

Steve Coles

Steve Coles is the Chief Executive Officer of Spitalfields Crypt Trust (SCT), an addictions recovery and homelessness charity in east London. Prior to that, he founded and ran Intentionality CIC, a social enterprise and well-being consultancy that worked with 600 social enterprises over 6 years. Steve has an MBA from Imperial College, London with a dissertation on social entrepreneurship and the well-being of NEET young people.

Nathan Critchlow

Nathan Critchlow is a researcher at the Institute for Social Marketing. He is a graduate of Manchester Metropolitan University and the University of Liverpool, and completed his PhD studies at the University of Stirling. His primary research interests are alcohol and tobacco marketing, consumer behaviour, and health policy. His recent research includes digital alcohol marketing, new media, sport sponsorship, and tobacco pricing. He has previously worked with the Salvation Army UK and Ireland and teaches on postgraduate and professional development courses through the UK Centre for Tobacco and Alcohol Studies.

Rosalind Fallaize

Dr Rosalind Fallaize is a Lecturer in Nutrition and Dietetics at the University of Hertfordshire and Research Fellow at the University of Reading. She is a registered dietician and member of the British Dietetic Association (BDA). Her research interests include dietary assessment, eating behaviour, e-health, nutritional genomics and health inequalities. Dr Fallaize has collaborated with Crime Reduction Initiatives, the Salvation Army (SA) and Good Food Oxford in order to advance the development of a UK-wide strategy for the improvement of nutritional status in the homeless community.

Deborah Fortescue

Deborah Fortescue is a consultant and previously Head of Foundation at the Disabilities Trust. Deborah has designed and led programmes to support people with acquired brain injury (ABI) within prisons and the community, and supported research in the field of ABI in the homeless, prison and veteran populations.

Jon Foster

Jon Foster is a Senior Research and Policy Officer at the Institute of Alcohol Studies and leads on the Institute's work on alcohol licensing.

Kayleigh Garthwaite

Dr Kayleigh Garthwaite is a Birmingham Fellow in the School of Social Policy, University of Birmingham. Kayleigh explores issues of health inequalities, welfare reform, and austerity through ethnographic research. She is author of *Hunger pains: Life inside foodbank Britain* (Policy

Press, 2016) and co-author of *Poverty and insecurity: Life in 'low-pay, no-pay' Britain* (Policy Press, 2012).

Neil Hamlet

Dr Neil Hamlet is a Consultant in Public Health Medicine NHS, Fife (Scotland). He has worked as an International Consultant for the World Health Organization (WHO), studying at the University of Glasgow, Liverpool School of Tropical Medicine and the Research Institute of Tuberculosis, Kiyose (Japan). Neil is currently leading the development of Scottish government policies aimed at reducing the impact of health and social inequalities on public health.

Jean Hannah

Dr Jean Hannah (MBChB, DRCOG, MSc, FRCGP) works as a general practitioner. Currently, she is undertaking PhD research at the University of Stirling into the use of Realist Evaluation in a community programme for people accessing Salvation Army services in three communities in Scotland, with a particular focus on people with Alcohol Related Brain Damage (ARBD).

Katy Hetherington

Katy has worked for NHS Health Scotland for 10 years. Prior to NHS Health Scotland, Katy worked in the Scottish government, including in education policy and in the Minister for Health's private office, where she developed a keen interest in the causes of health inequalities. She has a MA(Hons) Psychology and a MSc in Human Resource Management.

Nigel Hewett

Dr Nigel Hewett (OBE, MB, ChB, DRCOG, DCH, FRCGP) is a general practitioner who has worked with homeless people since 1990. In 2006, he was awarded an OBE for services to homeless people. In 2009, he launched University College London Hospital's Pathway homeless team. In 2010, he was a founder member of the Faculty for Homeless and Inclusion Health of the College of Medicine, and in 2011, he became Medical Director of Pathway – a new charity formed to improve the health care of homeless people and other excluded groups and to support the faculty.

Kirstin Kerr

Dr Kirstin Kerr is a Senior Lecturer in Education at the Manchester Institute of Education, University of Manchester (UK). Her research explores how educational inequalities arise and are sustained over time

in neighbourhood and community contexts, with a particular focus
on how policymakers and practitioners can intervene more effectively
in the link between education, disadvantage and place. Much of her
work is in active partnership with schools, local authorities and third
sector organisations who are seeking to develop and evaluate complex,
localised responses to educational disadvantage.

Julie Lovegrove

Julie Lovegrove is a Professor of Human Nutrition, Director of the
Hugh Sinclair Unit of Human Nutrition and Deputy Director of
the Institute of Cardiovascular and Metabolic Research (ICMR) at
the University of Reading. Her research focuses on investigations
into nutritional influences of metabolic syndrome development and
increased cardiovascular risk, including nutrient–gene interactions, and
she is currently developing UK-wide research into nutrition and health
and social inequalities. She is a registered nutritionist and member of
the UK government's Scientific Advisory Committee on Nutrition
(SACN), the Saturated Fat Working Group and Rolling National Diet
and Nutrition Survey (NDNS) Programme Committee, and Deputy
Chair of the Council for the Association for Nutrition (Afn).

Claire Luscombe

Claire Luscombe has a PhD from the University of Kent based on a
large diagnostic study into the mental health needs of homeless people
using Salvation Army services. She currently manages the Salvation
Army's National Monitoring and Evaluation Scheme.

Nick Maguire

Dr Nick Maguire is Deputy Head of Psychology within the
Department of Psychology at the University of Southampton. As a
qualified clinical psychologist, he previously worked for the NHS,
focusing on reducing antisocial behaviours and concomitant eviction
rates in homeless people. He is a member of the All Party Parliamentary
Group for complex needs and mental health. He is a founding member
of the Faculty of Homeless and Inclusion Health.

Barbara McIntosh

Barbara studied Social Work and Anthropology at McMaster University
(Canada), then an MSc in Health and Social Policy at the LSE
(London). She was Commissioner for Learning Disability Services in
the London Borough of Sutton, then National Programme Manager
for Learning Disabilities at the Kings Fund. Until 2014, Barbara was

Director at the Mental Health Foundation, working in children's mental health and in developing new community-based services for people with learning disabilities.

Joyce Melican
Joyce Melican is a local authority councillor and currently Deputy Mayor of the London Borough of Sutton. She lives in and engages with her local community, and has a grounded insight into the lives of people who are precariously placed in the community. Before becoming involved in politics, she was a local authority senior housing officer. Joyce is a certified member of the Chartered Institute of Housing.

Gayle Munro
Dr Gayle Munro has held research and teaching positions at the Salvation Army (London), Lemos&Crane (London), the European Centre for Minority Issues (Germany), the Organisation for Security and Cooperation in Europe (Bosnia) and Sichuan University (China). Her doctoral work explored the transnational and diasporic experiences of migrants from the former Yugoslavia in the UK. She also has an MA in Politics, Security and Integration (School of Slavonic & East European Studies, 2002).

Amy Greer Murphy
Amy Greer Murphy is a PhD student in the Department of Geography, Durham University. Amy has a BA in Sociology & Social Policy from Trinity College, Dublin, and an MA in Gender, Media & Culture from Goldsmiths College, University of London. Her research focuses on the experiences of austerity and welfare reform for mothers living in Stockton-on-Tees.

Michael Oddy
Professor Michael Oddy has worked in brain injury rehabilitation for more than 30 years and was Director of Clinical Services for the Disabilities Trust. A former Chair of the British Psychological Society Divisions of Neuropsychology, he is Honorary Professor of Psychology at the University of Wales. An authority on brain injury, Professor Oddy was the clinical lead on the first UK study into the prevalence of traumatic brain injury in the homeless community.

Andrew Parnham
Dr Andrew Parnham trained and worked as a medical doctor for some years before spending most of the next 30 years in community work in

South London and abroad. He trained as a life coach and now works independently and with the charity Livability as a well-being trainer, coach and advisor.

Sara da Silva Ramos

Dr Sara da Silva Ramos is a chartered psychologist. She joined the Disabilities Trust in 2011, where she is currently focusing on the outcome of Acquired Brain Injury rehabilitation and is evaluating the usefulness of technology to support independent living.

Katherine Smith

Dr Katherine Smith is a Reader in the Global Public Health Unit at the University of Edinburgh, where she analyses policies impacting on public health (especially health inequalities) and processes of advocacy, lobbying and knowledge translation in public health.

Jenny Svanberg

Dr Jenny Svanberg is a consultant clinical psychologist working in the NHS Forth Valley Alcohol and Drug Partnership. She became a principal clinical psychologist in 2007, working in Glasgow Addiction Service, and specialised in the assessment and treatment of adults with Alcohol Related Brain Damage (ARBD).

Charles West

Charles West has spent over 30 years as a general practitioner (GP) in Shropshire, where he also taught and assessed new doctors and appraised established GPs. He also spent five years as an NHS General Manager and led a directorate at the NHS Information Authority. He served as a local councillor and stood for parliament. Nationally, he is well known for his critical commentary on the regulatory framework of the Health and Social Care Act 2012 and management of the NHS at this time of economic austerity.

Acknowledgements

The term 'expert by experience' is often given to service users and the beneficiaries of statutory and voluntary services provided for those in need of support. This term could be used for each one of us when we enter this world and depend so much on others for support. From my earliest memories, I have so many rich experiences provided by Bram and Olive, my parents, who, at a time of limited food and domestic resources in the post-war years of the 1950s, provided a safe and secure environment, giving me a good start to life that has been enriched by many people and relationships over the years. Gill, my wife, continues to provide an insight into the social determinants of health from 30 years of providing educational leadership and wisdom for the many staff and children at a school in South London, where social deprivation is not uncommon. My children have been instrumental in showing me the complexities of human development in this changing and increasingly technology-dependent world. My son, Adam, inspiring people by his commitment to leading and being immersed in community development, and his wife, Gemma, with her artistic skills, work at local and national levels in contributing to the development of healthy communities. My daughter, through her training as a general practitioner, works with people with a wide range of physical and psychosocial issues, some at the edge of life, and her husband, Jake, is personally and professionally committed to making this a more sustainable world through increasing the use of renewable energy. Their role models as good parents are nurturing the next generation. Hope, Thea, Cassian and Freya are maturing into a very different world, with unpredictable living and working conditions. This functioning family unit, living in a healthy community, is self-supporting to a large degree and has little reliance on the statutory services described in this book but is very much aware of the need for effective health and care services in the community.

My life experience has benefited from friends and professional colleagues, all of whom have contributed unknowingly to the concept of this book. I am deeply grateful to Colonel Alan Burns for his significant impact on the management and organisational change of the wide-ranging services of the Salvation Army (SA) in the UK, making it 'Fit for Mission' in the 21st century. Major Paul Kingscott has journeyed with me in attempting to understand the nature of social exclusion. He continues to provide leadership of the addiction, homelessness, older persons and other social services provided by the SA. Jacqui King,

Director of the SA Research and Development Unit, with her critical analytical skills in supporting the organisation in the use of its resources in the development of new projects, has provided opportunities to discuss approaches to measuring impact and developing an evidence-based approach to programme-building developments across the UK. Some insights into the SA's work are highlighted in Chapters Eight, Nine, Twelve, Seventeen and Twenty-one.

Councillor Ruth Dombey OBE, Leader of Sutton Borough Council, has provided inspirational political and managerial leadership of a local authority attempting to maintain and develop services for local people in the face of decreasing funding from central government. Her underlying approach to developing an open, tolerant and fair society has promoted a stable, effective council providing housing, health and social care, and other services (see Chapter Fifteen). She represents a 'Flagship Borough' that has impacted on national policy via the community-based activities of former local MP, Paul Burstow (see Chapter Twenty-two).

An important contribution to local health and social care has been influenced by Pete Flavell and other Directors of HealthWatch Sutton, including Barbara McIntosh (see Chapter Ten).

I am indebted to Professor Alison Bowes and her colleagues at the University of Stirling, who have provided an academic base for the application of social science through the development of a Salvation Army-funded research centre within the university. This evidence-based approach to understanding the needs of people with problematic alcohol and other lifestyle issues will hopefully provide a unique insight into the development of community-based approaches for vulnerable people who need support beyond that which can be provided by their families and social networks. Some examples of this collaboration are given in Chapters Four, Seven and Twelve.

I am indebted to the enthusiasm and insight of the contributors to this book. A combination of many years of practical and academic support for people experiencing social inequality and poor well-being has resulted in this interdisciplinary perspective.

People at the edge of the community, to some extent, are the victims of a range of complex societal changes, and have low political priority in this time of austerity budgets and increasingly right-wing social policies that increase social and health inequalities. Hopefully, increased understanding and communication between service providers and family members will support those in need and help to empower them to make or regain their contribution to a healthy society.

As a humble expert by experience, my intention in bringing this edited volume together is to provide an interdisciplinary perspective on the interlinked domains of Dahlgren and Whitehead's model of social determinants of health, focused on the needs of people with multiple complex needs, in order to inform appropriate community responses.

Professor Adrian Bonner, April 2017

Preface

In the UK general election of May 2015, the main political parties pledged to develop economic growth and encourage a fairer society. In the snap general election of 2017, the main focus was on the withdrawal of the UK from the European Union (EU). The direct and indirect consequences of a hard or soft 'Brexit' will have significant consequences for individuals and the health of the community. From public health, economic, political and social justice perspectives, *health inequalities* are bad for individuals and bad for society. Concern about the escalating costs of the health and welfare systems in this diverse and ageing UK society should be addressed by considerations of upstream prevention strategies, mainly directed at lifestyle choices, and evidence-based approaches aimed at supporting people who are vulnerable to poor *health* and limitations in their *quality of life*.

The impact on the health of people in the UK following the passing of the National Health Services Act 1946, financed by general taxation, was a major breakthrough in public health that has laid the foundation for a healthy society in the UK. However, despite concerns about health and social class inequalities highlighted in the Black Report (1980), there was no political response to the Black recommendations to reduce social class inequalities by improving housing conditions and child benefit. In recent years, there have been attempts to deal with the health consequences of social inequalities and lifestyle choices; however, the most significant change in understanding these issues was clearly evidenced in the Marmot Report (2010). This analysis of extensive epidemiological data showed the strong links between the social gradient and the physical and mental health of people. This report highlighted the wide variations in social gradients in various countries and population health in those countries. Early childhood experiences, living conditions and employment all contribute to the quality of health and well-being across the life cycle.

It is widely understood that early childhood experiences and the development of social networks have a major impact on later-life health and well-being, which are mediated by the development of *pro-social* behaviour, resilience, coping skills and optimal cognitive functioning. These complex social behaviours require a healthy mind and body and the motivation to benefit and learn from a supportive environment. The complex biological and psychological factors needed for successful development and maturation will be significantly influenced by appropriate nutrition, exercise, support from primary caregivers and engagement with family and the community. Becoming a member of an identifiable group has health benefits, socialisation being dependent on communication and learning to respond to threats. This is best done within a group and family network. The role of schools and related policies to support disadvantaged children is important in 'giving children a good start in life' (Marmot, 2010). Young people who are not in education, employment or training (NEETs) are at particular risk of becoming marginalised. In adult life, financial independence and having a secure role in the world of work have previously provided stability for the individual and for his/her family. Across the world, job insecurity is becoming the norm for many people. The high demands and reduced long-term security of modern business models increase personal stress and anxiety, which impact on health and well-being. Reducing anxiety over life's challenges is a core element of health and social vitality and is the essence of a happy, healthy community. Threats and adverse life experiences are experienced by all, starting with the process of birth. Post-Traumatic Stress Disorder (PTSD) can result from events in early life, domestic abuse, accidents and being in a war zone. This type of brain damage is often associated with alcohol abuse, which can reduce cognitive function and, in some situations, lead to Alcohol-Related Brain Damage (ARBD). Cognitive and behaviour dysfunction can mitigate against a person reaching their potential. The presentation of, and how we deal with, these challenges has been explored within a range of disciplines, which have contributed to our understanding of the social determinants of health, as presented in the Marmot Review (2010). The implications of the increasingly widespread use of social media on the individual and their social networks, and links with health and well-being, are currently being questioned, particularly in relation to body image, personal identity and the mental health of young people.

The trajectory into homelessness often begins with problematic substance use (primarily alcohol and other drugs), adopting a street lifestyle and then being confirmed as officially homeless. Key risk factors for becoming homeless are: being a survivor of abuse or neglect during childhood; being arrested or charged with anti-social behaviour; and living in the care system (Bramley et al, 2015: footnote). Other routes into social exclusion include learning disabilities and related issues that reduce effective communication and integration into social groups.

The organisation of this book maps the contents onto the 'rainbow' model presented by Dahlgren and Whitehead (1991), which provides a perspective on the social determinants of health. The interconnectedness and interdependence of socio-economic, cultural, environmental, living and working conditions, social and community networks, and lifestyle choices contribute to a person's health and well-being.

Figure 0.1: Sections of this book mapped on to the 'rainbow model' of social determinants of health

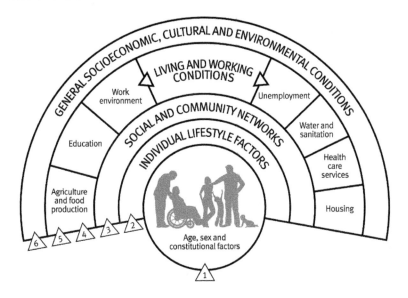

Source: Adapted from Dahlgren and Whitehead (1991).

The main aim of this book is to provide an interdisciplinary approach to an understanding of the key social, psychological and biological factors that impact on the *quality of life*, particularly of those people who are most vulnerable to a high burden of physical and mental ill health and social dysfunction. This will hopefully provide an introduction to specific research methods to inform the planning and funding of the most appropriate health, social and economic interventions to support those at the edge of the community and the promotion of their inclusion in society. This collection of chapters from experts in a wide range of disciplines, within a socio-political-economic context, will provide contemporary insights at this time when the UK and other countries are emerging from a major global economic recession. Although the main political parties are committed to developing economic growth and encourage a fairer society, reducing the UK deficit by more austerity for some and reducing the size of the welfare state is currently being debated by central and local government. The unintended consequences of reductions in welfare budgets, and the move to abolish social housing, could result in higher health and social care costs due to the negative economic impact of widening social inequalities, as highlighted in the Marmot Review (2010).

At this moment in time (September 2016), the UK is on the brink of exiting the EU following a referendum in June 2016 in which 52% of the voting UK electorate voted to leave the EU. Prior to the legal declaration by the UK government of this intention, there is considerable uncertainty about the economic and social consequences of leaving the European common market, which would be linked to controls over the free movement of people in the EU. Those people who voted for 'Brexit' are predominantly located in socially deprived areas, are thought to have been motivated by concerns about immigration and are considered to be alienated from the political establishment. This societal response is in line with the link between social gradient, health and well-being, as highlighted in the Marmot Reviews into health inequalities.

Reference

Bramley, G., Fitzpatrick, S., Edwards, J., Ford, D., Johnsen, S., Sosenko, F. and Watkins, D. (2015) 'Hard edges: mapping severe and multiple disadvantage', The LankellyChase Foundation. Available at: http://lankellychase.org.uk/multiple-disadvantage/publications/hard-edges/

Dahlgren, G. and Whitehead, M. (1991) *Policies and strategies to promote social equity in health*, Stockholm, Sweden. Institute for Futures Studies

DHSS (1980) *The Black Report. Inequalities in Health: Report of Working Group*, London: Department for Health and Social Security.

Marmot, M. (2010) *Fair society, healthy lives: The Marmot Review. Strategic review of health inequalities in England post-2010*, London: UCL Institute of Health Equity.

Part One
Life chances

The interconnectedness and interdependence of socio-economic, cultural, environmental, living and working conditions, social and community networks, and lifestyle choices contribute to a person's health and well-being. Social and health strategies, in the community, clearly need to focus on individual needs and vulnerabilities. As indicated in the 'rainbow' model of social determinants of health, age, sex and constitutional factors should be at the centre of these considerations. This section on 'Life chances' offers an introduction to some of the key biological, psychological and social drivers that lead to social exclusion in some disadvantaged people, necessitating support from outside the family and involving statutory and voluntary agencies, as reviewed in subsequent sections of this book.

ONE

The individual: growing into society

Adrian Bonner

Dahlgren and Whitehead's model of the social determinants of health (Dahlgren and Whitehead, 1991; Dahlgren, 2007) provides a framework from which we can begin to understand the complex interaction of genetic factors and prenatal, perinatal and postnatal events in influencing the development of the individual from childhood, through adolescence and into adult life. The early life stages lay the foundation for adult life and successful ageing. The biological processes of natural selection operate at each of these stages, starting before birth, the outcomes of which are significantly influenced by external factors such as the supply of adequate nutrition, a secure environment and nurturing by parents and others supporting the individual on their journey through life (see Parts Three, Four and Five, this volume). The maturation of the human nervous system, musculature and metabolic processes are essential for independent living; however, the social environment provides the external drivers that shape behaviour, cognitive functioning and decision-making. The primary determinants important in social development include levels of sensory stimulation and prosocial learning, which support communication and the shaping of appropriate behavioural responses, such as positive (eg human bonding) and negative (eg aggressive) relationships, which are prerequisites for healthy relationships within the family, the workplace and the community.

The well-being of children and the safeguarding of vulnerable people generally involves protecting them from abuse, exploitation and physical and psychological damage. Sexual abuse and exploitation, sadly, are not uncommon in modern society. These adverse early life experiences not only affect an individual's relationships with others and mental health in later life, but also impact directly and indirectly on physiological status via the immune system (Baumeister et al, 2016), leading to increased vulnerability to communicable and non-communicable diseases, including childhood cancers (Anon, 2016a). This vulnerability is exacerbated by psychological factors that undermine self-esteem and self-image (see Chapter Sixteen). An overview of the positive aspects of the psychological environment within the wider health context is provided in Chapter Three.

Early childhood experiences and the development of social networks have a major impact on later-life health and well-being, which are mediated by the development of prosocial behaviour, resilience, coping skills and optimal cognitive functioning. These complex issues require a healthy mind and body and the motivation to benefit and learn from a supportive environment. This chapter provides an overview of the main developmental processes underlying future emotional and social behaviours. The key risk factors for becoming homeless, being a survivor of abuse or neglected during childhood, having a learning disability, being arrested or charged with anti-social behaviour, and living in the care system are explored in later parts of this book.

Neuropsychological development

Problems of cognitive dysfunction and mental ill health, as reviewed in Part Five, begin in the early developmental stages as a result of cumulative developmental issues such as poor nutrition and the presence of harmful substances in the prenatal blood supply. The impact of external stress in the mother, resulting in higher levels of the stress hormone cortisol, has an important influence on cognitive functioning. This series of threats increases the vulnerability of the child, adding to a vicious circle of events exacerbated by alcohol misuse in the later years, possibly leading to alcohol dependence or dependence on other drugs that increase the probability of brain damage (see Chapters Five, Six, Seven and Eighteen). The maximum rate of brain growth occurs during the first two years of life. Genetic information, inherited from the parents, directs growth and the development of the nervous system, as is the case with other systems in the body. This information, encoded in DNA molecules, is *translated* and *transcribed* into a diverse range of proteins that form the material basis of body structures, such as skin, muscle and nervous tissue, and (protein) enzymes that control the body's metabolism, some of which are produced on a regular basis and others are induced briefly for specific purposes. These processes are dependent on adequate nutrition (see Chapter Four).

Although the basic infrastructure of the brain is genetically preprogrammed, an overproduction of neurons occurs in some regions such as the olfactory and hippocampal regions, where the fine neuronal structure is tuned by the *pruning* of neuronal axons, dendrites and synapses that are not utilised. This process is influenced by sensory stimulation and increasing efficiency of specific neuronal pathways,

4

an aspect of the process of learning. Neuronal pathways not used will degenerate according to the concept of Neural Darwinism (Edelman, 1987), which provides an explanation, based on the principles of natural selection, of the way by which neurones are influenced by brain stimulation via sensory inputs from the environment. This physiological process of learning is perceived as a behavioural output originating from neurobiological mechanisms at cellular and molecular levels. The concept of Long Term Potential (LTP) provides a useful conceptual framework for understanding the cellular basis of learning (Okada et al, 2003). Emotional behaviour, a specific form of learning, results from sensory inputs, which are assimilated and processed in association within existing memories within the limbic system. Prenatally and postnatally, the development and maintenance of this neuronal infrastructure is significantly influenced by the internal biochemical status of the brain.

Affection, fear and anxiety in early development

The role of stress and anxiety in mental health will be explored in Part Five, but in view of the role of developmental stressors in children and their impact on later-life mental health, a brief review of social anxiety and the links between anxiety and the physiological events in mother–infant relationships will be given here.

At the time of puberty, gender identity, gender role and sexual orientation become incorporated into the formation of and maintenance of emotional relationships, and sexual orientation becomes organised and relatively fixed. The origins of affection and trust begin in the secure nurturing relationship between the infant and its mother. In both males and females, affectionate relationships in these early years and later stages of childhood lay the foundations of later sexual relationships between adults. Various studies indicate that fearful children are at a high risk of later emotional distress. Kagan and colleagues (1988) have shown that a child who is profoundly shy at the age of two years is more likely to suffer from anxiety and depression later in life than a less inhibited child. Children who become severely inhibited in unfamiliar places produce high levels of stress hormones, including cortisol from the adrenal gland. Cortisol, a stress-related hormone, is produced at elevated levels at times of crisis and is part of the 'fight or flight' reaction, which includes maximising energy for use by the muscles. Cortisol results in a number of other physiological changes occurring at times of 'fight or flight'; however, long-term elevations of this stress hormone may contribute to gastric ulcers, cardiovascular disease and neurotoxicity. Fearful children enter a vicious circle leading from isolation and lowered self-esteem, through underachievement, to possibly anxiety and depression.

There is some evidence that unusually fearful children are prone to physical illness, for example, fearful children and their families are more likely to suffer from allergic disorders. In animal studies, the persistent elevation of cortisol increases the vulnerability of neurons in the hippocampus to damage by other substances. This region is involved in memory, motivation and emotion and so fear-related responses involving chronic elevated levels of cortisol are thought to have a negative effect on brain function.

Brain regions, primarily the limbic system, regulate fearfulness and are thought to develop at 9–12 weeks. This system is linked to the 'prefrontal cortex', which is an area of the brain concerned with cognitive and emotional responses, brought about by the interpretation of sensory stimuli. This is possibly the site where potential danger is assessed. The 'amygdala', part of the limbic system, is involved in generating fear, which is expressed via the 'hypothalamus', which secretes cortico releasing hormone (CRH) stimulating the pituitary to produce adrenocorticotropic hormone (ACTH), which, in turn, causes the adrenal gland to release cortisol and prepares the body to defend itself.

In human maturation, when an infant reaches 12 months of age, the 'prefrontal cortex' increases in activity and enables the child to distinguish between threatening cues. During this developmental stage, children begin to show marked fear of strangers and become skilled at social referencing. They regulate their level of fear based on interpretation of the expressions they observe on a parent's face. Animals have been used to explore mother–infant relations, and the effects of maternal deprivation (Bowlby, 1977). The work by Kagan (Kagan et al, 1988) provides an important insight into the physiological mechanisms that underpin mother–infant bonding and anxiety produced by disruption of the bond as a result of maternal separation. The conclusion from animal studies is that *opiate-using neural pathways* regulate affiliative (mother–infant) behaviours. In summary, when a young monkey is separated from its mother, *opiate-releasing* and *opiate-sensitive* mechanisms become inhibited. This gives rise to yearning for the mother and a generalised vulnerability and resulting vocalisations. This reduction of activity in *opiate-sensitive* systems enables motor systems in the brain to produce *cooing*, an outward expression of fear. When a potential predator appears, neurons that secrete endogenous benzodiazepine become suppressed to some degree. This leads to elevated anxiety and the appearance of behaviours and hormones that accompany fear. As a sense of alarm grows, the system prepares for *fight or flight*. The benzodiazepines thus alter opiate systems, which results in *cooing* behaviour during threatening situations.

Social anxiety

An insight into the linkage between anxiety and exclusion from social groups in the early years is provided by Gazelle and Ladd (2003). In studying 388 children, equal numbers of boys and girls, the authors observed social behaviour, peer exclusion and emotional adjustment at kindergarten (primary school). Observations, primarily by the teacher, were made at entry and every spring thereafter through to the fourth year. These observations indicated that soon after joining the primary school, anxiety (due to solitude) and peer exclusion co-occur in the children. Anxious solitude became more entrenched in those anxious solitary children who were excluded early on, in comparison with their non-excluded anxious solitary counterparts. The *diathesis-stress* model proposed by the authors indicated that the joint forces of individual vulnerability (anxious solitude) and interpersonal adversity (peer exclusion) were strongly associated with symptoms of depression, noted in the children and young people (Griffin, 2010). In Chapter Eight, Nathan Critchlow reviews social anxiety in relation to digital social media.

Communication and socialisation

The term '*prosocial behaviour*' is used to describe 'voluntary actions that are intended to help or benefit another individual or group of individuals' (Dennis, 1975). These anthropological studies have suggested that *prosocial behaviours* may be motivated by selfish reasons, for example, to gain a reward or gain approval, or he/she may be displaying sympathy and caring (Dennis, 1965: 3). These apparently empathetic behaviours are sometimes described as *altruistic*, driven by internal values, which include a belief in the importance of the welfare or social justice of others. An inability of a child to conform to learned social norms may result in inappropriate responses in particular situations (Eisenberg, 1989). Moral *judgement* could be considered to be a cognitive aspect of morality involving reasoning about moral issues and conceptualisations and is quite distinct from *prosocial behaviour*. Learning *social norms*, having moral concepts, being able to make moral judgements and being motivated to act in certain ways are important contributions to an individual's capacity to become a member of the functional community.

Biological factors, noted earlier in this chapter, contribute to the process of socialisation; these include the genetic vulnerability to prenatal exposure to alcohol (Ungerer and Ramsey, 2013) and hyperactivity (Elia, 2007). Genetic influences on the development and maturation of the sensory systems, and hormonal influences on emotional behaviour, contribute to the process of socialisation. Both genetic and cultural factors influence the development of *social behaviour* and *prosocial behaviour*. A child's capacity to interact with parents, teachers and siblings, as well as the influence of cultural and religious institutions, plays a major role in socialisation.

The changing views of prosocial behaviour can be seen in emerging literature. Extensive studies into moral development in the 1920s (Anon, 1928) led to an incorrect conclusion that the prosocial behaviour of school-age children was situation-specific and not influenced by moral behaviours such as generosity. In the 1980s, studies on delinquency and violence showed that these antisocial behaviours had their roots in parental rejection. A focus on injustice suffered by women, minority ethnic groups and the disabled, leading to positive action programmes, was a major theme during 1969–89. In the 1970s, a consolidation of ideas from developmental and social psychologists resulted in a greater understanding of social learning and related cognitive processes (Eisenberg, 1989).

The well-being of children

Many childcare policies are aimed at supporting children in health and social care, day care, and education, and approaches to the care and custody of young children are based on adverse effects of early life separation (from his/her mother) on the child's mental well-being and subsequent emotional development. These negative views of separation are informed by the work of Bowlby (1977), and reviewed by Rutter (1979). However, there is increasing evidence that *protect–despair–detachment* is far less predictable than originally described. Helen Barret (1998) has drawn attention to the variable responses of children and that they are not always dominated by separation anxiety and the need to 'attach' to one key care provider. Some may be capable of forming multiple attachments and being competent in skills to form new attachments. This positive experience for some children will be mediated by the child's perception of security. Emotional vulnerability or shyness in others will be challenged by relatively short separation experiences. Children and young people in care are most likely to have suffered extreme and recurrent losses in their formative years. The death of parents or parental issues relating to mental illness or problematic alcohol or drug use are not uncommon in this group of 'looked-after 'children. Physical, sexual or emotional abuse all contribute to a strong sense of stigma, shame and victimisation, often related to parental and family relationships and their own feeling of rejection.

Poverty, child abuse and neglect

The estimated cost of poverty in the UK is £78 billion. This accounts for £1 in every £5 spent on public services (Anon, 2016b). These costs are attributed to: education (£10 billion = 20% of the schools budget), health care (25% of total spend), child and adult social services (£7.5 billion = 40% of early years budget, 60% of children's social care) and justice (£9 billion). Despite a large body of statistical reports, there is a significant challenge to reduce poverty as 'Interventions to reduce poverty have been piecemeal, poorly understood, and rarely had the sense of shared endeavour' (Julia Unwin, Chief Executive of the Joseph Rowntree Foundation, quoted in Anon, 2016b).

The intergenerational cycles of family poverty and achievement in children is linked to nutritional deficits, as discussed in Chapter Four, and contributes to individuals and families being excluded from society (Bonner, 2006). There is a need to reframe poverty. Knight (2015) has suggested that we need to understand the nature of a 'good society' and work backwards from there. In reviewing the rise and fall of the 'planned society', from Aristotle to modern philosophers, Knight has highlighted the market-driven Washington Consensus, which promotes the concept of small state safety nets, leaving gaps in which civil society (note the role of volunteering reviewed in Chapter Nine) would provide support for the most vulnerable. Clearly, the balance between 'a good society' and what people want is subject to political influences. Geopolitical factors and welfare reform have been critically analysed by Clare Bambra in ongoing research within a health inequalities framework developed from the Marmot Reports (see Chapter Twenty). Geographical variation in England regarding young people's profiles has been published by Public Health England (Anon, 2014). Regrettably, in addition to philosophical and socio-economic discourses, there is much hardship and despair in contemporary UK society, this includes child abuse and neglect (CAN). The association between socio-economic status and CAN has been noted across developed countries; however, there does not appear to be a binary divide between families in poverty and those that are not. A gradient in the relationship between CAN and socio-economic status has been reported. This gradient is also found in relation to child health and educational attainment. Poverty seems not to be necessary or solely linked to CAN. Understanding these relationships is problematic due to a range of methodological issues. Bywaters et al (2016) have undertaken a rapid evidence review of papers published during the last 10 years, and concluded that direct and indirect impacts of poverty on CAN, in consideration of parenting, can be summarised as follows:

• Parental capacity: problematic mental and physical illness, and learning disabilities.
• Family capacity for investment: financial resources to purchase care, respite or better environmental conditions.
• Negative adult behaviour: domestic violence/substance use, exacerbated by family stress.
• Positive adult and child behaviours: facilitating social support and resilience.
• External neighbourhood factors: social and physical environment.

Social inclusion strategies

In 1997, the New Labour government established a Social Exclusion Unit, within the Office of the Deputy Prime Minister (Anon, 2004). A number of new initiatives were developed, including Sure Start children's centres, funded via local authorities, providing a 'one-stop shop' to support disadvantaged families in their communities. These were well embedded and popular in local communities and appeared to be an effective way of delivering services to transform the lives of children, and disengage them from intergenerational cycles of social disadvantage. Since 2010, expenditure on children's centres has been significantly reduced. In this age of austerity, when local authorities are subjected to continued decreases in the revenue grant from central government, there is a greater need for them to make better use of children's centres and other services, and to close the gap between the rich and poor. Early intervention is essential to reduce the risks to childhood well-being (Waldegrave, 2008). Many local authorities can no longer fund children's centres.

Troubled families

Following the riots in 2011, Prime Minister David Cameron announced plans to 'turn around the lives of the 120,000 most troubled families in the country' (HMG, 2011). The initial intervention was costed at £400 million, a further allocation of £900 million was set aside for a second wave aimed at a further 400,000 families in 2015. Each local authority was given a target number of families to identify and recruit to the scheme, each family receiving £3,200. These large-scale interventions across the UK were focused on unemployment, antisocial behaviour and truancy, and have been evaluated by a consortium of analysts led by a consultancy, Ecorys (Anon, 2015). Despite upbeat outcome reports from the government, the analysis of data from 56 local authorities showed 'no obvious effect from the first eighteen months of the programme. There was no measurable impact on families, and no detectable impact on child offending' (Jameson, 2016). The various debates regarding the focus on 'trying too hard to fix dysfunctional families ... [rather] than making care a decent and stable place', Martin Narey, Head of Barnardos, stated that 'many of the children come from deprived backgrounds and may have been severely neglected before being removed into care' (quoted in Jameson, 2016). These fundamental area of support needs to be addressed by new government initiatives to reform the care system.

Deviant and anti-social behaviour

Being arrested or charged with anti-social activities and living within the care system during childhood are key predictors of later-life homelessness (Bramley et al, 2015; News, 2015). Notwithstanding the preceding discussion on the variability of a child's response to adversity, social and emotional adjustments are clearly important in the development of prosocial and antisocial behaviour. Parental bonding, divorce, family structure, family size, ordinal position, parental style, marital discord, parental mental illness, life events and parental criminality will all contribute to a child's perception of the world and his/her responses to the challenges of life. In the preschool period, middle childhood and adolescence, progress at school will be affected positively or negatively by this wide range of influences (see Chapter Two). At this time, individual behavioural and intellectual issues become noticeable, offering a window of opportunity to address problematic issues. Some children will be clinically diagnosed with one or more emotional problems such as anxiety disorders, fears and phobias, depression, suicide and self-harm, school refusal, obsessive-compulsive disorders, elective mutism, hysteria, post-traumatic stress disorder, conduct disorder, hyperactivity, hyperkinesis and attention deficit disorder, autism, eating disorders, psychoses, and sexual problems. Conduct disorder is a description of antisocial behaviour, in which social norms are broken, and often includes excessive fighting, disobedience, tantrums, stealing, destruction of property, arson, cruelty (mainly to animals) and truancy. Both *socialised conduct disorder*, involving a peer group, and *unsocialised conduct disorder* are more likely to be displayed by boys, though girls are increasingly likely to become antisocial, particularly when alcohol is involved. 'Delinquency' is a legal term referring to those forms of antisocial behaviour that involve breaking the law. Conduct disorder in children is associated with delinquency in adults. Hyperactivity, hyperkinesis, attention deficit disorder and autism are not directly linked to deviant and criminal behaviour; however, limitations on educational attainment and the related impact on social capacity increase the likelihood of social exclusion and the possible displaying of antisocial behaviours (Black, 1993; Campbell, 2016).

Mental health and human distress

The 'complex trauma' often found in homeless people, as discussed in Chapters Sixteen, Seventeen and Nineteen, results from a reaction to ongoing and sustained traumatic experiences, associated with adverse childhood experiences and the cumulative effect of difficult life events.[1] People with a history of complex trauma may display a range of emotions that undermine building and maintaining relationships, increase the likelihood of self-harm and have the possibility of uncontrolled alcohol and/or drug problems. A recent survey by the National Health Service (NHS) has found increases in post-traumatic stress disorder (PTSD) (12.6%) and self-harm (28.2%) in women aged 16–24 (Campbell, 2016). These anti-social behaviours mitigate against positive educational performance, getting into employment and increased criminal behaviour (see Chapter Thirteen). Emotional and behavioural problems are particularly acute in 16–17 year olds who may have had traumatic childhoods. This is a period when high levels of impulsivity and sensation-seeking behaviour are significantly elevated. At this time, 'courting behaviour' involves behavioural activities, fundamentally important in seeking out a sexual partner, an important set of events, rituals and decision-making that will lead to life relationships or social isolation. Increased vulnerability to risky behaviour occurs during drinking alcohol (White and Labouvie, 1989).

In summary, many lifestyle non-communicable diseases (NCDs) have their origins in the early years. It is therefore important to ensure that 'every child should have the best start in life' (Marmot, 2010).

Note

1. See: http://www.jrf.org.uk/publications/tackling-homelessness-and-exclusion

References

Anon (1928) 'Moral development'. Available at: http://isites.harvard. edu/fs/docs/icb.topic823420.files/morality Extension 2010 - Handout.pdf

Anon (2004) 'The Social Exclusion Unit', London. Available at: http:// webarchive.nationalarchives.gov.uk/+/http:/www.cabinetoffice. gov.uk/media/cabinetoffice/social_exclusion_task_force/assets/ publications_1997_to_2006/seu_leaflet.pdf

Anon (2014) 'Health behaviours in young people – What about YOUth? survey'. Available at: http://fingertips.phe.org.uk/profile/ what-about-youth

Anon (2015) '2010–2015 government policy: support for families'. Available at: http://www.gov.uk/government/publications/2010- to-2015-government-policy-support-for-families/2010-to-2015- government-policy-support-for-families

Anon (2016a) 'Behind the headlines is modern life really killing our children?', Children's Cancer and Leaukemia Group.

Anon (2016b) 'We can solve poverty'. Available at: https://www.jrf. org.uk/report/we-can-solve-poverty-uk

Barret, H. (1998) 'Protest-despair-detachment: Questioning the myth' in I.M. Hutchby and J. Moran-Ellis (eds) *Children and social competence: Areas of action*, London: Falmer Press.

Baumeister, D., Akhtar, R., Ciufolini, S., Pariante, C.M. and Mondelli, V. (2016) 'Childhood trauma and adulthood inflammation: a meta-analysis of peripheral C-reactive protein, interleukin-6 and tumour necrosis factor-alpha', *Mol Psychiatry*, 21(5): 642–9.

Black, D.C.D. (1993) 'Child and adolescent psychiatry', Royal College of Psychiatrists.

Bonner, A.B. (2006) *Social exclusion and the way out: An individual and community perspective on social dysfunction*, Chichester: John Wiley.

Bowlby, J. (1977) 'The making and breaking of affectional bonds. I. Aetiology and psychopathology in the light of attachment theory. An expanded version of the Fiftieth Maudsley Lecture, delivered before the Royal College of Psychiatrists, 19 November 1976', *Br J Psychiatry*, 130: 201–10.

Bramley, G., Fitzpatrick, S., Edwards, J., Ford, D., Johnsen, S., Sosenko, F. and Watkins, D. (2015) 'Hard edges: mapping severe and multiple disadvantage', The LankellyChase Foundation. Available at: http:// lankellychase.org.uk/multiple-disadvantage/publications/hard-edges/

Bywaters, P., Bunting, L., Davidsosn, G., Hanratty, J., Mason, W., McCartean, C. and Steils, N. (2016) 'The relationship between poverty, child abuse and neglect: an evidence review', Joseph Rowntree Foundation.

Campbell, D.S.H. (producer) (2016) 'Mental illness soars among young women in England – survey'. Available at: http://www.theguardian.com/lifeandstyle/2016/sep/29/self-harm-ptsd-and-mental-illness-soaring-among-young-women-in-england-survey

Dahlgren, G.W.M. (2007) *European strategies for tackling social inequalities in health: Leveling up Part 2 (Studies on social and economic determinants of population health, No.3 ed.)*, Denmark: World Health Organisation Regional Office for Europe.

Dahlgren, G. and Whitehead, M. (1991) *Policies and strategies to promote social equity in health*, Stockholm, Sweden: Institute for Futures Studies.

Dennis, W. (1965) *The Hopi child*, Chichester: Wiley.

Edelman, G.M. (1987) *Neural Darwinism*, New York, NY: Basic Books.

Eisenberg, N.M.P.H. (1989) 'The roots of prosocial behavour in children', Google Books.

Elia, J.D.M. (2007) 'ADHA genetics: 2007 update', *Current Psychiatric Reports*, 9(5): 434–9.

Gazelle, H. and Ladd, G.W. (2003) 'Anxious solitude and peer exclusion: a diathesis-stress model of internalizing trajectories in childhood', *Child Dev*, 74(1): 257–78.

Griffin, J. (2010) 'The lonely society', Mental Health Foundation.

HMG (Her Majesty's Government) (2011) *Tackling troubled families*, Department for Communities. https://www.gov.uk/government/news/tackling-troubled-families (retrieved 10 08 2017).

Jameson, H. (2016) 'Troubled Families scheme had no "discernible impact" claims suppressed report'. Available at: https://www.localgov.co.uk/Troubled-Families-scheme-had-no-discernible-impact-claims-suppressed-report/41414 (retrieved 10 08 2017).

Kagan, J., Reznick, J.S. and Snidman, N. (1988) 'Biological bases of childhood shyness', *Science*, 240(4849): 167–71.

Knight, B. (2015) *The society we want*, London: Webb Memorial Trust.

Marmot, M. (2010) *Fair society, healthy lives: The Marmot Review. Strategic review of health inequalities in England post-2010*, London: UCL Institute of Health Equity.

News, B. (producer) (2015) 'Offending rates among children in care investigated'. Available at: http://www.bbc.co.uk/news/uk-33221247

Okada, T., Yamada, N. and Tsuzuki, K. (2003) 'Long-term potentiation in the hippocampal CA1 area and dentate gyrus plays different roles in spatial learning', *Eur J Neurosci*, 17: 341.

Rutter, M. (1979) 'Maternal deprivation, 1972–1978: new findings, new concepts, new approaches', *Child Development*, 50(2): 282–305.

Ungerer, M.K.J. and Ramsey, M. (2013) 'In utero alcohol exposure, epigenetic changes, and their consequences', *Alcohol Research*, 35(1): 37–46.

Waldegrave, H. (2008) *The role of children's centres in early intervention*, London: Policy Exchange.

White, H.R. and Labouvie, E.W. (1989) 'Towards the assessment of adolescent problem drinking', *Journal of Studies on Alcohol*, 50(1): 30–7.

TWO

Addressing inequalities in education: parallels with health

Kirstin Kerr

Introduction

There are striking similarities in patterns of inequality in education and in health. In education, as in health, the poorest outcomes accrue systematically to the most disadvantaged (DfE, 2016). Moreover, just as health outcomes are not simply a product of access to, or the practices of, health-care providers, educational outcomes are not simply products of access to particular schools or of schools' internal practices – important though these are. In both fields, to start to understand why this is so requires an explanatory framework that considers the 'social determinants' that shape these outcomes (see, for instance, the 'rainbow model' of the social determinants of health outlined in the Preface). This, as Sir Michael Marmot has argued, requires a focus on 'the causes' and 'the causes of the causes' of poor outcomes; as he explains in relation to health:

> Inequalities … are closely linked to the conditions in which we raise our children, the education we get, the neighbourhoods we live in, the work we do, whether we have the money to make ends meet, our social relationships and our care for the elderly. (Marmot, cited in ABC News, 2016)

Much the same could be said of inequalities in education, which, as will be explored later in this chapter, are also known to be affected by where children live, family income and local employment prospects, among other factors.

Given these strong similarities, this chapter will argue that a central part of efforts to address educational inequalities must be for education, as a field, to think and act more comprehensively in ways that parallel thinking about the social determinants of health. Taking England as an illustrative case, the chapter will outline broad patterns of educational inequality and recent policy responses to these, arguing that there is a need for greater understanding of, and engagement with, the underlying causes of educational inequalities. It will then argue that it is possible for schools to lead the development of innovative responses to educational inequalities at a local level by engaging in children's family and community contexts alongside internal school reforms – with this highlighting overlaps between educational and health inequalities and the responses needed to address these. To illustrate this, an empirical example of an initiative to develop children's speech, language and communication skills is reported. The chapter concludes that initiatives which more clearly engage with the wider social determinants of education can form an important part of responses to educational inequality. They may, furthermore, open opportunities for new synergies between education and health to emerge conceptually, as well as in policy and practice, and so better tackle inequalities in both fields.

Patterns of inequality in educational outcomes

Children enter the education system from very unequal backgrounds, have very unequal experiences within the system and leave with very unequal outcomes. In England, for example, pupils receiving free school meals (FSM) (state-funded meals for pupils from low-income backgrounds) are systematically more likely to underperform compared to their more advantaged peers. For instance, in the English school-leaving examination (the General Certificate of Secondary Education [GCSE]) in 2015, 33.1% of FSM pupils achieved the benchmark of five top grade GCSEs (A★–C), including maths and English, compared to 60.9% of all other pupils (DfE, 2016). The impacts of economic disadvantage are, moreover, present throughout children's school careers and compounded by a range of familial factors. For example, Hills et al (2010: 22) report that 'looking from age 3 to age 14, differences in assessment related to family income, father's occupation and mother's education widen at each stage'. These factors are also cut across by a combination of gender and ethnicity; in 2015, only 24% of white British FSM boys achieved five A★–C GCSEs, including maths and English, the lowest of any ethnic-gender FSM group, the highest attaining being Chinese FSM girls, at 80.6% (DfE, 2016).

Such inequalities are also spatially distributed. Poorer outcomes are concentrated predominantly in deindustrialised urban areas in town and cities, and also increasingly in seaside towns and former coalfield sites – places that typically also have poor outcomes across a range of other domains, including health, employment and community safety. Such concentrations are also likely to compound the challenges faced by the children and families living in these areas, and can make it harder for schools in these areas to achieve the conditions needed for pupils to learn effectively (Dyson et al, 2011). Chapter Twenty provides an insight into the geopolitical dimensions of inequality.

The processes through which these contextual factors shape educational outcomes are hugely complex and imperfectly understood, appearing to originate deep within children's family, community and social backgrounds – for instance, in the ways in which their families engage (or otherwise) in learning, or in community expectations, or in the physical and psychological constraints created by where they live (Kerr et al, 2014). Family incomes, housing quality, nutrition, educational resources, parenting practices and the quality and accessibility of local schools, for example, are all likely to play a role. Echoing Marmot's earlier arguments about health, Dyson et al (2009: ii) suggest that it is the 'nurturant' quality of children's interconnected environments (ie how well these support the achievement of good outcomes) that are of particular importance:

> Children live, grow up and learn through their interactions with a wide range of interconnected environments – including the family, residential communities, relational communities, and the environment of child development services (such as the childcare centres or the schools that children attend). Each of these environments is situated in a broad socioeconomic context that is shaped by factors at the local, national, and global level. Whether children do well depends to a very significant extent on the 'nurturant' quality of these environments.

The question this poses is whether it is possible to strengthen the 'nurturant' qualities of children's environments in ways that can disrupt educational inequalities by addressing at least some of the underlying local (or proximal) causes of poor outcomes. Indeed, that some children, schools and communities in disadvantaged circumstances nonetheless achieve good educational outcomes would seem to suggest that this is possible. This, in turn, raises questions for policy and practice about how schools, in particular, might help to create high-quality 'nurturant' environments, as they engage directly with children and families, are amenable to policy reform, and, alongside their explicitly educational role, have the potential to partner with other agencies to intervene in children's wider environments.

Policy responses to educational inequalities

Over the last 30 years especially, English education policy has been preoccupied with finding ways to narrow gaps in educational outcomes between the most and least advantaged pupils. Central to this, it has maintained a consistently strong focus on internal school improvement measures – reforming curricular content, improving the quality of teaching and learning, and promoting the use of evidence-based interventions to raise attainment – with schools being held to account for their pupils' progress through punitive accountability and inspection regimes.

This range of activity has made some improvements in attainment overall, and has had some benefits for the most disadvantaged. However, it has arguably also done little to actually narrow the attainment gap (see, eg, 'Trend in the disadvantaged pupil attainment gap index', in DfE, 2016). Indeed, reflecting on the achievements of the international school improvement movement, Levin (2006: 401) notes that 'actually improving achievement has proven to be an extraordinarily difficult and badly underestimated challenge, even when vastly greater resources are devoted to it'.

A central challenge is undoubtedly the impact of out-of-school factors on in-school improvement processes. As Mujis (2010: 89) reflects:

> even if we found all the factors that make schools more or less effective, we would still not be able to affect more than 30 per cent of the variance in pupils' outcomes. It has therefore become increasingly clear that a narrow focus on the school as an institution will not be sufficient to enable work on more equitable educational outcomes to progress.... Interventions will need to impact more directly on pupils' environment.

Simply, while internal school reforms can make an important difference, they ultimately appear limited in what they can achieve.

Importantly, therefore, English education policy has, at times, seen serious efforts to develop the 'nurturant quality' of children's out-of-school environments. For instance, the development of Full Service Extended Schools (FSES) between 2005 and 2010 typically involved locating additional services in schools, with the expectation that, by 2010, all schools should provide:

- a varied menu of activities for children, including access to sport, cultural and leisure opportunities;
- wraparound childcare, from 8.00am to 6.00pm;
- parenting support;
- swift and easy access to targeted and specialist support services, including health services; and
- community access to school facilities, including adult education opportunities.

The then Department for Education and Skills (DfES, 2005) suggested that this should lead to improvements in attainment, community cohesion, health and employment outcomes, among other benefits.

The national evaluation of FSES (see Cummings et al, 2011) suggests that these had some positive impacts, seen most strongly in relation to provision that FSES put in place to provide personal support, practical advice and access to new opportunities for those pupils and families facing greatest difficulties. However, there was much less evidence of widespread impacts. There was, for instance, little to suggest that an extended offer *per se* improved school-level attainment, or improved a wider range of outcomes at a neighbourhood level. Such findings raise important questions about how effective a simple additive model – of adding disconnected services to an otherwise un-reconstituted school day – can be in addressing educational inequalities. Indeed, as Dyson and Raffo (2007) argue, extended approaches often (tacitly) assume that professionals can 'fix' deficits in the children and families they work with, and can do so through rafts of single-issue interventions that separately target the 'symptoms' of educational inequality, without having any deeper engagement with underlying causal issues.

Whatever the strengths and limitations of such extended approaches, it also remains the case that pressures on schools to raise attainment year on year have tended to cut across opportunities to develop more complex and holistic responses to educational inequalities. This can be seen in relation to the current Pupil Premium (PP) policy, which replaced FSES as the government's flagship policy for supporting disadvantaged pupils. PP provides additional funding to schools for every pupil on their roll who is known to be eligible for FSM, or who has received FSM in the previous six years, or who is or has been looked after.

There are two central challenges associated with this (see Carpenter et al, 2013). First, while schools have flexibility over how they spend PP to meet the needs of disadvantaged pupils (and there is no required 'offer', as with FSES), they are also held to account for demonstrating that PP funds are being used to raise FSM pupils' attainment. This raises significant questions about what constitutes a legitimate use of PP funds. For example, should a school use some PP funds to purchase winter coats, provide a free breakfast, offer parenting support or otherwise intervene in children's wider environments if there is no immediate and direct correlation between this and improved attainment? A 'safer' investment could, for instance, be in a targeted short-term mathematics intervention that impacts directly (if unsustainably) on attainment.

Second, schools often operate with a much broader understanding of the range of disadvantages in pupils' environments that could make them vulnerable to underachievement than eligibility for FSM. This might include, for instance, pupils who have: a chronic health condition; a close family member serving a custodial sentence; experience of bereavement; or caring responsibilities – all of whom may be more prevalent in communities where outcomes across a range of domains are poor. Even in terms of economic disadvantage, schools often identify families whose income is slightly above the FSM threshold as struggling most materially.

As this brief overview demonstrates, important though school improvement, targeted interventions and 'extended' approaches may be, they appear limited in what they can achieve, tending to encourage schools to look inwards and to focus on narrowly defined attainments, even when offering a range of extended provision. This suggests that there is a need to find ways to intervene in educational inequalities that can more fully acknowledge and respond to their underlying complexity, as well as focus attention on the 'causes' and 'causes of the causes' of poor outcomes. As the next section will illustrate, the emergence of localised models of intervention that seek not only to tackle 'symptomatic' poor outcomes, but also to address some of their underlying causes as grounded within particular neighbourhood contexts, may offer an important additional approach – and one that can also promote synergies with efforts to address health inequalities.

Complex local responses to educational inequalities

There is a growing body of evidence detailing local initiatives – often led by schools and their partners from other services and third sector organisations – which are starting to act on complex understandings of how poor outcomes arise and are sustained in children's environments (see Kerr et al, 2014). One such example, of an initiative to improve speech, language and communication skills (SLCS), arising out the 2011 national year of communication supported by the Department for Education and Department of Health (commonly known as the 'Hello' campaign), is briefly outlined here (for more information, see Ainscow et al, 2012).

This one-year initiative, supported by a national speech, language and communication charity and a National Health Service (NHS)-seconded speech and language therapist (SLT), was designed to lay the foundations for a long-term strategy for improving children's SLCS in a disadvantaged urban neighbourhood with a majority white British population. It involved a partnership of four schools (three primaries and one secondary), where the electoral ward most closely corresponding to the schools' locations was ranked 240 in the ward-level indices of deprivation. A rank of 1 is most deprived and 8,414 is least deprived.

As a baseline measure, the SLCS of 105 children in the primary schools' foundation stage classes (pupils aged five) was assessed by SLTs using nationally recognised tests. The overwhelming majority were found not to be school ready in terms of SLCS, scoring below normal for their age range, with 47 children having an age-equivalent score of less than 36 months – the youngest age at which a child would normally be admitted to a pre-school nursery class. The secondary school also considered the long-term implications of these findings, noting, for instance, that at least 60% of young people in the youth justice system have specific SLCS difficulties, compared to about 10% of the general population of young people (TCT, no date).

These baseline measures were of considerable concern to the schools, where, before working with the NHS SLT, staff had had little knowledge of children's typical SLCS development, viewing this instead in terms of what was typical for their school. The schools' immediate priorities were to introduce a series of targeted, evidence-based interventions – for instance, around phonological awareness – as well as universal within-school strategies to improve teaching and learning around SLCS. For the purposes of this chapter, however, the work that the schools undertook to identify what was happening in children's environments outside school to create SLCS delays is of particular interest. For instance, through their own research, the teachers identified a number of underlying issues relating to the nature of child–parent relationships, including:

- the number of young, typically single, mothers, who were often quite isolated and had poor support networks, rarely leaving their housing estate or sometimes their home, and thereby limiting children's exposure to language in different contexts;
- the number of children starting school not weaned off dummies and/or bottles, with this creating a physical obstruction to the development of speech sounds;
- limited interaction between parents and children, for example, many parents were noted to listen to music on headphones when out with their children; and
- when communicating with the school, parents were also noted to often lack good SLCS, confidence and self-esteem.

The schools then started to explore how they could intervene effectively in these proximal causal issues – mindful, as one teacher put it, that *"people don't like to be told they need help. It's different to be told your child needs an intervention from being told you need help to support your child's communication"*.

One primary school, for instance, developed a range of SLCS activities for parents that were not dependent on parents' own literacy skills or high-level SLCS. For example, one activity involved sessions where parents could make a puppet with their child. Staff then modelled how to act out a story with the puppet that could be repeated at home, helping to develop children's narrative skills. The school also started to identify other professionals working with pre-school children with whom it might work in partnership. For instance, it started to work with health visitors to address the continued use of bottles and dummies, as well as with staff from its local Sure Start children's centre to help develop the children's centre's teaching and learning offer and so build school-readiness. The school also began to develop its own accessible self-assessment questionnaires for parents to give them a better understanding of age-related SLCS milestones, with signposting to school and Sure Start-based SLCS activities.

In addition, to address issues of parent isolation, the school started to explore different models of peer mentoring for parents (for instance, the National Literacy Trust's Parent Ambassador Programme). It planned to invite parents who had been involved in school-based SLCS sessions to train as mentors, with the school, health visitors and Sure Start working together to identify parents who could benefit from mentoring. Plans had been proposed to allow births to be registered at the local Sure Start centre, and it was felt that this could help with identifying and engaging new, potentially vulnerable parents, who might otherwise be hard to identify.

An example like this suggests that while schools and their partners may not be in a position to address macro- and meso-level factors (notably, those originating at global and national levels) that help to create educational inequalities – for instance, by concentrating young, vulnerable, single mothers in social housing in highly disadvantaged neighbourhoods – they can nonetheless do something to engage with some of the factors grounded in local neighbourhood contexts, such as how people parent within the community, and the opportunities, supports and services available to them. They can also do so in ways that start to cross traditional service boundaries, notably, in the case of SLCS, between health and education. In doing so, it appears important that rather than simply adding disconnected services to schools – be it hosting health visitor clinics or a befriending service for vulnerable parents – any additional activities or services need to be aligned in such a way as to create a coherent response to an analysis of the local causes of poor outcomes. It is also important to note that this is not at the expense of using high-quality, evidence-based interventions and universal strategies to improve outcomes; however, these need to operate alongside efforts to engage with underlying causal issues.

Concluding comments

This chapter has argued that there is a need for education to start to mirror, more comprehensively, thinking in health about the importance of 'social determinants' in shaping outcomes. Strategies to improve the quality of schools, of course, remain an important element of efforts to address educational inequalities, as do high-quality targeted interventions. However, alone, these are not sufficient, and it is also necessary to think about how best to intervene in the causes of poor education outcomes. It is promising, therefore, that opportunities are also beginning to emerge for the locally led development of contextualised initiatives, which seek to understand what is happening locally to produce poor outcomes, to identify those factors that schools and their partners can act upon, and to do so in ways that can begin to form part of a wider strategic response to developing the 'nurturant quality' of children's environments.

Recognising the value of a social determinants model to education as well as to health could, therefore, mark an important forward step for both fields. Although the precise nature of the relationship between education and health remains uncertain (beyond higher attainment being linked to better health [Karas Montez and Friedman, 2015]), a shared focus on social determinants could help to foster new synergies between these related fields. There are, moreover, increasingly urgent policy imperatives that could be captured and used to drive this; for instance, the wider services that schools have typically accessed (such as school nursing and child and adolescent mental health services) are coming under increasing threat, and the commissioning of public health services is now entering a period of change, enabling strategic and operational reform.

These shifts, while underpinned in part by economic necessity, are nonetheless also beginning to create a space where relationships between sets of professionals – from education, health and other services – can potentially be reconfigured around shared thinking about social determinants. Initiatives like Public Health England's 'Healthy Child Programme' may have an important role to play in stimulating activity, its aims including to ensure that every child is school-ready and 'supported to thrive in school years, gaining maximum benefit from education', and that children, young people and families are helped 'with problems that might affect their chances later in life, including building resilience' (Public Health England, 2016: 7). As the SLCS initiative outlined in this chapter suggests, even if only locally in the first instance, opportunities are likely to emerge for boundaries between services to be challenged, and for community members to be actively involved in addressing inequalities as mutual concerns are identified and acted upon. Research that can capture and learn from these developments will have an important role to play in helping to shape future responses to both education and health inequalities.

References

ABC News (2016) 'Boyer lectures: Sir Michael Marmot highlights health inequalities and "causes of the causes"', 11 September. Available at: http://www.abc.net.au/news/2016-09-03/boyer-lecture-sir-michael-marmot-highlights-health-inequalities/7810382

Ainscow, M., Gallannaugh, F. and Kerr, K. (2012) 'An evaluation of the Communication Trust's "talk of the town" project, 2011–12', Centre for Equity in Education, University of Manchester.

Carpenter, H., Papps, I., Bragg, J., Dyson, A., Harris, D., Kerr, K., Todd, L. and Laing, K. (2013) Evaluation of pupil premium: Research report, London: DfE.

Cummings, C., Dyson, A. and Todd, L. (2011) Beyond the school gates. Can full service and extended schools overcome disadvantage?, London: Routledge.

DfE (Department for Education) (2016) 'Revised GCSE and equivalent results in England, 2014 to 2015', SFR 01/2016. Available at: https://www.gov.uk/government/uploads/system/uploads/attachment_data/file/494073/SFR01_2016.pdf

DfES (Department for Education and Skills) (2005) *Extended schools: Access to opportunities and services for all. A prospectus*, London: DfES.

Dyson, A. and Raffo, C. (2007) 'Education and disadvantage: the role of community-oriented schools', *Oxford Review of Education*, 33(3): 297–314.

Dyson, A., Hertzman, C., Roberts, H., Tunstill, J. and Vaghri, Z. (2009) 'Childhood development, education and health inequalities'. Available at: https://view.officeapps.live.com/op/view.aspx?src=http%3A%2F%2Fhummedia.manchester.ac.uk%2Finstitutes%2Fcee%2Fearly_years_and_education.doc

Dyson, A., Jones, L. and Kerr, K. (2011) 'Inclusion, place, and disadvantage in the English education system', in A.J. Artiles, E.B. Kozleski and F.R. Waitoller (eds) *Inclusive education: Examining equity on five continents*, Cambridge, MA: Harvard Education Press.

Hills, J.C., Brewer, M., Jenkins, S., Lister, R., Lupton, R., Machin, S., Mills, C., Modood, T., Rees, T. and Riddell, S. (2010) *An anatomy of economic inequality in the UK: Report of the National Equality Panel*, London: Government Equalities Office and Centre for Analysis of Social Exclusion.

Karas Montez, J. and Friedman, E. (2015) 'Introduction: educational attainment and adult health: under what conditions is the association causal?', *Social Science & Medicine*, 127(February): 1–7.

Kerr, K., Dyson, A. and Raffo, C. (2014) *Education, disadvantage and place: Making the local matter*, Bristol: The Policy Press.

Levin, B. (2006) 'Schools in challenging circumstances: a reflection on what we know and what we need to know', *School Effectiveness and School Improvement*, 17(4): 399–407.

Mujis, D. (2010) 'Effectiveness and disadvantage in education', in C. Raffo, A. Dyson, H. Gunter, D. Hall, L. Jones and A. Kalambouka (eds) *Education and poverty in affluent countries*, Abingdon: Routledge, pp 85–96.

Public Health England (2016) *Best start in life and beyond: Improving public health outcomes for children, young people and families*, London: Public Health England.

The Communication Trust (no date) 'Youth justice programme'. Available at: https://www.thecommunicationtrust.org.uk/projects/youth-justice/

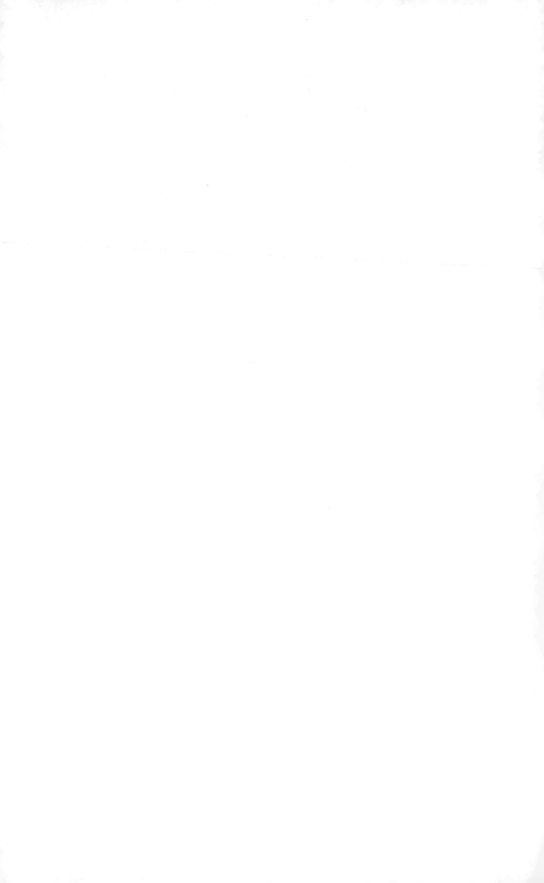

THREE

Wholistic well-being and happiness: psychosocial-spiritual perspectives

Andrew Parnham

21st-century living

By most measures, the UK is a wealthy society, possessing resources and facilities of which previous generations might only have dreamt. However, most of these measures are material and physical, with gross domestic product dominating other perspectives. If mental, emotional, relational and social dimensions are examined, this nation's 'wealth' is not so impressive. One recent national study found that nearly half of the population reported at least one adverse childhood experience and over 8% reported four or more (Bellis et al, 2014). Vulnerable families continue to face acute ongoing economic pressures.

Health professionals speak of social 'epidemics' in society. One of these is stress, which affects one in five of the working population and is the single largest cause of sickness absence, accounting for 37% of all work-related illnesses and 45% of all working days lost (Buckley, 2016). Only 17% of employees are engaged with their work, with 63% not engaged and 20% disengaged (Kular et al, 2008). One in six people experience a mental health problem each year (McManus et al, 2014). Depression is now the second most burdensome disorder in the world (Ferrari et al, 2013). Ironically, National Health Service (NHS) workers, charged with responsibility for the care of people with illness, experience some of the highest sickness absence rates in the country, with an annual cost of £2.4 billion (Horan, 2016).

Lifestyle choices have a profound effect on our health, as discussed in Section Two. Alcohol misuse disorders, drug dependency and lack of exercise are widespread concerns. The top five causes of premature death in this country are cancer, heart disease, stroke, respiratory disease and liver disease (Murray et al, 2013). All of these are strongly affected by lifestyle. These conditions, as well as being causes of pain and suffering in themselves, are also symptoms of a deeper malaise.

Unhealthy habits like excessive alcohol intake and overeating point to psychological, emotional and existential issues of discontent and dissatisfaction. It is these underlying problems that should concern us, as well as the physical maladies.

All of this comes at a time when state care provision is under great strain. Cuts in services are exerting a major impact on individuals and communities. However, there is an underlying, longer-term societal phenomenon, which transcends shorter-term political changes. The post-war welfare state was designed to deliver physical, material support but assumed that social 'shock absorbers' like family, neighbours, churches and community groups would provide the relational underpinning that all needed. However, these have atrophied in the intervening decades, leaving many to struggle with loneliness and depression (Young Foundation, 2009). Arguably, today, our social, communal and existential needs are greater than our physical and material deficiencies. This calls for a profound review of our priorities.

This point is emphasised by the 'epidemic' of loneliness. Humans are profoundly social beings and one of the most robust findings in well-being research is that strong relationships are by far the most significant factor in promoting life satisfaction (Economic and Social Research Council, 2013; Lyubomirsky, 2007). So, if our relationships are not healthy, our well-being will be damaged. Loneliness is a clear indicator that something is wrong. With nearly 8 million people living alone in Britain, this is an epidemic that is showing no signs of relenting (Campaign to End Loneliness, 2012).

Life in 21st-century Britain, then, is a mixed experience, with challenges that are not likely to go away in the near future. For those on the margins of society, the problems outlined earlier are especially acute. So, how might the tide be turned? Current and previous UK governments have taken considerable interest in the subject of happiness and well-being, stimulated by economic and political interests supported by the 'new science of happiness'. The Behavioural Insights Team, sometimes referred to as the Nudge Unit, was set up by the cabinet with a view to understanding and influencing people's behaviour (Behavioural Insights Team, 2016).

What is well-being?

Many definitions of well-being have been devised, and yet such is its complexity that 'the search for a generally accepted definition is fruitless, frustrating and ultimately impossible' (McNaught, 2011: 10). The reason is clear: 'well-being' encompasses all aspects of life, from physical to spiritual, from individual to global, reaching into every sphere of human existence.

Anne-Marie Bagnall (Chapter Eleven) quotes the helpful and workable Office for National Statistics (ONS) definition, which encompasses 10 broad categories. Her emphasis on personal and community well-being is welcome, since both perspectives are vital. The definitions that she quotes are highly relevant to my work with the Happiness Course (see later), which though focusing primarily on personal well-being, inevitably also impacts on community well-being.

Positive psychology has significantly expanded our understanding of what makes for human thriving, recognising, for example, that expressing gratitude, undertaking acts of kindness, nurturing relationships and practising spirituality all make a measurable difference to well-being (Seligman and Csikszentmihalyi, 2000; Seligman et al, 2005).

Yet, simply promoting a number of 'helpful interventions' risks the emergence of anecdotal, fragmentary living, lacking an underlying, whole-life framework. A deeper question arises: how does all this work out across the whole of life? How may we live a joined-up, integrated life? Such questions are especially relevant to socially marginalised people, for whom anecdotal, isolated interventions are of limited long-term value. This leads on to a consideration of whole-life well-being.

Wholistic living

For many people today, an underpinning foundation of meaning and purpose is often lacking. In Seligman's (2003) words, 'when an entire lifetime is taken up in the pursuit of the positive emotions … authenticity and meaning are nowhere to be found'. One of our most pressing challenges today is to discover a more joined-up, whole-life paradigm. This is 'the wholistic life', which encompasses and integrates all aspects: physical, mental, emotional, relational, societal and spiritual. It requires a mindset that integrates rather than fragments these dimensions. Kirstin Kerr reflects this view when she refers to the vital '"nurturant" quality of children's interconnected environments' (Chapter Two, p 19). Later, she speaks of statutory educational interventions seeking to 'separately target the "symptoms" of educational inequality, without having any deeper engagement with underlying causal issues' (**p 21**). These 'underlying issues' impact on later-life emotional health and the whole spectrum of people's lives.

Aaron Antonovsky's term 'salutogenesis' is of value here (see Figure 3.1). For him, three beliefs are necessary for a 'sense of coherence' that produces resilience under stress:

1. Comprehensibility: life's events occur in an orderly, predictable fashion.
2. Manageability: one's skills and resources permit control over life's experiences.
3. Meaningfulness: life has purpose and satisfaction, giving reasons to care about what happens (Antonovsky, 1979).

Of these elements, Antonovsky considered meaningfulness to be the most crucial. If someone lacks an awareness of meaning, their weakened sense of coherence will bring vulnerability to illness and disease. Others concur. Victor Frankl (2004), in his classic autobiography of life, death and survival in Nazi death camps, writes: 'Life is never made unbearable by circumstances, but only by lack of meaning and purpose'. Martin Seligman's (2004) description of the Full Life comprises: the Pleasant Life (positive emotions); Engagement (relationships, occupation, hobbies); and Meaning (living in the service of something larger than oneself).

For those living on the margins of society, there can surely be no greater need than to discover and develop a sense of meaning and

Figure 3.1: A simplified model of salutogenesis

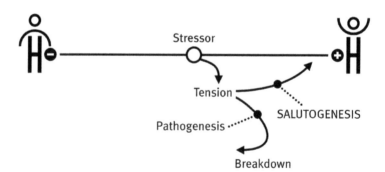

Notes: Stressor may be internally or externally generated. H– = poor health; H+ = good health.

Source: Adapted from Lindstrom and Eriksson (2010).

purpose in life. Such considerations were, for me, foundational in formulating and developing the Happiness Course (see later).

This paradigm of wholism has profound outworkings. State health and welfare service-based approaches are proving inadequate, as recognised by the incorporation of salutogenesis within the current Scotland NHS strategy (Taylor, 2004). A different emphasis is required, based less on us/them programmes and more on integrated, joined-up strategies, focusing on relationships, community and meaning. Research has shown conclusively that networks of healthy personal relationships and strong social capital in communities bring profound all-round benefits (Office for National Statistics, 2001). Robert Putnam (2000) notes that if you belong to no groups but decide to join one, 'you cut your risk of dying over the next year in half'. The most disadvantaged groups in society stand to gain enormously from such an approach.

Spiritual and faith dimensions

The definition of 'well-being' is problematic because of its complexity. Alternative words cannot easily express the necessary depth and breadth of meaning. However, the Hebrew concept of 'shalom' is a candidate for such a challenge. Often translated as 'peace' (which is usually construed as 'lack of conflict' but, like 'health', has concrete reality in itself), its true meaning is 'completeness' or 'wholeness'. It has three main dimensions: the state of wellness in the material or physical domain; relational and social well-being between friends, communities or nations; and moral and ethical integrity in all areas of life. No arena is excepted since shalom is the consequence of life lived 'as it should be lived' (Yoder, 1987).

This framework lies at the heart of the Judaeo-Christian worldview. Notwithstanding much that has muddied the water, faith-based spirituality and practice have a long history, including the development of hospitals, schools, the probation service, hospices, political and philanthropic initiatives, and many more. The first hospitals were often founded and funded by religious orders or through Christian donors. In the 12th and 13th centuries, hundreds of leper houses and hospitals for the sick and poor were established across Europe, health care was provided by organisations providing charitable mutual support, and monasteries and penitential groups were complemented by hospitaller and military groups, which were developed to provide care for wounded soldiers. Faith and psychology have been uneasy bedfellows since Freud but, more recently, this conflict has been re-evaluated (Ellison and Levin, 1998; Koenig, 2009).

Today, faith communities make a significant contribution to individual and social well-being, often providing long-term 'community within the community', filling in the gaps left by statutory provision and developing specific initiatives in youth work, aid for homeless people, financial advice, parent-and-toddler groups, help for the elderly, street pastors, food banks, and many more.

The Happiness Course

With this context in mind, it may be instructive to relate my own experience. For many years, I worked with faith communities in South-East London and developed a variety of approaches to community engagement. The most successful initiative was called 'Healthy Brockley'; it combined larger community events with accessible courses focusing on key life issues such as money and stress management, parenting, and relationships. However, although this met with a positive response among the local community, it still lacked the joined-up dimension outlined earlier.

Drawing on my experience in community engagement over many years, coupled with insights from positive psychology and other well-being research, I developed a well-being course that aimed to engage participants in a deeper, more wholistic way. 'The Happiness Course' emerged as a four-session programme, with each session focusing on one aspect of well-being.

The course

The course explores the meaning of happiness and well-being and enables participants to both reflect on and make progress in their lives. During each session, members reflect on a wide range of topics, including how success, relationships and a sense of purpose can contribute to happiness.

The course is fashioned around three recognised levels of well-being (Seligman, 2003):

1. Pleasure: with the emphasis on the material and life via our five senses.
2. Engagement: the more demanding dimension of relationships, career and hobbies.
3. Meaning: what enables us to live meaningful and purposeful lives.

Each session employs a number of means and approaches, including videos, readings, plenary discussion, small group work and personal reflection. In this way, participants are enabled to go on a journey: starting with the relatively superficial experience of 'pleasure'; progressing to an understanding of 'success'; then to the challenges and joys of relationships; and on to the deeper dimensions of meaning and purpose. The sessions follow this pattern:

1. 'A Happy Life' asks what makes us happy, what holds us back and whether we can become happier.
2. 'A Successful Life' examines what true success is, whose narrative about success we are following and what can take us beyond pleasure alone.
3. 'A Relational Life' recognises the profound importance of relationships in determining our well-being, how they can go wrong and how they can be restored.
4. 'A Meaningful Life' emphasises the importance of discovering meaning and purpose in life, and of finding practical avenues to pursue them.

The first course ran in 2008, facilitated by a grant from the local council. Early responses from participants were encouraging, including feedback such as:

> *The course enabled me to look for the good things rather than dwelling on the bad.*

> *I was able to be more aware of my thinking and influences. Aware of wanting to focus more on positives and happiness and practising this.*

Over the following years, I have run the course across the UK and beyond, in schools, colleges, children's centres, hospitals and other NHS contexts, community centres, and churches, working with a variety of ages, cultures and backgrounds. In the church setting, I currently work with the charity Livability, but in the wider context, I work as an independent trainer.

Participants consistently observe that they have been enabled to grasp those things that make for well-being and satisfaction, many of which are simple and doable. Others remark that it has helped them to both review their lives to date and project forwards into the future. Examples of feedback include:

It made me consider how to make myself more happy by just appreciating simple things in my life. It made me think about deeper things that matter in life.

It will make a great difference to know who I am and realise the choices that I make for my own life and other people.

Thank you, I have taken loads of notes from you which I will reflect on in changes to my life. You explained these views like a life coach.

It made a very big difference. I'll think more carefully about the decisions that I make and I'll always keep in mind how these decisions can affect others.

It has changed my life.

Evaluation

At the end of the course, each participant completes a standardised evaluation. Some questions enable a quantitative assessment, but even the more qualitative questions yield valuable information. The averages of participants' responses from 10 courses, with a total of 80 participants, are outlined in Table 3.1.

Table 3.1: Evaluation of the Happiness Course

1. Were your **expectations** met?	**96%** say 'yes'
2. How useful did you find the course materials? (10 = very; 0 = not at all)	**8.3**
3. Which parts were **most valuable**?	25% say 'relationships'
4. Which parts were **least valuable**?	65% say 'none'
5. To what extent would you agree with the following statements (10 = very; 0 = not at all): I better **understand** things that affect my happiness I feel better **equipped** to develop my happiness The course has **changed** my outlook on life	 8.4 8.2 7.7
6. Would you recommend the course to a friend or attend a **follow-up** course yourself?	**92%** say 'yes'

Lessons learned

After several years of running the course, a number of conclusions are discernible. The course has proved to be very accessible. Language such as 'happiness', 'success' 'relationships' and 'meaning' is viewed by most people as both everyday and significant.

The variety of training approaches enables people with different learning styles and dispositions to benefit. In particular, time spent in personal reflection can lead to deeper insights. Often, people's busy lifestyles do not provide such opportunities.

The course takes a wholistic approach to life, exploring physical, emotional, relational and existential dimensions, from both an individual and corporate perspective. This is not common in well-being education and training, which often focuses on one or the other domain. Participants are therefore enabled to encounter more profound areas of their lives, despite the short time available.

For this reason, objections are sometimes raised concerning people's mental health – are those with depression not troubled by the more challenging encounters? In practice, this has not proved to be the case. At the end of a course, one woman said: "*I've suffered from moderate depression for 20 years, but if this course had been available back then, perhaps I wouldn't have had to take so many antidepressants!*".

This resonates with an asset-based approach to community well-being, as Anne-Marie Bagnall records (Chapter Eleven), since participants gain insights into their strengths and capabilities through the course.

Kirstin Kerr (Chapter Two, p 21) asserts that statutory service provision often assumes that 'professionals can "fix" deficits ... through rafts of single-issue interventions'. The recipients of such help may perceive it as being 'done to' them. The Happiness Course takes a co-production approach, in which no one is the 'expert' and all participants have a significant contribution to make.

The third session, on relationships, consistently proves to be the most popular and impactful. Many say that the work they have done on forgiveness and the healing of relationships was most significant for them. This finding should not surprise us since healthy relationships are at the heart of well-being (Lyubomirsky, 2007).

Bagnall (Chapter Eleven) rightly emphasises both personal and community well-being, stressing, among other conducive elements, socio-economic factors, relationship with others, neighbourliness and community cohesion. 'What works' for community well-being includes strengthening communities, collaborations and partnerships, and volunteer and peer approaches. The Happiness Course engages with all these dimensions, and has brought both personal and corporate benefit.

After completing the course, participants are encouraged to access further pathways to well-being through signposting to a range of statutory and voluntary services, including mental health services, counselling, mentoring and life coaching. More commonly, friendships flourish during the course and beyond. The course therefore provides a helpful foundation for personal growth and well-being.

The development, maintenance and repair of relationships are of great relevance to people experiencing social exclusion. Healthy relationships are a vital ingredient for them since they often experience isolation and stigma. The course can be both a space to develop deeper and more meaningful relationships and a launching pad for longer-term help and support. The host community providing the course can be an effective servant to people in need of friendship and support.

The province of the Happiness Course is not limited to faith communities. People of diverse faiths and no faith have profited much from it. However, churches have hosted the course many times, benefitting people in their local community. It is clear that faith communities still have an important place in community engagement today.

Conclusion

There is a great need in our nation to help people discover those things that generate whole-life health and well-being, and then journey with them in that process. The principles and practice outlined in this chapter can enable many more to make that journey, especially at the margins of our society.

References

Antonovsky, A. (1979) *Health, stress and coping*, San Francisco, CA: Jossey-Bass.

Behavioural Insights Team (2016) 'Update report 2015–16'. Available at: https://www.gov.uk/government/organisations/behavioural-insights-team (accessed 30 January 2017).

Bellis, M.A., Hughes, K., Leckenby, N., Lowey, H. and Harrison, D. (2014) 'Adverse childhood experiences: retrospective study to determine their impact on adult health behaviours and health outcomes in a UK population', *Journal of Public Health*, 36: 81–91.

Buckley, P. (2016) 'Work related stress, anxiety and depression statistics in Great Britain 2016', Health & Safety Executive. Available at: http://www.hse.gov.uk/statistics/causdis/stress/stress.pdf (accessed 27 January 2017).

Campaign to End Loneliness (2012) 'Summit on tackling loneliness in older age'. Available at: http://www.campaigntoendloneliness. org/wp-content/uploads/downloads/2012/03/15.03.12-Summit-on-Tackling-Loneliness-Report.pdf (accessed 6 September 2016).

Economic and Social Research Council (2013) 'Mental health and social relationships'. Available at: http://www.esrc.ac.uk/news-events-and-publications/evidence-briefings/mental-health-and-social-relationships (accessed 7 September 2016).

Ellison, C. and Levin, J. (1998) 'The religion–health connection: evidence, theory and future directions', *Health Education & Behavior*, 25(6): 700–20.

Ferrari, A.J., Charlson, F.J., Norman, R.E., Patten, S.B., Freedman, G., Murray, C.J. et al (2013) 'Burden of depressive disorders by country, sex, age, and year: findings from the Global Burden of Disease Study 2010', *PLoS Med*, 10: 11.

Frankl, V. (2004) *Man's search for meaning*, London: Rider.

Horan, B. (2016) 'NHS sickness absence rates April 2016–June 2016', NHS Digital, p 1. Available at: http://www.content.digital.nhs.uk/catalogue/PUB22226/nhs-sick-abs-rate-apr2009-jun2016-report.pdf (accessed 27 January 2017).

Koenig, H. (2009) 'Research on religion, spirituality and mental health: a review', *The Canadian Journal of Psychiatry*, 54(5). Available at: https://hivdatf.files.wordpress.com/2011/01/research-on-religion-spirituality-and-mental-health-a-review.pdf (accessed 1 September 2016).

Kular, S., Gatenby, M., Rees, C., Soane, E. and Truss, K. (2008) 'Employee engagement: a literature review', Kingston University, p 13. Available at: http://eprints.kingston.ac.uk/4192/1/19wempen.pdf (accessed 27 January 2017).

Lindstrom, B. and Eriksson, M. (2010) *The hitchhiker's guide to salutogenesis*, Helsinki: Folkhälsan Research Centre.

Lyubomirsky, S. (2007) *The how of happiness*, London: Sphere.

McManus, S., Bebbington, P., Jenkins, R. and Brugha, T. (2014) 'Mental health and wellbeing in England. Adult Psychiatric Morbidity Survey 2014, executive summary', p 2. Available at: http://content.digital.nhs.uk/catalogue/PUB21748/apms-2014-exec-summary.pdf (accessed 27 January 2017).

McNaught, A. (2011) 'Defining wellbeing', in A. Knight and A. McNaught (eds) *Understanding wellbeing*, Lantern: Banbury.

Murray, C., Richards, M., Newton, J. et al (2013) 'UK health performance: findings of the Global Burden of Disease Study 2010', *The Lancet [Online]*, 381(9871): 997–1020.

Office for National Statistics (2001) *Social capital: A review of the literature*, London: Socio-economic Inequities Branch, Social Analysis and Reporting Division.

Putnam, R. (2000) *Bowling alone*, New York: Simon and Schuster.

Seligman, M. (2003) *Authentic happiness*, London: Nicholas Brealey.

Seligman, M. (2004) 'A balanced psychology and a full life', *Phil. Trans.R.Soc.Lond.B*, 359: 1379–81.

Seligman, M. and Csikszentmihalyi, M. (2000) 'Positive psychology', *American Psychologist*, 55(1): 5–14.

Seligman, M.E., Steen, T.A., Park, N. and Peterson, C. (2005) 'Positive psychology progress', *American Psychologist*, 60(5): 410–21.

Taylor, J. (2004) 'Salutogenesis as a framework for child protection: literature review', *Journal of Advanced Nursing*, 45(6): 633–43.

Yoder, P. (1987) *Shalom: The Bible's word for salvation, justice and peace*, Evangel: Nappanee.

Young Foundation (2009) 'Sinking and swimming: understanding Britain's unmet needs'. Available at: http://youngfoundation.org/wp-content/uploads/2012/10/Sinking-and-swimming.pdf (accessed 2 August 2016).

FOUR

Nutrition in marginalised groups

Rosalind Fallaize and Julie Lovegrove

Introduction

The nutritional intake of the homeless and other marginalised groups, including those surviving on limited income, is inadequate. This chapter gives an overview of key nutritional issues and contemporary advances in human nutrition in marginalised groups and provides insight from primary research into the nutritional needs of vulnerable groups. There is evidence to suggest that the dietary choices of communities on low income, including the homeless and families residing in temporary accommodation, are compromised. This chapter will examine the potential benefit and community responses to dietary intervention, food banks and voucher systems, within the context of complex nutritional needs, food insecurity and marginalised housing scenarios. UK policies and guidelines, including the National Institute of Clinical Excellence (NICE) and specialist groups, will also be discussed. It is concluded that further research is required to develop effective nutritional strategies to address the complex nutritional and physical requirements of disadvantaged groups on low income.

Homelessness is associated with increased physical and mental health needs. The absence of a nutritionally adequate diet, in combination with a marginalised housing situation, is likely to exacerbate this further (Luder et al, 1989). The average age of death for homeless adults is 47 years (CRISIS, 2011); thereafter, cardiovascular disease (CVD) is the leading cause of mortality (aged 45–65 years) (Hwang et al, 1997). With up to 80% of chronic diseases such as CVD attributed to poor dietary and lifestyle choices (eg smoking) (Alwan et al, 2011), there is a clear role for adequate nutritional intake in enhancing health.

Determinants of food choice include sociological, psychological and physiological factors, with food availability being a key issue in the homeless community. In a review of health promotion needs, *Big Issue* vendors rated 'nutritional deficiencies' as the third most common health concern for vulnerably housed individuals, following 'drug and alcohol use' and 'the effects of the cold weather' (Power and Hunter, 2001). In children, health, hunger and dietary intake were primary concerns; inadequacies in these areas have been associated with developmental delays (speech delay and impaired cognitive ability) (Rafferty and Shinn, 1991).

This chapter considers the evidence for the nutritional requirements, dietary intake and associated health and lifestyle factors in homeless individuals. Single homeless adults (living 'rough' or in temporary accommodation) and homeless families (residing in temporary or bed-and-breakfast [B&B] accommodation) will be considered, including the unique challenges faced by each community and possible interventions to overcome these.

Nutritional requirements

In 2012, the Queen's Nursing Institute (QNI) produced specific guidance for practitioners on recognising and screening for nutritional need in single homeless adults and homeless families (Coufopoulos and Mooney, 2012). The guidance is based on the 'eatwell plate', recently replaced by *The eatwell guide* (Public Health England, 2016), and includes standard tailored dietary recommendations for pregnant women (eg 400μg supplement of folic acid), young children, adolescents and adults (18–65 years). Key barriers faced by single homeless adults and homeless families are also described (eg the reliance of single homeless people on day centres for food).

In contrast to many government institutions, including schools, prisons and residential care facilities, which receive guidance to ensure meals provided meet dietary reference values, homeless institutions are mostly charity-funded. Thus, the provision of food at soup kitchens and catered living hostels is largely unregulated. Nutrient and food-based guidance for UK institutions is provided by the Food Standards Agency (FSA, 2007), although these are not enforced and may not meet the needs of single homeless adults using these facilities, who present with a complex range of psychological and clinical conditions.

Factors affecting nutritional requirements

Factors affecting nutritional requirements in the homeless include substance misuse, alcoholism and chronic and acute physical and mental health conditions. In a 2014 health audit by Homeless Link ($n = 2,590$), 73% of UK homeless people reported physical health problems, of whom 41% identified a chronic condition (Homeless Link, 2015).

Chronic medical conditions, such as CVD and type-2 diabetes, are likely to impact on the nutritional needs of a homeless individual (eg a low-salt diet in the management of hypertension). However, adherence to dietary guidance may be unachievable for those relying on charity meal provision. Limited food choice was noted as a key 'barrier' to adequate glucose control in homeless diabetics ($n = 50$) (Hwang and Bugeja, 2000), suggesting that while nutritional requirements may differ in those with chronic conditions, these may not be achievable via existing housing scenarios.

Higher rates of health issues, in addition to high hospital admissions, have been observed in homeless children (Bassuk et al, 1986; Alperstein et al, 1988), although this research is over 25 years old. An independent association between severe hunger and adverse physical health and mental health outcomes among low-income children was reported more recently (Weinreb et al, 2002). Yet, the sacrifice of parental food intake to ensure that children have three meals per day has also been reported in the US (Rafferty and Shinn, 1991). There is a distinct lack of research on factors that influence nutritional requirements in homeless children in the UK.

High levels of mental illness, including depression, anxiety and bipolar disorders, have repeatedly been observed in the homeless. In addition to a negative impact of depression on appetite and subsequent food intake (FSA, 2006), psychiatric medications may also increase appetite and promote weight gain (Basson et al, 2001). Depression has been associated with low-plasma omega-3 fatty acids (Riemer et al, 2010), vitamin D (Kerr et al, 2015) and selenium (Conner et al, 2015). However, evidence is limited and it is unknown whether the increased dietary intake or supplementation of these nutrients would be beneficial. Health needs are further complicated by the frequent occurrence of alcohol and substance misuse (Homeless Link, 2015). In a 2008 systematic review and meta-regression analysis ($n = 5,684$), the most commonly identified mental disorders were alcohol and drug dependence (Fazel et al, 2008).

Chronic alcohol intake can affect both nutrient intake and/ or absorption (De Timary et al, 2012) and homeless individuals who misuse alcohol are more likely to be malnourished due to the substitution of food with alcohol (Langnäse and Müller, 2001). Thiamin absorption is impaired in chronic alcoholism and prophylactic oral thiamine is advised for harmful or dependent drinkers at risk of malnutrition (National Institute of Clinical Excellence, 2010). Thiamin deficiency causes the alcohol-linked neurological disorder Wernicke–Korsakoff syndrome, and a high prevalence of dietary, biochemical and clinical features to indicate early clinical thiamin deficiency have been observed in homeless men (Darnton-Hill and Truswell, 1990).

Smoking can also impact on the nutritional needs of the individual, as evidenced by the increased vitamin C requirements in smokers (Lykkesfeldt et al, 2000). The abuse of illicit substances is an additional issue for some homeless individuals. The effects on nutrient absorption/status vary in accordance with the type of drug (eg hypercholesterolemia with morphine use) (Mohs et al, 1990), although this, in addition to the likelihood that drug addicts will use money to feed their drug habit in preference to feeding themselves, and postpone seeking advice for medical conditions (Kushel et al, 2006; Baggett et al, 2010), highlights the detrimental effect of this behaviour on nutrient intake.

Nutritional status of homeless individuals

Homelessness has been frequently associated with hunger, food insecurity and malnutrition. Skin fold thickness and muscle measurements have demonstrated evidence of 'wasting' in the homeless community (Luder et al, 1989; Wolgemuth et al, 1992; Langnäse and Müller, 2001). The QNI suggests the assessment of nutritional status using the Malnutrition Universal Screening Tool, although this is unlikely to detect nutritional deficiencies in the absence of a low body mass index (BMI).

Several researchers have identified homeless individuals who, according to their BMI, are overweight or obese (BMI $\geq$ 30 kg/m^2) (Koh et al, 2012; Tsai and Rosenheck, 2013). In a large group (n = 5,632) of homeless adults in Boston, significantly more adults were obese (32.3%) than underweight (BMI < 18.5 kg/m^2) (1.6%), characterising a situation whereby food insecurity and hunger coexist with obesity (Koh et al, 2012). Limited income often results in the purchase of energy-dense, nutrient-poor, low-cost convenience foods and food insecurity may result in high–energy intake during periods of food availability. Physiological adaptation (eg the increased efficiency of storing energy as fat) to chronic fluctuations in dietary intake may also predispose homeless adults to gain weight (Center on Hunger and Poverty, 2003).

Nutritional status is typically assessed using anthropometric measures, such as weight and waist circumference. Biochemical measurement of fatty acids, lipids and nutrients may provide additional insight. It also avoids the inherent bias of questionnaire techniques and accounts for individual variation in absorption. However, venous sampling in transient homeless populations is challenging. To date, elevated serum cholesterol (Luder et al, 1989) and low-plasma vitamin C levels (Malmauret et al, 2002) have been described in the homeless, although the samples sizes were small ($n = 17$ and $n = 71$, respectively). Based on their research, Malmauret et al suggested a target of 140mg/d vitamin C in homeless adults, which is significantly higher than the UK reference nutrient intake (RNI) (40mg/d) (Malmauret et al, 2002).

To overcome the detrimental health effects of malnutrition, a nutritionally balanced diet is vital. The hunger–obesity paradox demonstrates the importance of assessing dietary intake as opposed to relying on anthropological measurements when determining nutritional status.

Dietary intake in homeless individuals

Dietary intake has been assessed by a number of studies using questionnaire methods: the food frequency questionnaire (FFQ) and 24-hour recall. Analysis of these questionnaires provides estimates of food, energy and nutrient intake and can be used to identify deficiencies and develop nutrition intervention strategies (Seale et al, 2016).

Reported intakes of food, energy and nutrients

Food insecurity, defined as 'limited or uncertain availability of nutritionally adequate and safe food or limited or uncertain ability to acquire food in socially acceptable ways' (Olson and Holben, 2002) is prevalent in the homeless community. For example, homeless adults have reported consuming significantly fewer meals per day than housed adults (Fallaize et al, forthcoming). Sources of food include catered hostel accommodation, charity- or council-funded soup kitchens, and food banks. In a study of the food acquisition practices of young homeless people in Australia ($n = 149$), the majority of food (45%) was obtained from hostel/emergency accommodation, although food theft was high (65%), suggesting that welfare services were inadequate (Booth, 2006). In Canada, street-youths obtained food mostly through purchases (inexpensive, portable and ready to eat) and charitable meal provision (Dachner and Tarasuk, 2002).

Food insecurity has a detrimental impact on nutrient intake, and questionnaire data have repeatedly found insufficient intakes of fruit and vegetables (F&V) in the homeless community (Rushton and Wheeler, 1993; Langnäse and Müller, 2001; Hickey and Downey, 2003). Low intakes of milk and milk products have also been reported, with rough sleepers particularly vulnerable due to the absence of food storage facilities (Fallaize et al, forthcoming). In addition, high saturated fat (SFA) intakes have been observed in the UK (Evans and Dowler, 1999; Fallaize et al, forthcoming), New York (Luder et al, 1989) and Paris (Darmon et al, 2001).

Micronutrient intakes are also deficient in homeless populations. For example, low levels of vitamin B6, calcium and iron were reported in homeless families residing in temporary accommodation in Boston, USA (Wiecha et al, 1993). In this study, clear differences were also observed between families residing in hotels and shelters, with lower vitamin B6, iron and zinc intake, as well as diet satisfaction, reported in those placed in hotel accommodation (Wiecha et al, 1993). Insufficient intakes of vitamin B6, zinc and calcium were also reported in adults ($n = 277$) residing in an overnight shelter in Florida (Wolgemuth et al, 1992). However, in Sheffield ($n = 24$) (Sprake et al, 2014) and Paris ($n = 97$) (Darmon et al, 2001), vitamin B6 and niacin intakes exceeded the recommended nutrient intake levels.

In the UK, homeless pregnant women ($n = 10$) were found to have folate intakes significantly lower (100mg/d) than the RNI (300mg/d) (Dowler and Calvert, 1995). This group is particularly vulnerable given that requirements increase during pregnancy and deficiency of folate is associated with the risk of neural tube defects. Food insecurity has also been found to be higher in children from families with low socio-economic status (SES) where the mother is experiencing mental health issues (Melchior et al, 2009).

Trends in low F&V, vitamin B6 and calcium, as well as high SFA intake, appear consistent across homeless populations in developed countries; however, the severity of nutrient inadequacy may differ according to housing status, physiological condition (eg pregnancy) and food access. This, in addition to the complex physical and mental health needs mentioned, suggests that 'standard' guidelines are unlikely to be sufficient for the homeless community.

Factors affecting food choice

Food insecurity has a profound effect on food choice, particularly in street homeless people. Research conducted on street-youths in Canada revealed that food access was contingent upon conditions of health, shelter and income, and, therefore, acquisition strategies (purchase or charitable meal provision) varied meal to meal. Furthermore, when purchased, 'choice' was severely limited by food preparation facilities and cost, with street-youths reporting a reliance on inexpensive, portable, ready-to-eat foods (eg sandwiches, pizza, hamburgers) and snack foods (Dachner and Tarasuk, 2002). These food purchase habits have also been reported in low-SES families. In a UK study of homeless mothers (n = 66), over 50% of women reported higher takeaway, sweet and chocolate consumption in their children since living in a hostel. Snacking was also associated with boredom and lack of play facilitates (Coufopoulos et al, 2009).

Key barriers to purchasing raw and perishable food items in homeless men (n = 12) residing in Sheffield, UK, were limited cooking and storage space (Sprake et al, 2014). A quarter of women living in hostels identified poor cooking facilities as a barrier to eating green vegetables. These shared cooking facilities were often located several floors away and 77% of women reported sharing these with six or more other families (Dowler and Calvert, 1995). Dependency upon benefits to purchase food and inadequate cooking facilities are also key issues for homeless families residing in B&B accommodation.

Further to the absence of food storage facilities, a lack of nutritional and cooking knowledge has been reported in the homeless community (FSA, 2006). While lacking resources, several researchers have identified that homeless individuals aspire to consume a 'healthy' diet containing F&V (Jenkins, 2014; Sprake et al, 2014). Several methods of improving dietary intake in homeless communities have been proposed, including education, although research in this area is lacking.

Improving dietary intake in the community

Interventions to improve dietary and nutritional intake in the homeless community range from direct food provision to health education. Hostels and soup kitchens provide ideal access points for intervention in this group (Power and Hunter, 2001), and several education programmes have been developed to provide information on nutrition and cooking skills (Yousey et al, 2007; Johnson et al, 2009). Although these have mostly been targeted at women and young children, and while engagement has been demonstrated (Johnson et al, 2009), their efficacy is yet to be determined. Sustained nutrition education is also likely to be costly and challenging given the transient nature of this population. It is unclear whether there is a demand for nutritional education in single homeless groups.

Catered homeless hostels and soup kitchens enable the direct provision of a nutritionally balanced diet. However, analysis of foods provided by these premises has often identified them as inadequate. In Canada, charitable meal provision was considered to be of poor quality and associated with food sickness in homeless youths (Dachner and

Tarasuk, 2002). A survey of meals (n = 22) provided to the homeless in San Francisco revealed high SFA and low fibre, potassium, calcium and vitamins E and A compared to the US Department of Agriculture standards (Lyles et al, 2013). High SFA and low fibre intakes have also been demonstrated elsewhere (Sisson and Lown, 2011; Pelham-Burn et al, 2014; Frost et al, 2016).

In the UK, 'subtle' changes were made to lunch recipes (n = 12) provided by a food aid organisation, such as using wholemeal flour, to improve the nutritional content. Despite strong preconceived ideas from kitchen staff that the new foods would be rejected, the meals were well received by the homeless participants during taste tests (Pelham-Burn et al, 2014). The authors highlight the need to consider kitchen capabilities, financial resources and food donations. Food donations may be particularly challenging given that they are unstable, and issues have been raised regarding the food safety and storage of perishable food (Frost et al, 2016).

Another method of improving dietary intake is via food banks; the increased use and reliance of which has recently been reported in the UK (Loopstra et al, 2015). In the US, the Supplemental Nutrition Assistance Program (SNAP) provides benefits to food-insecure households to purchase nutrient-rich food items. However, the extent to which this programme improves dietary intake is unclear. Recently, researchers have also trialled financial incentives to further improve F&V intake in SNAP participants. Food storage facilities and cooking capabilities remain an issue with both food banks and products purchased via the SNAP programme.

In the UK, the government 'Healthy Start' scheme provides vouchers (£3.10) to pregnant women and children between one and four years old to purchase unflavoured cow's milk, plain fresh or frozen F&V, and infant formula; children younger than one year old are entitled to two vouchers per week (£6.20). The scheme is means-tested based on receipt of income support or age (< 18 years). Healthy start vitamins are also available free to pregnant women and children under one year old. Women using the scheme have reported increases in the quantity of F&V and the quality of family diets (McFadden et al, 2014).

The provision of supplements to homeless people at risk of one or more nutrient deficiencies provides a means of specifically targeting those in need. For example, researchers in France fortified a chocolate-flavoured spread with calcium and potassium (Darmon, 2009). However, it may be challenging to detect such deficiencies (eg thiamin deficiency) and fortification requirements will differ for each individual.

Conclusion

Homeless adults and families residing in temporary accommodation are at high risk of food insecurity and nutritional deficiencies. Adequate dietary intake is further exacerbated by limited income, a lack of nutritional knowledge, poor food storage and a lack of cooking facilities. To date, limited interventions and initiatives to improve the quality of dietary intake have been conducted. Interventions have focused on direct food provision and the promotion of healthy food choices via benefits and food vouchers. In the future, clear guidance for charity-funded organisations will be paramount, alongside full consideration of nutritional issues in UK policies aimed at supporting individuals at the edge of the community.

References

Alperstein, G., Rappaport, C. and Flanigan, J.M. (1988) 'Health problems of homeless children in New York City', *American Journal of Public Health*, 78: 1232–3.

Alwan, A., Armstrong, T., Bettcher, D., Branca, F., Chisholm, D., Ezzati, M., Garfield, R., MacLean, D., Mathers, C., Mendis, S., Poznyak, V., Riley, L., Tang, K.C. and Wild, C. (2011) *Global status report on noncommunicable diseases 2010*, Geneva: World Health Organization.

Baggett, T.P., O'Connell, J.J., Singer, D.E. and Rigotti, N.A. (2010) 'The unmet health care needs of homeless adults: a national study', *American Journal of Public Health*, 100: 1326–33.

Basson, B.R., Kinon, B.J., Taylor, C.C., Szymanski, K.A. and Tollefson, G.D. (2001) 'Factors influencing acute weight change in patients with schizophrenia treated with olanzapine, haloperidol, or risperidone', *The Journal of Clinical Psychiatry*, 62: 231–8.

Bassuk, E.L., Rubin, L. and Lauriat, A.S. (1986) 'Characteristics of sheltered homeless families', *American Journal of Public Health*, 76: 1097–101.

Booth, S. (2006) 'Eating rough: food sources and acquisition practices of homeless young people in Adelaide, South Australia', *Public Health Nutrition*, 9: 212–18.

Center on Hunger and Poverty (2003) 'The paradox of hunger and obesity in America'. Available at: https://olliasheville.com/sites/default/files/LAS/LAS_26/day2_hungerandobesity.pdf (accessed 2 August 2016).

Conner, T.S., Richardson, A.C. and Miller, J.C. (2015) 'Optimal serum selenium concentrations are associated with lower depressive symptoms and negative mood among young adults', *The Journal of Nutrition*, 145: 59–65.

Coufopoulos, A. and Mooney, K. (2012) *Food, nutrition and homelessness: Guideance for practitioners*, London: The Queen's Nursing Institute.

Coufopoulos, A.M., Hackett, A.F., Dykes, F. and Moran, V. (2009) 'Homeless mothers and their children: two generations at nutritional risk', in F. Dykes and V.H. Moran (eds) *Infant and young child nutrition: Challenges to implementing a global strategy*, Chichester: Wilry-Blackwell, 146–62.

CRISIS (2011) 'Homelessness: a silent killer'. Available at: https://www.crisis.org.uk/media/237321/crisis_homelessness_a_silent_killer_2011.pdf

Dachner, N. and Tarasuk, V. (2002) 'Homeless "squeegee kids": food insecurity and daily survival', *Social Science & Medicine*, 54: 1039–49.

Darmon, N. (2009) 'A fortified street food to prevent nutritional deficiencies in homeless men in France', *Journal of the American College of Nutrition*, 28: 196–202.

Darmon, N., Coupel, J., Deheeger, M. and Briend, A. (2001) 'Dietary inadequacies observed in homeless men visiting an emergency night shelter in Paris', *Public Health Nutrition*, 4: 155–61.

Darnton-Hill, I. and Truswell, A. (1990) 'Thiamin status of a sample of homeless clinic attenders in Sydney', *The Medical Journal of Australia*, 152: 5–9.

De Timary, P., Cani, P.D., Duchemin, J., Neyrinck, A.M., Gihousse, D., Laterre, P.F., Badaoui, A., Leclercq, S., Delzenne, N.M. and Stärkel, P. (2012) 'The loss of metabolic control on alcohol drinking in heavy drinking alcohol-dependent subjects', *PloS one*, 7: e38682.

Dowler, E. and Calvert, C. (1995) *Nutrition and diet in lone-parent families in London*, London: Family Policy Studies Centre.

Evans, N.S. and Dowler, E.A. (1999) 'Food, health and eating among single homeless and marginalized people in London', *Journal of Human Nutrition and Dietetics*, 12: 179–99.

Fallaize, R., Seale, J.V., Mortin, C., Armstrong, L. and Lovegrove, J.A. (forthcoming) 'Dietary intake, nutritional status and mental wellbeing of homeless adults in Reading, UK', *British Journal of Nutrition*.

Fazel, S., Khosla, V., Doll, H. and Geddes, J. (2008) 'The prevalence of mental disorders among the homeless in Western countries: systematic review and meta-regression analysis', *PLoS Med*, 5: e225.

Frost, C., Pelham-Burn, S., Russell, J. and Barker, M. (2016) 'Improving the nutritional quality of charitable meals for homeless and vulnerable adults: A mixed method study of two meals services in a large English city', *Journal of Hunger & Environmental Nutrition*, 11: 14–28.

FSA (Food Standards Agency) (2006) *Research into food poverty and homelessness in Northern Ireland – final report*, London: Food Standards Agency.

FSA (2007) *FSA nutrient and food based guidelines for UK institutions*, London: Food Standards Agency.

Hickey, C. and Downey, D. (2003) *Hungry for change: Social exclusion, food poverty and homelessness in Dublin; a pilot research study*, Dublin: Focus Ireland.

Homeless Link (2015) The unhealthy state of homelessness: health audit results 2014, London: Homeless Link.

Hwang, S.W. and Bugeja, A.L. (2000) 'Barriers to appropriate diabetes management among homeless people in Toronto', *Canadian Medical Association Journal*, 163: 161–5.

Hwang, S.W., Orav, E.J., O'Connell, J.J., Lebow, J.M. and Brennan, T.A. (1997) 'Causes of death in homeless adults in Boston', *Annals of Internal Medicine*, 126: 625–8.

Jenkins, M. (2014) 'An assessment of homeless families' diet and nutrition', *Community Practitioner*, 87: 24–8.

Johnson, L.J., Myung, E., McCool, A.C. and Champaner, E.I. (2009) 'Nutrition education for homeless women – challenges and opportunities: a pilot study', *Journal of Foodservice Business Research*, 12: 155–69.

Kerr, D.C., Zava, D.T., Piper, W.T., Saturn, S.R., Frei, B. and Gombart, A.F. (2015) 'Associations between vitamin D levels and depressive symptoms in healthy young adult women', *Psychiatry Research*, 227: 46–51.

Koh, K.A., Hoy, J.S., O'Connell, J.J. and Montgomery, P. (2012) 'The hunger–obesity paradox: obesity in the homeless', *Journal of Urban Health*, 89: 952–64.

Kushel, M.B., Gupta, R., Gee, L. and Haas, J.S. (2006) 'Housing instability and food insecurity as barriers to health care among low-income Americans', *Journal of General Internal Medicine*, 21: 71–7.

Langnäse, K. and Müller, M.J. (2001) 'Nutrition and health in an adult urban homeless population in Germany', *Public Health Nutrition*, 4: 805–11.

Loopstra, R., Reeves, A., Taylor-Robinson, D., Barr, B., McKee, M. and Stuckler, D. (2015) 'Austerity, sanctions, and the rise of food banks in the UK', *BMJ*, 350: h1775.

Luder, E., Boey, E., Buchalter, B. and Martinez-Weber, C. (1989) 'Assessment of the nutritional status of urban homeless adults', *Public Health Reports*, 104: 451.

Lykkesfeldt, J., Christen, S., Wallock, L.M., Chang, H.H., Jacob, R.A. and Ames, B.N. (2000) 'Ascorbate is depleted by smoking and repleted by moderate supplementation: a study in male smokers and nonsmokers with matched dietary antioxidant intakes', *The American Journal of Clinical Nutrition*, 71: 530–6.

Lyles, C.R., Drago-Ferguson, S., Lopez, A. and Seligman, H.K. (2013) Peer reviewed: nutritional assessment of free meal programs in San Francisco', *Preventing Chronic Disease*, 10.

Malmauret, L., Leblanc, J., Cuvelier, I. and Verger, P. (2002) 'Dietary intakes and vitamin status of a sample of homeless people in Paris', *European Journal of Clinical Nutrition*, 56: 313.

McFadden, A., Green, J.M., Williams, V., McLeish, J., McCormick, F., Fox-Rushby, J. and Renfrew, M.J. (2014) 'Can food vouchers improve nutrition and reduce health inequalities in low–income mothers and young children: a multi-method evaluation of the experiences of beneficiaries and practitioners of the Healthy Start programme in England', *BMC Public Health*, 14: 1.

Melchior, M., Caspi, A., Howard, L.M., Ambler, A.P., Bolton, H., Mountain, N. and Moffitt, T.E. (2009) 'Mental health context of food insecurity: a representative cohort of families with young children', *Pediatrics*, 124: e564–e572.

Mohs, M.E., Watson, R.R. and Leonard-Green, T. (1990) 'Nutritional effects of marijuana, heroin, cocaine, and nicotine', *Journal of the American Dietetic Association*, 90: 1261–7.

National Institute of Clinical Excellence (2010) *Alcohol-use disorders: Diagnosis and management of physical complications [CG100]*, London: NICE publications.

Olson, C.M. and Holben, D.H. (2002) 'Position of the American Dietetic Association: domestic food and nutrition security', *Journal of the American Dietetic Association*, 102: 1840–7.

Pelham-Burn, S.E., Frost, C.J., Russell, J.M. and Barker, M.E. (2014) 'Improving the nutritional quality of charitable meals for homeless and vulnerable adults. A case study of food provision by a food aid organisation in the UK', *Appetite*, 82: 131–7.

Power, R. and Hunter, G. (2001) 'Developing a strategy for community-based health promotion targeting homeless populations', *Health Education Research*, 16: 593–602.

Public Health England (2016) *The Eatwell Guide*, London: Public Health England.

Rafferty, Y. and Shinn, M. (1991) 'The impact of homelessness on children', *American Psychologist*, 46: 1170.

Riemer, S., Maes, M., Christophe, A. and Rief, W. (2010) 'Lowered ω-3 PUFAs are related to major depression, but not to somatization syndrome', *Journal of Affective Disorders*, 123: 173–80.

Rushton, C.M. and Wheeler, E. (1993) 'The dietary intake of homeless males sleeping rough in Central London', *Journal of Human Nutrition and Dietetics*, 6: 443–56.

Seale, J.V., Fallaize, R. and Lovegrove, J.A. (2016) 'Nutrition and the homeless: the underestimated challenge', *Nutrition Research Reviews*, 29(2): 143–51.

Sisson, L.G. and Lown, D.A. (2011) 'Do soup kitchen meals contribute to suboptimal nutrient intake and obesity in the homeless population?', *Journal of Hunger & Environmental Nutrition*, 6: 312–23.

Sprake, E.F., Russell, J.M. and Barker, M.E. (2014) 'Food choice and nutrient intake amongst homeless people', *Journal of Human Nutrition and Dietetics*, 27: 242–50.

Tsai, J. and Rosenheck, R.A. (2013) 'Obesity among chronically homeless adults: is it a problem?', *Public Health Reports*, 128: 29.

Weinreb, L., Wehler, C., Perloff, J., Scott, R., Hosmer, D., Sagor, L. and Gundersen, C. (2002) 'Hunger: its impact on children's health and mental health', *Pediatrics*, 110: e41–e41.

Wiecha, J.L., Dywer, J.T., Jacques, P.F. and Rand, W.M. (1993) 'Nutritional and economic advantages for homeless families in shelters providing kitchen facilities and food', *Journal of the American Dietetic Association*, 93: 777–83.

Wolgemuth, J.C., Myers-Williams, C., Johnson, P. and Henseler, C. (1992) 'Wasting malnutrition and inadequate nutrient intakes identified in a multiethnic homeless population', *Journal of the American Dietetic Association*, 92: 834–9.

Yousey, Y., Leake, J., Wdowik, M. and Janken, J.K. (2007) 'Education in a homeless shelter to improve the nutrition of young children', *Public Health Nursing*, 24: 249–55.

Part Two
Lifestyle challenges

Part One provided an introduction to individual development, focusing on neuropsychological and behavioural changes that are mediated by early environments within the family and the education system. Good psychosocial and nutritional support and exercise are important for a person to experience good health and a sense of well-being. This part reviews the need to understand the impact of legal and illegal drug use and the increasing use of the internet on various social groups. Although risks of alcohol and other drug use are widespread across society, the impacts on health and increased vulnerability to addictive behaviours are greater in disadvantaged groups. The underlying psychological factors of stigma and exclusion from society, combined with a more sedentary lifestyle related to increasing use of computers, are resulting in modern epidemics such as obesity. Although a wide range of interventions are being developed to support individuals, upstream policies relating to welfare and community infrastructure are needed.

FIVE

Alcohol-related harm and health inequalities

Katherine Smith, Jon Foster and Katherine Brown

Introduction

Health inequalities between social classes and neighbourhoods have been a persistent feature of the health landscape of the UK for many decades, with more disadvantaged communities suffering greater and earlier morbidity and mortality. These unequal health experiences have remained in spite of multiple policy interventions implemented under the Labour governments in power from 1997 to 2010. The relationship between alcohol and health inequalities is, however, under-studied. In this context, this chapter starts by providing an overview of evidence and theories concerning health inequalities in morbidity and mortality before moving on to consider evidence and theories that specifically relate to the role of alcohol within these broader inequalities. The available evidence suggests that alcohol-related harms follow the expected social gradient, with more disadvantaged groups suffering greater harms, at least for men and for younger women. However, some statistics suggest that people living in deprived communities consume less alcohol than more advantaged communities. This apparent tension is often referred to as the 'alcohol harm paradox' and the chapter provides a brief overview of potential explanations for this paradox before considering evidence concerning the impact of alcohol-related interventions on inequalities. It concludes by setting out a range of relevant research and policy recommendations.

What are 'health inequalities'?

The term 'health inequalities' refers to systematic differences in health between different social groups that are 'socially produced' and, therefore, 'potentially avoidable and widely considered unacceptable in a civilised society' (Whitehead, 2007, p 473). In the UK, research and policy tends to focus on health differences between people classed as being in different socio-economic classes or people living in different geographical areas. The 2010 government-commissioned Marmot Review of health inequalities in England (Marmot, 2010) provided a snapshot of the impact that health inequalities have across a wide range of health and social issues. It found, for example, that in the UK, infant mortality rates were 16% higher in children of routine and manual workers as compared to professional and managerial workers, and that alcohol-related hospital admissions were 2.6 times higher among men and 2.4 times higher among women in the 20% most deprived areas compared to the 20% least deprived areas (Marmot, 2010). Perhaps the most shocking statistic on UK health inequalities came from the 2008 World Health Organization (WHO) Commission on Social Determinants of Health, which reported that men living in the Calton area of Glasgow (Scotland) live, on average, 28 years less than men living in Lenzie, just a few kilometres away. The impact of health inequalities has clear public policy implications, including an estimated UK economic cost of £31–33 billion per year in terms of illness and lost taxes and productivity, in addition to £20–32 billion per year in social security payments that are due to poor health (Marmot, 2010).

There is a significant consensus within available research that such inequalities are related to material and environmental factors, such as financial resources and housing (Bartley, 2004; Graham, 2009; Marmot, 2010). There is also agreement that it is important to consider the whole life course, with evidence highlighting how individuals who are exposed to adverse conditions in one respect, such as work, are also more likely to encounter disadvantage in others, such as poor and damp housing, or inadequate nutrition (Bartley, 2004). These factors influence health both directly and indirectly, via psychological factors such as stress (Marmot, 2010). Finally, lifestyle-behavioural factors, such as alcohol consumption, smoking, exercise and diet, play a role.

Studies consistently find a socio-demographic gradient in the prevalence of multiple lifestyle-behavioural risk factors, with men, younger age groups and those in lower socio-economic groups all more likely to experience multiple risks (Buck and Frosini, 2012). However, health inequalities in the UK can only partially be explained by differences in lifestyle-behaviours (Marmot, 2010). Moreover, these factors are generally regarded by researchers as symptoms, as well as causes, of health inequalities because such behaviours are themselves shaped by the socio-economic contexts in which people live and work (Bartley, 2004; Commission on Social Determinants of Health, 2008). The following section explores the relationship between alcohol and health inequalities in the UK in more detail before the chapter moves on to consider policy responses to health inequalities, the inequalities impacts of alcohol-focused policy interventions and directions for future research.

The relationship between alcohol and health inequalities

There is strong evidence that alcohol is a factor underlying higher mortality risks in more disadvantaged populations, although its impact can be seen across the social gradient (Marmot, 2010). Alcohol also seems to have a greater impact on male health than female health (Probst et al, 2015). In Scotland, where alcohol-related harms are particularly high, the cumulative cost of alcohol-related harm is estimated at £7,457 million per year (Johnston et al, 2012), with 40.41% of the total costs arising from the 20% most deprived areas. These costs are not purely economic; people living in deprived areas experience first-hand the burden of alcohol harms, including alcohol-related violence, more than any other group.

While there has been relatively little research exploring the relationship between health inequalities and alcohol in the UK, the data that are available back up the international evidence. Indeed, one study covering the West of Scotland undertaken by Batty and colleagues (2008), concluded that 'exposure to disadvantaged social circumstances across the lifecourse, but particularly in adulthood, is associated with detrimental patterns of alcohol consumption and problem drinking in late middle age'. In addition, a consistent feature of available studies is that the association of deprivation with alcohol-related deaths appears to be greater among men than women (Probst et al, 2015).

Patterns of alcohol-related mortality have also been found to be associated with age, particularly within certain socio-economic groups. For example, Harrison and Gardiner (1999) found that alcohol-related mortality rates are higher for British men in manual occupations than in non-manual occupations. However, the strength of the relationship depends on age:

> men aged 25–39 in the lowest class are 10–20 times more likely to die from alcohol-related causes than those in the professional class, whereas men aged between 55 and 64 in the unskilled manual class are about 2.5–4 times more likely to die. (p 1871)

The authors propose that this could be because alcohol-related mortality for younger men is more likely to be due to death from acute causes, such as alcohol poisoning, and that this could have a particularly steep class gradient. For women in paid employment, they found no consistent class gradient; younger women in manual classes are more likely to die from alcohol-related causes, but for older women, it is those in the professional class who suffer elevated mortality (Harrison and Gardiner, 1999).

Geographically, Breakwell et al (2007, p 21) report a strong association between alcohol-related death rates and deprivation in England and Wales, 'with alcohol-related death rates more than five times higher in males and more than three times higher in females for those living in the most deprived areas compared to those in the least deprived areas'. As already mentioned, Johnston and colleagues (2012) also found that there are greater costs associated with alcohol consumption in deprived areas of Scotland, with 40.41% of the total costs arising from the 20% most deprived areas. Similarly, a large-scale ecological study covering England and Wales found 'a clear association between alcohol-related mortality and socioeconomic deprivation, with progressively higher rates in more deprived areas' (Erskine et al, 2010). However, as with other studies, the authors note that the strength of the association varied with age (Erskine et al, 2010). This study also notes that people 'living in urban areas experienced higher alcohol-related mortality relative to those living in rural areas, with differences remaining after adjustment for socioeconomic deprivation' (Erskine et al, 2010).

The 'alcohol harm paradox'

As noted earlier, compared to other 'lifestyle-behavioural' factors, the relationship between alcohol and health inequalities seems particularly complicated. Whereas for smoking, for example, rates of smoking increase with levels of deprivation, and smoking-related harms mirror this (Marmot, 2010), alcohol *consumption* does not appear to increase with deprivation (see Bellis et al, 2016). Nonetheless, alcohol-related harms do follow a social gradient, with the most alcohol-related harms experienced by deprived socio-economic groups, despite the fact that they generally consume no more, or perhaps less, alcohol than the most affluent groups (Bellis et al, 2016). This creates something of a paradox: why should some groups experience worse alcohol-related harms despite consuming less alcohol?

Consumption patterns

One explanation could be that people living in more difficult circumstances consume alcohol in more harmful ways. For example, light to moderate drinkers have been found to have higher mortality risks when they reported heavy drinking occasions, rather than more regular lighter sessions (Rehm et al, 2001). This could potentially explain the paradox if it were the case that people living in more deprived situations also tended to have greater levels of occasional heavy drinking (Bellis et al, 2016). However, the evidence supporting this explanation is mixed. A number of studies have found that men classed as being in higher socio-economic groups tend to drink smaller amounts of alcohol more frequently, while men classed as being in lower socio-economic groups are more likely to drink large amounts on fewer occasions (Fone et al, 2012). However, some studies have found that women classed as being in higher socio-economic groups are more likely to consume heavily than those classed as being in middle or lower socio-economic groups (Probst et al, 2015).

Moreover, research using data from 25 countries found that 'lower educated men and women were more likely to report negative consequences than higher educated men and women *even after controlling for drinking patterns*' (Grittner et al, 2012: 597, emphasis added). So, while consumption patterns may play a role in alcohol-related health inequalities, other factors seem to be involved.

Inaccurate consumption reporting

Given that both levels and patterns of alcohol consumption do not appear to fully explain the alcohol harm paradox, there are a number of other potential explanations that require further research (Bellis et al, 2014). These include the possibility that the consumption of alcohol is under-reported in more deprived groups (relative to less deprived groups), possibly because key groups are missed, such as people living in particularly stressful circumstances (eg people experiencing homelessness and working in the military). Consumption on holiday and on special occasions is also often not included when people estimate their average weekly intake, but can add a significant amount to their total annual consumption. This seems unlikely to explain the paradox, though, since poorer groups tend not to be able to afford to go on holidays and have less to spend on special occasions (Shildrick and MacDonald, 2013).

Alcohol and other unhealthy behaviours

Some research has looked at alcohol consumption as part of a complex system of interactions with other 'poly-behaviours', such as a diet and exercise, which account for the relatively greater harms that are experienced by more deprived groups. Research by the Kings Fund, for example, explores how patterns of multiple lifestyle risks (smoking, excessive alcohol use, poor diet and low levels of physical activity) are spread across different socio-economic groups (Buck and Frosini, 2012). It found that people with no qualifications were five times more likely to engage in all four unhealthy behaviours as those with higher education. It also found that engaging in all four unhealthy behaviours resulted in a 14-year reduction in life expectancy compared with those who engaged in none of them.

Other research has gone further and investigated how some of these unhealthy behaviours might interact with each other. For example, there is some evidence that the uptake of vitamins and proteins can be affected by alcohol, and that malnutrition and heavy alcohol use can result in immunosuppressant effects (as well as evidence that people in lower socio-economic groups tend to have less healthy diets) (Buck and Frosini, 2012), while researchers looking at obesity and alcohol consumption have found a 'supra-additive interaction' between the two, particularly in relation to liver disease (Hart et al, 2010a).

It is also known that a combination of smoking and drinking accelerates the risk of mouth and throat cancers, and that premature mortality is particularly high in smokers who drink more than 15 units a week (Hart et al, 2010b). Evidence such as this could go some way in explaining the social gradient in alcohol-related harms, as well as broader health inequalities.

Access to health care

There is some evidence that those living in more deprived circumstances face greater barriers to accessing health and alcohol-related services and interventions than those in less deprived circumstances. Barriers include factors such as costs, distance, transport and availability, and stigmatisation (Probst et al, 2014). To take one example, those from a more deprived background with insecure employment may be less able to take time off work when they get ill (Shildrick and MacDonald, 2013), compounding the problem. These kinds of factors seem likely to exacerbate inequalities in alcohol-related health problems.

Materialist explanations

As noted earlier, one of the most well-supported explanations for overall health inequalities relates to the material (social, economic and environmental) circumstances in which people live and work (Bartley, 2004; Marmot, 2010). These factors also seem likely to contribute to explaining alcohol-related inequalities and, potentially, the alcohol harm paradox. For example, in reflecting on why lower-educated groups are more likely to report negative consequences of alcohol than higher-educated groups, even after controlling for drinking patterns (see earlier), Grittner and colleagues (2012, p 597) suggest that 'those of fewer resources are less protected from the experience of a problem or the impact of a stressful life event'.

Health inequalities: the UK policy context

The need to reduce health inequalities has been recognised by governments across the UK since Labour won the 1997 UK general election with a manifesto that included a commitment to reducing health inequalities. Since this time, there has been a lot of policy activity, with English efforts being described by one European researcher as 'historically and internationally unique' (Mackenbach, 2011: 1249). Yet, despite the raft of policies intended to reduce health inequalities introduced between 1997 and 2010, the UK's health inequalities have continued to widen by most (though not all) measures (see Bambra, 2012; Barr et al, 2012). A 2010 review by the National Audit Office stated that it was hard to see an obvious link between spending and improvements (National Audit Office, 2010). This review found that the number of policy pronouncements about health inequalities had been too numerous for local National Health Service (NHS) bodies to keep up with and highlighted the conflicting central government demands faced by local bodies. Some have suggested that we simply do not yet know 'what works' in reducing health inequalities, but others argue that the policy approaches to health inequalities taken in the post-1997 period did not reflect available evidence and placed too much emphasis on interventions aiming to change people's lifestyles and behaviours and not enough on trying to change the circumstances in which people live and work (see Garthwaite et al, 2016).

Since 2010, the Coalition (Conservative–Liberal Democrat) government (in power during 2010–15) transferred responsibility for public health in England to local authorities, which means that central government now has far less ability to performance-manage public health issues. While a broad policy commitment to reducing health inequalities remained in place under the Coalition government (Secretary of State for Health, 2010), specific targets were dropped (Gregory et al, 2012). Whether the current Conservative government has any interest in health inequalities seems unclear – there have been very few national policy pronouncements about health inequalities in England since 2015. (For an update on the outcome of the snap general election in June 2017, see the Conclusion at the end of the book.)

Interventions to address alcohol-related inequalities

Given the significant health and economic burden associated with alcohol, particularly for communities least able to afford it, the role of alcohol needs to be considered in strategies aiming to reduce overall health inequalities (Marmot, 2010). This does not mean, however, that efforts to reduce the harms relating to alcohol, or alcohol consumption, will necessarily lead to reductions in health inequalities. Indeed, many health interventions focusing on so-called 'lifestyle-behavioural' issues (alcohol, diet, exercise and tobacco) inadvertently increase health inequalities because those living in more affluent, less stressful circumstances are often better placed to change those behaviours (this leads to what Lorenc et al [2013] call 'intervention-generated health inequalities'): 'This reflects one of public health's most difficult dilemmas: unless consciously designed not to, policies and actions that work for populations as a whole often inadvertently entrench inequalities' (Buck and Frosini, 2012: 13).

This means that policymakers and advocates concerned with health inequalities ought to consider very carefully how potential policy changes and interventions might impact differentially on social groups and areas. While few alcohol-related interventions have been assessed from an inequalities perspective, there is evidence that some policies designed to reduce alcohol-related harm overall are more likely to reduce alcohol-related inequalities than others. A recent assessment of relevant systematic reviews concludes that public health interventions that rely on individuals to change, such as public education campaigns, are likely to increase health inequalities, while more 'upstream' public health interventions (eg price increases and restrictions on the availability of health-damaging products) are most likely to help reduce health inequalities (Lorenc et al, 2013). In terms of alcohol-related policies, the evidence suggests that minimum unit pricing (MUP) and further restrictions on the availability of alcohol are more likely to be effective in tackling health inequalities than education campaigns.

These kinds of 'upstream' interventions more effectively target heavy drinkers in lower socio-economic categories. The rest of this section explores specific policy interventions in more detail.

Alcohol price and minimum unit pricing

There is strong evidence that reducing the affordability of alcohol by raising prices leads to a reduction in alcohol consumption and associated harms, including reductions in mortality from liver cirrhosis, accidents, suicide, homicide and heart disease (Norstrom and Skog, 2001), as well as a reduction in levels of violence and crime (Matthews et al, 2006). One such price-related policy is MUP, which sets a level below which retailers are not allowed to sell alcohol, depending on the number of units it contains. From an inequalities perspective, scenario modelling suggests that poorer heavy drinkers would benefit the most from MUP in terms of health improvements, with 80% of avoidable deaths and hospital admissions linked to MUP coming from low-income groups (Meier et al, 2016). Research by the University of Sheffield indicates that MUP would be more effective than alcohol tax increases at reducing health and social harms, especially among lower-income groups, while having a minimal impact on moderate drinkers. This policy could therefore contribute to reducing alcohol-related inequalities (Holmes et al, 2014).

Alcohol availability, outlet density and alcohol licensing

Research in Scotland suggests that more hospitalisations and deaths occur in areas with greater outlet availability and that off-sales outlets are more important for health than on-sales outlets (Richardson et al, 2015). This same body of work also demonstrates that more deprived areas have a higher density of off-sales alcohol outlets (Shortt et al, 2015).

All this suggests that the differences in the availability of alcohol, particularly from off-sales suppliers, may play a role in explaining alcohol-related health inequalities in the UK. However, addressing the density of premises is not an easy task. In England and Wales, cumulative impact policies (CIPs) can be introduced in areas where the cumulative effect of licensed premises on the four licensing objectives is sufficient to suggest that the growth of similar premises in that area needs to be controlled. While it introduces an assumption that no further licences will be granted unless the applicant can show that it will not add to the existing problems, it does not allow for the current density to be reduced, even if it is already a problem.

In Scotland, licensing boards have had public heath as a fifth licensing objective since 2005, which (in theory) allows licensing boards to be proactive in assessing the oversupply of both off- and on-licences. This kind of public health licensing objective seems to offer opportunities for contributing to reducing the inequalities in access to alcohol described earlier. However, the impact of this objective has not yet been assessed from an inequalities perspective and emerging evidence suggests that while it has succeeded in increasing the use of health evidence in licensing board discussions, the impact on licensing decisions has been more limited (Gillan et al, 2014). Nonetheless, groups such as the Local Government Association (LGA) have called for the addition of a public health licensing objective in England so that local authorities can better implement their public health responsibilities (LGA and Alcohol Research UK, 2013).

Reducing the strength schemes

Reducing the Strength (RTS) schemes, also known as super-strength schemes, developed as a response to street drinking and associated problems of anti-social behaviour. They involve restricting the availability of high-strength beer, lager and cider, typically of 6.5% alcohol by volume (ABV) and above. To achieve this, newsagents, off-licences and sometimes supermarkets are encouraged by the local authority not to stock these products. There are thought to be around 100 of these schemes in the UK at present, and if implemented well, by also engaging with and supporting the street-drinking community, they have the potential to reduce health inequalities.

Due to competition law, these schemes have to be voluntary, with no element of coercion, something that can greatly limit their effectiveness as businesses may choose not to take part. However, the LGA has produced guidance on how to implement this type of scheme legally by clearly explaining the potential benefits to businesses without compelling action (LGA, 2016).

The response from the licensed trade varies; in some areas, it can be hard to gain the voluntary support necessary and stores may benefit financially from being outside the scheme as there is less competition for the high-strength drinks they sell. Other retailers have reported reduced problems and a safer working environment for staff by taking part, in addition to community benefits (LGA, 2016).

Due to their relatively new status, the current literature has not been able to assess the long-term impacts of these schemes (Sumpter et al, 2016). Some schemes do seem to have produced positive results in the short term, particularly regarding crime rates and reductions in street drinking (Foster and Charalambides, 2016). Increased engagement with street drinkers and the improved likelihood of them receiving access to support services and treatment do seem likely to offer opportunities to reduce health inequalities.

Welfare spending

Reflecting the broader evidence base regarding health inequalities and the importance placed on upstream determinants of health (Marmot, 2010), general welfare spending has been found to impact positively on alcohol-attributable mortality. Stuckler and colleagues (2010) demonstrate that a rise in social welfare spending is associated with a decrease in alcohol-attributable mortality, whereas rising health-care spending was not. This coheres with qualitative studies in the UK which consistently find that people describe alcohol consumption as a 'coping mechanism' and form of 'escapism' when experiencing the stresses of socio-economic deprivation (Smith and Anderson, 2018).

Conclusion and ways forward

Despite improvements in health and life expectancy across most social groups in the UK in recent decades, health inequalities remain entrenched, with little sign of improving in the near future. There are clear moral, economic and policy implications of this situation. As well as influencing how long someone is likely to live, health inequalities affect how long they are likely to live without being affected by disability or a long-term illness. There is also evidence that alcohol plays a significant part in health inequalities, with low socio-economic groups being disproportionally affected by alcohol-related harms, despite appearing to have lower overall rates of consumption.

Researchers whose work focuses primarily on health inequalities tend to argue in favour of upstream policies to tackle the social and economic determinants of health that stretch well beyond the remit of the health sector (Marmot, 2010). However, from the perspective of trying to minimise alcohol-related health harms, it is worth considering what the impact of various alcohol-focused policy options might be on health inequalities. There do appear to be some synergies: the available evidence on effective means of reducing alcohol-related harms *and* health inequalities points to the need for upstream policy measures (Lorenc et al, 2013) addressing factors such as the availability, marketing, regulation and price of alcohol. In contrast, the kinds of interventions and policies promoted by alcohol industry interests in the UK have tended to involved voluntary, educational approaches, which research suggests are not only less effective overall, but also likely to increase health inequalities (Lorenc et al, 2013). The Scottish government has passed legislation to introduce MUP, which has been obstructed by a legal challenge from the Scotch Whisky Association; this is a clear example of business interests undermining public health goals and demonstrates the threat to health inequalities posed by producers of unhealthy commodities (see Hill and Collin, 2016 for further discussion).

There are also some obvious research gaps, including a need to examine how interventions intended to address alcohol-related harms impact on different social groups or areas. There is a need to rebalance the emphasis that public health researchers have placed on understanding tobacco industry efforts to influence policy with much more work to understand the influence of alcohol industry interests (Casswell, 2013). This is particularly so in light of the proven ineffectiveness of the English Public Health Responsibility Deal for tackling alcohol-related problems (Knai et al, 2015).

Finally, since determined action to address any policy issue requires public as well as political will, more attention needs to be paid to understanding the interaction of evidence and ideas about alcohol policy and health inequalities across the public, media, research, advocacy and policy spheres (Smith et al, 2016). This may require stronger links between research, advocacy and public engagement across sectors concerned with alcohol and with inequality and poverty.

References

Bambra, C. (2012) 'Reducing health inequalities: new data suggests that the English strategy was partially successful', *Journal of Epidemiology and Community Health*, 66(7): 662.

Barr, B., Taylor-Robinson, D. and Whitehead, M. (2012) 'Impact on health inequalities of rising prosperity in England 1998–2007, and implications for performance incentives: longitudinal ecological study', *BMJ*, 345: e7831.

Bartley, M. (2004) *Health inequality: An introduction to theories, concepts and methods*, Cambridge: Polity Press.

Batty, D., Lewars, H., Emslie, C., Benzeval, M. and Hunt, K. (2008) 'Problem drinking and exceeding guidelines for "sensible" alcohol consumption in Scottish men: associations with life course socioeconomic disadvantage in a population-based cohort study', *BMC Public Health*, 8(302).

Bellis, M.A., Hughes, K., Leckenby, N., Clare, P. and Lowey, H. (2014) 'National household survey of adverse childhood experiences and their relationship with resilience to health-harming behaviours in England', *BMC Medicine*. Available at: https://bmcmedicine.biomedcentral.com/articles/10.1186/1741-7015-12-72

Bellis, M.A., Hughes, K., Nicholls, J., Sheron, N., Gilmore, I. and Jones, L. (2016) 'The alcohol harm paradox: using a national survey to explore how alcohol may disproportionately impact health in deprived individuals'. *BMC Public Health*, 16(111).

Breakwell, J., Baker, A., Griffiths, C., Jackson, G., Fegan, G. and Marshall, D. (2007) 'Trends and geographical variations in alcohol-related deaths in the United Kingdom, 1991–2004', *National Statistics Quarterly*, 33: 6–24.

Buck, D. and Frosini, F. (2012) *Clustering of unhealthy behaviours over time: Implications for policy and practice*, London: The King's Fund.

Casswell, S. (2013) 'Vested interests in addiction research and policy. Why do we not see the corporate interests of the alcohol industry as clearly as we see those of the tobacco industry?', *Addiction*, 108(4): 680–5.

Commission on Social Determinants of Health (2008) *Closing the gap in a generation: Health equity through action on the social determinants of health. Final report of the Commission on Social Determinants of Health*, Geneva: World Health Organization.

Erskine, S., Maheswaran, R., Pearson, T. and Gleeson, D. (2010) 'Socioeconomic deprivation, urban–rural location and alcohol-related mortality in England and Wales', *BMC Public Health*, 10(99).

Fone, D., Dunstan, F., White, J., Webster, C., Rodgers, S., Lee, S., Shiode, N., Orford, S., Weightman, A., Brennan, I., Sivarajasingam, V., Morgan, J., Fry, R. and Lyons, R. (2012) 'Change in alcohol outlet density and alcohol-related harm to population health (CHALICE)', *BMC Public Health*, 12: 428. Available at: http://www.biomedcentral.com/1471-2458/12/428

Foster, J. and Charalambides, L. (2016) *The Licensing Act (2003): Its uses and abuses 10 years on*, London: Institute of Alcohol Studies.

Garthwaite, K., Smith, K.E., Bambra, C. and Pearce, J. (2016) 'Desperately seeking reductions in health inequalities: perspectives of UK researchers on past, present and future directions in health inequalities research', *Sociology of Health & Illness*, 38(3): 459–78.

Gillan, E., Mahon, L., MacNaughton, P., Bowie, L. and Nicholls, J. (2014) 'Using licensing to protect public health: from evidence to practice', Alcohol Insight Number 114, Alcohol Research UK. Available at: http://alcoholresearchuk.org/alcohol-insights/using-licensing-to-protect-public-health-from-evidence-to-practice-2/

Graham, H. (2009) 'Health inequalities, social determinants and public health policy', *Policy & Politics*, 37(4): 463–79.

Gregory, S., Dixon, A. and Ham, C. (2012) *Health policy under the Coalition government. A mid-term assessment*, London: The King's Fund.

Grittner, U., Kuntsche, S., Graham, K. and Bloomfield, K. (2012) 'Social inequalities and gender differences in the experience of alcohol-related problems', *Alcohol and Alcoholism*, 47(5): 597–605.

Harrison, L. and Gardiner, E. (1999) 'Do the rich really die young? Alcohol-related mortality and social class in Great Britain, 1988–94', *Addiction*, 94(12): 1871–80.

Hart, C.L., Morrison, D.S., Batty, G.D., Mitchell, R.J. and Davey Smith, G. (2010a) 'Effect of body mass index and alcohol consumption on liver disease: analysis of data from two prospective cohort studies', *The BMJ*, 340: c1240. Available at: http://doi.org/10.1136/bmj.c1240

Hart, C.L., Davey Smith, G., Gruer, L. and Watt, G.C. (2010b) 'The combined effect of smoking tobacco and drinking alcohol on cause-specific mortality: a 30 year cohort study', *BMC Public Health*, 10: 789. Available at: http://doi.org/10.1186/1471-2458-10-789

Hill, S.E. and Collin, J. (2016) 'Industrial epidemics and inequalities: The commercial sector as a structural driver of inequalities in non-communicable diseases', Chapter 13 in K.E. Smith, C. Bambra and S.E. Hill (eds) *Health inequalities: Critical perspective*, Oxford: Oxford University Press.

Holmes, J., Meng, Y., Meier, P.S., Brennan, A., Angus, C., Campbell-Burton, A., Guo, Y., Hill-McManus, D. and Purshouse, R.C. (2014) 'Effects of minimum unit pricing for alcohol on different income and socioeconomic groups: a modelling study', *The Lancet*, 383(9929): 1655–64.

Johnston, M.C., Ludbrook, A. and Jaffray, M.A. (2012) 'Inequalities in the distribution of the costs of alcohol misuse in Scotland: a cost of illness study', *Alcohol and Alcoholism*, 47(6): 725–31.

Knai, C., Pettigrow, M., Mays, N., Durand, M.A. and Eastmure, E. (2015) Knai and colleagues' response to comments of the Portman Group in news story about their research on "Responsibility Deal on Alcohol"', *BMJ (Clinical research ed)*, 350: h2063. Available at: http://researchonline.lshtm.ac.uk/2160169/1/bmj.h2063.full.pdf

LGA (Local Government Association) (2016) *Reducing the strength: Guidance for councils considering setting up a scheme*, London: Local Government Association.

LGA and Alcohol Research UK (2013) *UK briefing: Public health and alcohol licensing in England*, London: Local Government Association.

Lorenc, T., Petticrew, M., Welch, V. and Tugwell, P. (2013) 'What types of interventions generate inequalities? Evidence from systematic reviews', *Journal of Epidemiology and Community Health*, 67: 190–3.

Mackenbach, J.P. (2011) 'Can we reduce health inequalities? An analysis of the English strategy (1997–2010)', *Journal of Epidemiology and Community Health*, 65(7): 568–75.

Marmot, M. (2010) *Fair society, healthy lives: The Marmot Review. Strategic review of health inequalities in England post-2010*, London: UCL Institute of Health Equity.

Matthews, K., Shepherd, J. and Sivarajasingham, V. (2006) 'Violence-related injury and the price of beer in England and Wales', *Applied Economics*, 38(6): 661–70.

Meier, P., Holmes, J., Angus, C., Ally, A.K., Meng, Y. and Brennan, A. (2016) 'Estimated effects of different alcohol taxation and price policies on health inequalities: a mathematical modelling study', *PLos Medicine*, 13(2): e1001963.

National Audit Office (2010) *Healthy balance: A review of public health performance and spending*, London: National Audit Office.

Norstrom, T. and Skog, O.J. (2001) 'Alcohol and mortality', *Addiction*, 96(S1) S5-S17.

Probst, C., Roerecke, M., Behrendt, S. and Rehm, J. (2014) 'Socioeconomic differences in alcohol-attributable mortality compared with all-cause mortality: a systematic review and meta-analysis', *International Journal of Epidemiology*, 43(4): 1314–27.

Probst, C., Roerecke, M., Behrendt, S. and Rehm, J. (2015) 'Gender differences in socioeconomic inequality of alcohol-attributable mortality: a systematic review and meta-analysis', *Drug & Alcohol Review*, 34(3): 267–77.

Rehm, J., Greenfield, T.K. and Rogers, J.D. (2001) 'Average volume of alcohol consumption, patterns of drinking, and all-cause mortality: results from the US National Alcohol Survey', *American Journal of Epidemiology*, 153(1): 64–71.

Richardson, E.A., Hill, S.E., Mitchell, R., Pearce, J. and Shortt, N. (2015) 'Is local alcohol outlet density related to alcohol-related morbidity and mortality in Scottish cities?', *Health & Place*, 33: 172–80.

Secretary of State for Health (2010) *Healthy lives, healthy people: Our strategy for public health in England*, London: The Stationery Office.

Shildrick, T. and MacDonald, R. (2013) 'Poverty talk: how people experiencing poverty deny their poverty and why they blame "the poor"', *The Sociological Review*, 61(2): 285–303.

Shortt, N.K., Tisch, C., Pearce, J., Mitchell, R., Richardson, E.A., Hill, S. and Collin, J. (2015) 'A cross-sectional analysis of the relationship between tobacco and alcohol outlet density and neighbourhood deprivation', *BMC Public Health*, 15: 1014. Available at: http://doi.org/10.1186/s12889-015-2321-1

Smith, K.E. and Anderson, R. (forthcoming) 'Understanding lay perspectives on socioeconomic health inequalities in the UK: a meta-ethnography', *Sociology of Health & Illness*.

Smith, K.E., Bambra, C. and Hill, S.E. (eds) (2016) *Health inequalities: Critical perspectives*, Oxford: Oxford University Press.

Stuckler, D., Basu, S. and McKee, M. (2010) 'Budget crises, health, and social welfare programmes', *BMJ*, 341(7763): 77–9.

Sumpter, C., McGill, E., Dickie, E., Champo, E., Romeri, E. and Egan, M. (2016) 'Reducing the strength: a mixed methods evaluation of alcohol retailers' willingness to voluntarily reduce the availability of low cost, high strength beers and ciders in two UK local authorities', *BMC Public Health*, 16(448).

Whitehead, M. (2007) 'A typology of actions to tackle social inequalities in health', *Journal of Epidemiology and Community Health*, 61: 473–8.

SIX

Addiction, inequality and recovery

Jenny Svanberg

...addiction is unequally distributed among social groups, flourishing most where the power to resist it is weakest (Orford, 2012: xiii)

Introduction

In all societies, those in lower socio-economic positions experience worse physical and mental health (CSDH, 2008). Although health improvements have been seen in many countries, health inequalities mean that those in more disadvantaged positions experience slower improvements, widening the gap between those at the top and those at the bottom. The World Health Organization established the Commission on Social Determinants of Health in 2008 to 'marshal the evidence on what can be done to promote health equity, and to foster a global movement to achieve it' (CSDH, 2008: 1), recognising that equity in health and well-being gives an indication of the social development of a society.

As a result of this, the Marmot review was tasked with proposing strategies to reduce health inequalities in England (Marmot et al, 2010), and rightly recognised that health equality requires a debate about what kind of society we want to live in. A child born into a position of lower socio-economic status is more likely to experience problems with health, mental health, nutrition and education, have less stable employment, feel stigmatised, and experience a range of other difficulties (Griggs and Walker, 2008). However, poverty alone is not the most influential factor. When considering societies as a whole, there is a clearer relationship between poor health outcomes and societal inequality, meaning that rich countries with a steep social gradient do worse than poorer, but more equal, countries (Wilkinson and Pickett, 2010). This chapter will consider how addiction is influenced by health inequalities, and will reflect on how the recommendations of the Marmot review could influence recovery from addiction.

Health inequalities are seen across the field of addiction, although this is a field that is poorly defined. The Diagnostic and Statistical Manual of Mental Disorders, Version 5 (DSM V) has set criteria for substance use disorders, capturing the key, defining feature of addiction: continued use of a substance (or continued pursuit of a behaviour), despite negative consequences. Canadian Professor of Psychology Bruce Alexander (2008: 29) has described addiction as 'overwhelming involvement with any pursuit whatsoever (including, but not limited to, drugs or alcohol) that is harmful to the addicted person, to society, or to both'. Addiction can be seen as both a driver and a consequence of the widening health inequalities we see today. Drug and alcohol addiction occurs at every strata of society, but more unequal societies show higher levels of drug addiction (Wilkinson and Pickett, 2010). Within societies, those with lower socio-economic status, who are more marginalised and have less power, are more likely to become addicted to substances, more likely to use in a more risky way, more likely to suffer worse health consequences from their addictions and more likely to struggle to recover (Galea and Vlahov, 2002; Orford, 2013). At the other end of the socio-economic spectrum, those addicted to money and power are hastening increasing inequality and compounding societal difficulties (Alexander, 2008; Robertson, 2012).

Substance use and addiction

Around a quarter of Europe's adult population, including approximately a third of adults in the UK, have used an illicit drug at some point in their lives (EMCDDA, 2013), and over a fifth of the European population over the age of 15 drink heavily (five or more drinks in one go) at least once a week, making the European Union (EU) the heaviest drinking region in the world (Loring, 2014). However, the majority of people who use drugs and alcohol do not become addicted to them, just in the same way that the majority of people who gamble, shop, exercise, eat or have sex do not end up becoming addicted. In fact, for the majority of people using drugs, who tend to start in their late teens to early 20s, stopping or reducing drug use in the mid-20s is more common than starting to use (ACMD, 2006). Repeated use of some substances means that the body builds up tolerance, so that when use of the substance stops there is a physical withdrawal syndrome, but, again, this does not in itself lead to addiction, unless other factors come into play. Not all those who have experienced a hangover can be said to be addicted to alcohol. This is also true of behavioural addictions, illustrating a common underlying process to addictive behaviours

(Grant et al, 2010). It may be more accurate to say that we all have the potential to become addicted, and certain biological, psychological and social factors make that more or less likely for each of us at different times in our lives.

There are multiple routes into substance use, and the reason an individual begins to use a substance, whether licit or illicit, will depend on their motivations and social context, as well as the availability of particular substances (Orford, 2001), often beginning with the substance providing pleasure, or relief from pain. For the minority whose use becomes more problematic over time, the substance may begin to take over other functions in the person's life, for example, starting as a social bonding activity and moving into functions such as emotion regulation or relief from physical pain. For those who may have few other ways of finding pleasure or easing pain, the substance may become so valued that other parts of life lose their importance. As this path is repeated, compelling pathways are worn into the brain's motivation and reward centres, the addictive behaviour moves from being voluntary to being more habitual and automatic, and therefore less amenable to conscious control. Chronic substance use can lead to increasing chaos, and mounting losses, and facing this chaos, and the distress that comes with it, can become overwhelming. An easy and immediate answer may be to continue to 'block it all out', rather than face problems that may seem insurmountable.

This process is underpinned by our neurobiology, and research has outlined the key brain systems governing addiction. Some of the key components include: the insula, responsible for the internal sense of imbalance or craving; the amygdala/striatal areas, responsible for impulsive and automatic decision-making; and the prefrontal cortex, which governs slower, reflective decision-making and impulse control. Over time, and with repeated use of a substance, or repeated acting out of any addictive behaviour, the insula-mediated system learns to overrule the prefrontal cortex (in other words, the substance becomes so valued that other activities pale into insignificance, and the urge to take the substance becomes so strong that it prevents reflective decision-making), making it more likely that the behaviour will be impulsive, rigid and automatic (Noel et al, 2013). In theory, if the prefrontal cortex is already functioning below its optimal capacity, as is the case for those who experienced early life adversity (Anda et al, 2006), the compulsive behaviours associated with addiction may take hold more readily. 'Wanting' the substance becomes 'needing' the substance even when the person wants to stop, and when there are mounting costs to the use. Although there are similarities between drug and alcohol and other behavioural addictions, there may be additional difficulties for those trying to recover from substance addiction (Nutt, 2012; Orford, 2013), particularly for those with low socio-economic status, whose access to healthy diets and timely health and mental health care may be compromised. Prolonged use of most substances is associated with changes in episodic memory, emotional processing and executive processes, so, over time, the substances may directly influence the ability to control and change behaviour (Fernandez-Serrano et al, 2011).

Despite this, recovery from addiction is the norm. The majority of people addicted to substances recover naturally, and without seeking support from services (Heyman, 2013; Slutske, 2015). Factors supporting recovery include supportive social and family networks, access to meaningful activity in work and leisure time, practical factors like housing, and modifications to social networks and lifestyles, particularly for those deeply embedded within a drug-using culture (Best et al, 2008). In other words, recovery from addiction is about being able to choose more positive and healthy options over the addictive behaviour, and using available resources to change an old, ingrained habit. It will come as no surprise that there are more of these opportunities and choices available for those at the higher ends of the socio-economic spectrum. Those who struggle to recover and seek support from treatment services tend to have more severe difficulties with addiction, limited social support, poorer mental and physical health, and greater exposure to a number of life stresses (Grella and Stein, 2013). Risk factors for a greater severity of addictive behaviour include greater personal vulnerability, lower levels of resilience and social support, and genetic or biological vulnerabilities (White and Kelly, 2011; Nutt, 2012). If we all have the potential to become addicted to a particular behaviour, this potential sits on a continuum of severity, with the most severe addictions presenting in those who have experienced the greatest number of life's challenges, particularly if they begin in early life.

Early life adversity and addiction

Although not every child that faces early life adversity will become addicted to substances, children with adverse early experiences will grow up to be more likely to seek external means to regulate themselves (Blair, 2010). The specific means may depend to some extent on what is available from the environment and formative relationships. In environments where drugs or alcohol are readily available, it may be more likely that substances will come to be used as a form of self-regulation, particularly if this behaviour is modelled by others. Strategies that begin as intuitive attempts to cope may then become health risk behaviours themselves, or manifest as mental health disorders. This is illustrated by the Adverse Childhood Experiences Study, which found that those exposed to four or more adverse childhood experiences (including abuse, witnessing domestic violence or extreme household dysfunction) were 7.2 times more at risk of alcoholism, 4.5 times more at risk of illicit drug use and 11.1 times more at risk of injected drug use (Anda et al, 2006), as well as showing increased risk of a range of other health and mental health outcomes.

Early life adversity makes it harder to recognise and regulate our emotions and appetites (Briere and Spinazzola, 2005; Blair, 2010). This is a result of the brain adapting to the environment that it finds itself in after birth. Prolonged exposure to threat in early life alters the brain's stress response, inhibits the growth of parts of the brain involved in memory and alters the response of parts of the brain involved in social attachment and the regulation of mood (Anda et al, 2006), as well as leading to changes in multiple physiological systems. An infant's brain adapts to his or her environment, however dysfunctional it may be. Infants exposed to threat, neglect or deprivation may become skilled at scanning their environments for threat, being more reactive and less reflective in order to survive (Blair, 2010). These behaviours may become more problematic in the adolescent and adult, and present as difficulties controlling impulses, regulating emotions and finding balance in both the self and relationships (Felitti et al, 1998; Bellis et al, 2014). However, even among people who face the most risk factors, the majority do not become addicted, and the protective influence of strong social networks, peer and family attitudes and the availability of rewarding alternatives has been well documented (Hart, 2013). Even one stable and protective relationship in a child's life can provide enough security to counteract multiple and varied forms of adversity. The impact of early life adversity is explored more widely in Chapter One.

Inequality and addiction

'Early life adversity', as described earlier, includes deprivation and poverty, and there is a growing body of research illustrating the impact of deprivation on the developing brain. Deprivation is more likely to lead to reduced performance on complex cognitive tasks as a result of children being less likely to be exposed to complex language and enriched activities (McLaughlin et al, 2014), impacting on later life educational and occupational opportunities. Exposure to poverty in early life has been described as 'one of the most powerful risk factors for poor developmental outcomes' (Luby et al, 2013), and is associated with lower volumes of grey and white matter in the hippocampus and amygdala, parts of the brain associated with memory, learning, emotion and motivation. This relationship is mediated by caregiving, in other words, a nurturing and responsive caregiver will protect an infant from the risks associated with living in poverty (Luby et al, 2013).

Although there is not a direct link between substance use and socio-economic status, the consequences of using drugs or alcohol are not shared out in an equitable manner. Although people in lower socio-economic groups consume less alcohol than those in higher groups, and are more likely to abstain, they experience higher levels of alcohol-related harm (WHO, 2014). Across the UK, the likelihood of dying from factors related to alcohol increase sharply with decreasing socio-economic status, particularly for men, and particularly in Scotland (Scottish Government, 2008). Use of any drug is more likely for those in the most deprived areas, but class A drug use was found to be fairly equally distributed across areas of low and high deprivation (Home Office, 2015). However, in most cases, less healthy behaviours are more prevalent among socio-economically disadvantaged populations (Widome et al, 2013). Drug use among those from more deprived backgrounds is linked with more extreme problematic use, more risky types of drug use (such as injecting), a lower age of first use, greater criminal involvement and more health and social complications as a result of use (Galea and Vlahov, 2002; Orford, 2013). Hazardous and more problematic drug use has been found to be more associated with socio-economic status with increasing age, and in some communities, 'problem drug use has become an inescapable part of community life' (ACMD, 2006: 52). This is illustrated by many people presenting to drug treatment services who describe frequent offers of illicit substances from their local community, as well as fewer opportunities to consider alternatives to use, such as safe and healthy relationships, meaningful employment, and secure housing. Although the association between poverty and addiction is mixed, there is a much stronger association between economic inequality and addiction (Wilkinson and Pickett, 2010).

How do unequal societies generate addiction?

The majority of prevailing theories about addiction situate the problem with the individual, whether in their biology or their psychology.

However, if addiction is more common when society is less equal, and entrenched by social policies that stigmatise and criminalise those defined as 'addicts', then our interventions must expand to take in communities and our society if they are to be preventive rather than reactive. Wilkinson and Pickett (2010: 44) explain the problems of economic inequality as resulting from increased anxieties around social status: 'If inequalities are bigger, so that some people seem to count for almost everything and others for practically nothing, where each one of us is placed becomes more important'. Addiction then becomes a result of the way in which our global free market society has fractured cultural and social connections, resulting in 'dislocation' and a loss of psychosocial integration: belonging, meaning, purpose, identity and social connection (Alexander, 2012; Hari, 2015). Although it can be argued that addiction leads to the fragmentation of communities, damaging families and perpetuating problems, historical accounts of the spread of addiction across societies offer a compelling counter-argument that addiction comes as a consequence of societal disempowerment and dislocation, rather than a cause (Alexander, 2008; Hart, 2013).

The prevailing understanding of addiction as an individual problem also feeds stigma and prejudice against those struggling with addictive behaviours, particularly in relation to drugs and alcohol. This stigma is embedded in the dated view of addiction as a moral disorder, caused by personal weakness, which can still be illustrated by countless portrayals in the media of addiction stereotypes that glamorise or demonise drug users, but rarely promote recovery (White, 2014). In some cases, prejudice is experienced even from the services designed to help, and 'drug injecting is used as the cause, focus and explanation of all the drug user's difficulties in life' (Hammersley and Dalgarno, 2013: 7). Multiple problems may be attributed to an individual's substance use rather than pre-existing difficulties, including adverse experiences, poverty or social deprivation (Hart, 2013). This misattribution may have serious consequences. In the case of people presenting with difficulties relating to both addiction and post-traumatic stress disorder, misattribution or misdiagnosis of trauma symptoms may influence attendance and dropout rates, interfere with help-seeking, increase the risk of relapse, and reduce positive outcomes in substance misuse interventions (Brown et al, 1995; Ford et al, 2007). Stigma can reinforce the shame associated with both substance use and histories of trauma, which, in turn, has been shown to contribute to relapse (Randles and Tracy, 2013). Stigma and prejudice is further heightened if people using substances also have lower socio-economic status, as illustrated by politically driven media campaigns attacking people receiving welfare support. The most successful way to keep people isolated is to argue convincingly that they are a source of pollution (Harari, 2014), effectively carried out by waging a 'war on drugs' and those that use them. If dislocation and disconnection feed addiction, creating further divisions can only intensify the problem.

How can society support recovery from addiction?

Society creates the context in which recovery can occur. If society marginalises and stigmatises those using substances problematically, seeing them as 'separate' and 'other', it can only exacerbate and entrench addiction by reducing the choices available to those defined under that label. While health policies and interventions are effective for some individuals, the reduction and prevention of addiction at a population level require a societal shift right across the social spectrum. The Marmot review recognised that actions to reduce health inequality need to be universal, but described the need for 'proportionate universalism', in other words, by recognising that those from more disadvantaged backgrounds require interventions on a greater scale and intensity.

For the recommendations of the Marmot review to be met in the context of addiction, private suffering needs to move towards collective responsibility (Orford, 2013), and there needs to be recognition of social and economic inequality as a factor that drives and perpetuates addiction. This may involve further shifts away from the 'medical' or 'disease' model of addiction, which is helpful in describing the neurobiological changes associated with addiction, particularly for the small percentage of people who may experience lasting cognitive impairment as a result of long-term substance use and the associated lifestyle factors. However, it is also a model that can be damaging by emphasising helplessness and the need for specialist treatment, by emphasising the symptoms of the problem rather than the developmental causes, and by focusing on the severe end of the addiction spectrum (Hall et al, 2015; Lewis, 2015). While drugs and alcohol do change the brain, and repeated use changes it further, this is true of any repeated behaviour. When we know that one of the best predictors of addiction recovery is self-efficacy, or the belief in one's ability to make changes successfully (Bandura, 1977), a model that emphasises vulnerability rather than strength and personal agency may not be the best fit. However, many who have recovered from alcohol and drug addiction, particularly through the connections and community of the mutual aid fellowships, continue to find the disease model helpful in understanding their own experience, and rather than emphasise the separation between disease, learning and social models, finding the common ground between them may offer a new paradigm for the future.

Proportionate universalism indicates that addiction treatment centres serving areas of high deprivation should receive increased resources, reflecting the greater needs of the populations they serve, a recommendation already made for mental health services in the same areas (Delgadillo et al, 2015). Investment is required into early years and family services, recognising that substance misuse is one among many challenges faced by families in unequal societies (eg NTA, 2012a). A move towards a more evidence-based drug and alcohol policy would enable the creation of a social environment that promotes recovery rather than disconnection. The 'war on drugs' has not reduced supply or demand, and has increased harm in multiple ways, not least by creating a social environment that criminalises, stereotypes and stigmatises those addicted to alcohol and drugs (Nutt, 2012). UK drug and alcohol policies are moving towards a greater understanding of this, setting out the need to promote recovery in coordinated systems of care established across whole communities (Scottish Government, 2008, 2015; NTA, 2010, 2012b), although more work is necessary in integrating alcohol and drug policies, with the differing emphases on health versus criminal justice. Community approaches to addiction highlight the need to provide safe, non-stigmatising social environments to build the connections required to guide marginalised individuals back into mainstream society.

Ultimately, as the Marmot review highlights, if we are serious about reducing the impact of addiction, one of the factors influenced by health inequality, there needs to be a commitment to considering how society might transform to recognise that we are not born into equality, and must therefore redress imbalances to ensure that the environments that we are born into do not dictate our lives.

References

ACMD (Advisory Council on the Misuse of Drugs) (2006) *Pathways to problems: Hazardous use of tobacco, alcohol and other drugs by young people in the UK and its implications for policy*, London: Crown Copyright.

Alexander, B.K. (2008) *The globalisation of addiction: A study in poverty of the spirit*, New York, NY: Oxford University Press.

Alexander, B.K. (2012) 'Addiction: the urgent need for a paradigm shift', *Substance Use & Misuse*, 47(13/14): 1475–82.

Anda, R.F., Felitti, V.J., Bremner, J.D., Walker, J.D., Whitfield, C., Perry, B.D., Dube, S.R. and Giles, W.H. (2006) 'The enduring effects of abuse and related adverse experiences in childhood. A convergence of evidence from neurobiology and epidemiology', *European Archives of Psychiatry and Clinical Neuroscience*, 256(3): 174–86.

Bandura, A. (1977) 'Self efficacy: toward a unifying theory of behavioural change', *Psychological Review*, 84(2): 191–215.

Bellis, M.A., Lowey, H., Leckenby, N., Hughes, K. and Harrison, D. (2014) 'Adverse childhood experiences: retrospective study to determine their impact on adult health behaviours and health outcomes in a UK population', *Journal of Public Health*, 36(1): 81–91.

Best, D.W., Gufran, S., Day, E., Ray, R. and Loaring, J. (2008) 'Breaking the habit: a retrospective analysis of desistance factors among formerly problematic heroin users', *Drug and Alcohol Review*, 27(6): 619–24.

Blair, C. (2010) 'Stress and the development of self-regulation in context', *Child Development Perspectives*, 4(3): 181–8.

Briere, J. and Spinazzola, J. (2005) 'Phenomenology and psychological assessment of complex posttraumatic states', *Journal of Traumatic Stress*, 18: 401–12.

Brown, P.J., Recupero, P.R. and Stout, R. (1995) 'PTSD substance abuse comorbidity and treatment utilization', *Addictive Behaviour*, 20: 251–4.

CSDH (Commission on Social Determinants of Health) (2008) *Closing the gap in a generation. Health equity through action on the social determinants of health*, Geneva: World Health Organization.

Delgadillo, J., Asaria, M., Ali, S. and Gilbody, S. (2015) 'On poverty, politics and psychology: the socioeconomic gradient of mental healthcare utilization and outcomes', *The British Journal of Psychiatry*, Advance Online Article doi: 10.1192/bjp.bp.115.171017

EMCDDA (European Monitoring Centre for Drugs and Drug Addiction) (2013) *European drug report: Trends and developments*, Luxembourg: EMCDDA.

Felitti, V.J., Anda, R.F., Nordenberg, D., Williamson, D.F., Spitz, A.M., Edwards, V., Koss, M.P. and Marks, J.S. (1998) 'Relationship of childhood abuse and household dysfunction to many of the leading causes of death in adults: the Adverse Childhood Experiences (ACE) Study', *American Journal of Preventative Medicine*, 14(4): 245–58.

Fernandez-Serrano, M.J., Perez-Garcia, M. and Verdejo-Garcia, A. (2011) 'What are the specific vs. generalised effects of drugs of abuse on neuropsychological performance?', *Neuroscience and Biobehavioural Reviews*, 35: 377–406.

Ford, J.D., Hawke, J., Alessi, S., Ledgerwood, D. and Petry, N. (2007) 'Psychological trauma and PTSD symptoms as predictors of substance dependence treatment outcomes', *Behaviour Research and Therapy*, 45(10): 2417–31.

Galea, S. and Vlahov, D. (2002) 'Social determinants and the health of drug users: socioeconomic status, homelessness and incarceration', *Public Health Reports*, 117(1): S135–S145.

Grant, J.E., Potenza, M.N., Weinstein, A. and Gorelick, D.A. (2010) 'Introduction to behavioural addictions', *American Journal of Drug and Alcohol Abuse*, 36(5): 233–41.

Grella, C.E. and Stein, J.A. (2013) 'Remission from substance dependence: differences between individuals in a general population longitudinal survey who do and do not seek help', *Drug and Alcohol Dependence*, 133(1): 146–53.

Griggs, J. and Walker, R. (2008) *The costs of child poverty for individuals and society*, York: Joseph Rowntree Foundation.

Hall, W., Carter, A. and Forlini, C. (2015) 'The brain disease model of addiction: is it supported by the evidence and has it delivered on its promises?', *The Lancet Psychiatry*, 2(1): 105–10.

Hammersley, R. and Dalgarno, P. (2013) *Trauma and recovery amongst people who have injected drugs within the past five years*, Glasgow: Scottish Drugs Forum.

Harari, Y.N. (2014) *Sapiens: A brief history of humankind*, London: Harvill Secker.

Hari, J. (2015) *Chasing the scream: The first and last days of the war on drugs*, London: Bloomsbury.

Hart, C. (2013) *High price: Drugs, neuroscience and discovering myself*, London: Penguin.

Heyman, G.M. (2013) 'Addiction and choice: theory and new data', *Frontiers in Psychiatry*, 4(31): 1–5.

Home Office (2015) *Drug misuse: Findings from the 2014/2015 Crime Survey for England and Wales, second edition*, London: Home Office.

Lewis, M. (2015) *The biology of desire: Why addiction is not a disease*, New York, NY: PublicAffairs.

Loring, B. (2014) *Alcohol and inequities: Guidance for addressing inequities in alcohol-related harm*, Geneva: World Health Organization.

Luby, J., Belden, A., Botteron, K., Marus, N., Harms, M.P., Babb, C., Nishino, T. and Barch, D. (2013) 'The effects of poverty on childhood brain development: the mediating effect of caregiving and stressful life events', *JAMA Pediatrics*, 167(12): 1135–42.

Marmot, M. (2010) *Fair society, healthy lives: The Marmot Review. Strategic review of health inequalities in England post-2010*, London: UCL Institute of Health Equity.

McLaughlin, K., Sheridan, M.A. and Lambert, H.K. (2014) 'Childhood adversity and neural development: deprivation and threat as distinct dimensions of early experience', *Neuroscience and Biobehavioural Reviews*, 47: 578–91.

Noel, X., Brevers, D. and Bechara, A. (2013) 'A neurocognitive approach to understanding the neurobiology of addiction', *Current Opinion in Neurobiology*, 23: 632–8.

NTA (National Treatment Agency) (2010) *Commissioning for recovery*, London: NTA.

NTA (2012a) *Parents with drug problems: How treatment helps families*, London: NTA.

NTA (2012b) *Building recovery in communities: The transition to the new public health system*, London: NTA.

Nutt, D. (2012) *Drugs without the hot air: Minimising the harms of legal and illegal drugs*, Cambridge: UIT Cambridge.

Orford, J. (2001) *Excessive appetites: A psychological view of addictions* (2nd edn), New York, NY: John Wiley & Sons.

Orford, J. (2013) *Power, powerlessness and addiction*, Cambridge: Cambridge University Press.

Randles, D. and Tracy, J. (2013) 'Nonverbal displays of shame predict relapse and declining health in recovering alcoholics', *Clinical Psychological Science*, 1(2): 149–55.

Robertson, I.H. (2012) *The winner effect: How power affects your brain*, London: Bloomsbury.

Scottish Government (2008) *The road to recovery*, Edinburgh: Scottish Government.

Scottish Government (2015) *The quality principles: Standard expectations of care and support in drug and alcohol services*, Edinburgh: Scottish Government.

Slutske, W.S. (2015) 'Why is natural recovery so common for addictive disorders?', *Addiction*, 105(9): 1520–1.

White, W. (2014) 'Waiting for breaking good: the media and addiction recovery'. Available at: www.williamwhitepapers.com

White, W. and Kelly, J.F. (2011) 'What if we really believed that addiction was a chronic disorder?', in J.F. Kelly and W. White (eds) *Addiction recovery management: Theory, research and practice*, New York, NY: Humana Press.

Widome, R., Wall, M.M., Laska, M.N., Eisenberg, M.E. and Neumark-Sztainer, D. (2013) 'Adolescence to young adulthood: when socioeconomic disparities in substance use emerge', *Substance Use and Misuse*, 48: 1522–9.

Wilkinson, R. and Pickett, K. (2010) *The spirit level: Why equality is better for everyone*, London: Penguin Books Limited.

World Health Organization (2014) *Global status report on alcohol and health 2014*, Geneva: World Health Organization.

SEVEN

Health and exercise in the community

Naomi Brooks

Introduction

This chapter aims to detail the health benefits of exercise and physical activity (PA) in the community and provide some examples of successful public health and community interventions to increase PA and exercise programmes in the community. PA and exercise lead to improvements in a range of health outcomes. Although there are varying degrees of individual responsiveness, the benefits of PA and exercise include: reducing the risk of cardiovascular disease, type 2 diabetes and metabolic disorders, and some cancers; improving functional ability through strengthening muscle and bones; and improving psychological mood and well-being. Regardless of body mass index (BMI) and body weight, PA and exercise can improve fitness, which leads to healthy outcomes, regardless of weight loss. Skeletal muscle is important for maintaining functional ability, and is also an important metabolic tissue using glucose, fat and amino acids for energy production. Having muscle mass is important for strength as well as controlling blood glucose levels. As well as physiological health benefits, PA and exercise can provide social interactions, social support and reduced social isolation.

Health and exercise in the community

PA continues to be at the top of the government and health agendas throughout the world. Active lifestyles are important for the prevention of non-communicable diseases (NCDs), as well as for healthy ageing (Ding et al, 2016). Regular exercise improves physical and mental health, cognition, and general academic performance, reduces anxiety and depression, and adds to quality of life (Lee et al, 2012). Despite the known potential of PA to prevent NCDs and improve quality of life and mental well-being, public health campaigns have struggled to implement successful interventions on a large scale (Reis et al, 2016). It is essential to provide opportunities for PA and better health for all, not just those who can afford it. To successfully and sustainably address these pressing issues requires a coalition of policymakers and researchers, and involves social groups, the environment and policy to enable the maintenance and sustainability of health benefits (Reis et al, 2016).

Physical activity

Promoting PA for health is a high priority for government and other agencies as the prevalence of physical inactivity (PIA) continues to be a global concern for both children and adults. For the purposes of this chapter, we will define PA according to Caspersen and colleagues (Caspersen et al, 1985): skeletal movement resulting in energy expenditure that has a positive correlation with physical fitness. It is important to define PA separately to exercise and sport in order to recognise that exercise and sport are subcomponents of PA but PA comprises a wider spectrum, as highlighted by the definition. Frequency, intensity, volume and duration are key factors of PA (Caspersen et al, 1985). It is possible to estimate the energy expenditure of different PAs to classify the energy cost based on Metabolic Equivalents (Mets), where 1 Met represents $3.5ml/kg/min$ O_2 based on approximate value for resting metabolic rate (of quiet sitting). As such, the Compendium of Physical Activities, which quantifies the energy cost of different physical activities, takes into consideration the intensity of the activity, duration of the activity and volume of the activity (Ainsworth et al, 2000, 2011).

PA and exercise have consistently been shown to increase health outcomes in individual and group exercise programmes, albeit with varying degrees of individual responsiveness. Regular aerobic PA increases exercise capacity and physical fitness, which has long been known to have many health benefits (Fletcher et al, 1996; De Backer et al, 2003). PA has benefits for those with chronic disease; specifically, research shows benefits for patients with type 2 diabetes (Eriksson, 1999) and cancer (Courneya and Friedenreich, 1999; Byers et al, 2002), the prevention of hypertension (Petrella, 1998; Fagard, 2001) and obesity (Blair and Brodney, 1999; Seidell et al, 1999), and protection for individuals with ischaemic heart disease (Kavanagh et al, 2002). Figure 7.1 summarises the benefits of PA.

Although it is outside the scope of the chapter to discuss obesity, it is also important to mention that while there is consistent evidence that BMI is a predictor of all-cause mortality, and therefore reducing BMI is

Figure 7.1: Key outcomes and benefits from physical exercise

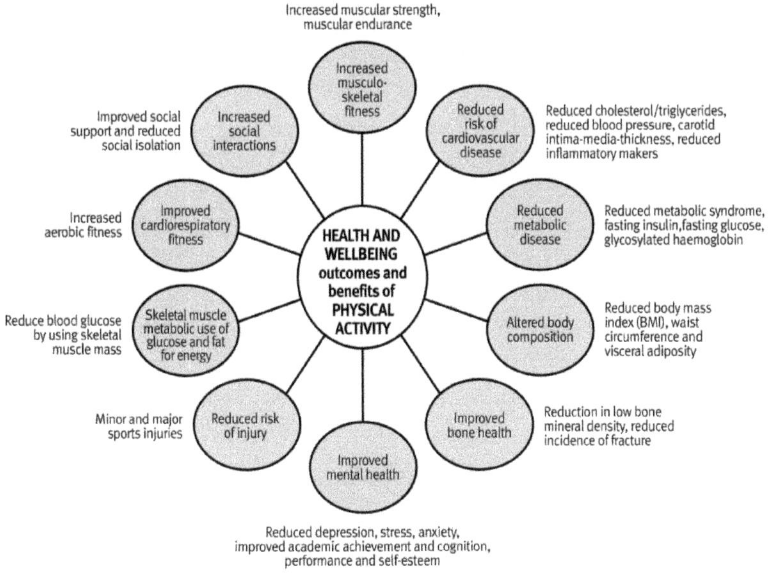

Increased muscular strength, muscular endurance

Increased musculo-skeletal fitness

Improved social support and reduced social isolation

Increased social interactions

Reduced risk of cardiovascular disease

Reduced cholesterol/triglycerides, reduced blood pressure, carotid intima-media-thickness, reduced inflammatory makers

Increased aerobic fitness

Improved cardiorespiratory fitness

HEALTH AND WELLBEING outcomes and benefits of PHYSICAL ACTIVITY

Reduced metabolic disease

Reduced metabolic syndrome, fasting insulin, fasting glucose, glycosylated haemoglobin

Reduce blood glucose by using skeletal muscle mass

Skeletal muscle metabolic use of glucose and fat for energy

Altered body composition

Reduced body mass index (BMI), waist circumference and visceral adiposity

Minor and major sports injuries

Reduced risk of injury

Improved bone health

Reduction in low bone mineral density, reduced incidence of fracture

Improved mental health

Reduced depression, stress, anxiety, improved academic achievement and cognition, performance and self-esteem

Source: Adapted from government guidelines (Department of Health, Physical Activity, Health Improvement and Protection, 2011).

of benefit health-wise, there are a number of paradoxes to this thinking. One of these is the 'FIT FAT' phenomenon, suggesting that obesity is not a risk factor for mortality if the individuals are also physically fit (McAuley and Blair, 2011). While weight loss is important for obese and overweight individuals, increasing PA and exercise to improve fitness is of importance to healthy outcomes regardless of weight loss. This is a key aspect often missed when interpreting results of exercise programmes and when planning interventions for improvements in health.

Physical inactivity

PIA is the fourth leading cause of death worldwide. Throughout recent history, there have been substantial changes in PA in our culture and society, and these contribute to health and well-being. During pre-agricultural and agricultural periods, there were high levels of PA and low-fat diets as humans lived as hunters and gatherers (Blair, 1988). During the industrial period (1800–45), there was a shift with industrialisation to overcrowding, poor diet and poor public health measures. The nuclear/technological period (1945 until the present) particularly reflects substantial improvements in medical and public health measures but increases in lifestyle-related health issues. These are associated with reductions in active transport, entertainment and energy expenditure in household activities and leisure time, and have contributed greatly to the increase in obesity and cardiovascular disease (Archer and Blair, 2011). Throughout the world, increasing urbanisation and economic development have been linked with reduced overall and occupational PA levels in adults (Ng et al, 2009), with the influences of rural to urban migration also being associated with reduced PA (Abubakari et al, 2009).

An important research study published in the 1950s brought to light the link between PA and cardiovascular health. The study compared coronary heart disease in bus conductors and bus drivers in London. The report concluded that bus conductors, who were active throughout their working day walking and climbing stairs on the bus, experienced half the coronary heart disease that their driving counterparts experienced (Morris et al, 1953a, 1953b). Many studies that have been conducted since these initial reports have provided similar results, highlighting that active people have lower rates of cardiovascular disease than inactive individuals.

Despite continued research results highlighting the importance of being physically active, recent evidence suggests that 31% of the world's population are not meeting minimal PA recommendations (Hallal et al, 2012). More than one third of all deaths can be attributed to five risk factors: PIA, high blood pressure, tobacco use, high blood glucose and obesity (WHO, 2009). PIA has a direct influence on NCDs and further influences on three of the top five risk factors (high blood pressure, high blood glucose and obesity). In the US, obesity and PIA account for nearly 20% of all deaths (Danaei et al, 2009) and contribute to portions of disability and the mortality of some cancers, diabetes and cardiovascular disease (WHO, 2000; LaMonte et al, 2005). Furthermore, NCDs tend to cause death over longer periods after initial diagnosis and can require extensive and expensive treatments that have profound economic consequences for individuals, families, communities and countries (Beaglehole et al, 2011). It is no surprise, then, to realise the importance of combating PIA.

International policy

Despite the benefits of PA being well known, and the rising global epidemic of PIA demonstrated in the continually rising statistics of increased mortality and morbidity, action on a national and international level has lagged behind other health improvements. Key organisations have released statements and policy documents to highlight the need to increase PA at a population level. It is important that international and national policies promote opportunities for whole populations to be active by adopting an intersectoral approach with international organisations, national governments and multiple strategic development plans (discussed in Bull et al, 2004).

In 2004, the World Health Assembly adopted the World Health Organization (WHO) global strategy on diet, PA and health (WHO, 2004). In 2011, the WHO met with health ministers from various countries and discussed the global crisis of the rise of NCDs and potential control efforts. They acknowledged that women, men and children in all countries and all income groups are at risk (UN, 2011). In 2010, the Global Advocacy Council for Physical Activity (GAPA) launched 'The Toronto Charter for Physical Activity: a global call for action' (Global Advocacy Council for Physical Activity and International Society for Physical Activity and Health, 2010). The aim of GAPA is to strengthen the advocacy, dissemination and capacity of PA promotion and policy (Kohl and Hootman, 2012). The Toronto Charter calls for an increase in action and greater investment in PA as a comprehensive approach, and calls for global action from governments to create policies and opportunities for everyone to lead physically active lives. The aim of the Toronto Charter is 'to elevate physical activity as a policy priority and develop, adequately resource, and implement cross-sector policies, plans and intervention programs to increase population levels of physical activity throughout the world' (Global Advocacy Council for Physical Activity and International Society for Physical Activity and Health, 2010). The charter provides guiding principles for a population-based approach to PA that coincide with the WHO's Global Strategy on Diet, PA and Health.

The charter provides a framework for action over five key areas that bring together governments, non-governmental organisations, professional associations and other agencies, including health professionals and the communities themselves. It provides a solid foundation and direction for the development and implementation of actions to increase population levels of physical activity adoption and implementation.

At a national level, the UK has ambitious targets for increasing the percentage of the population who are regularly active. For example, the goal outlined by the Scottish Executive is to have 50% of the adult population regularly active (30 minutes' moderate activity five times per week) by 2022 (Scottish Executive, 2003). England has a target for 70% of the adult population being regularly active by 2020

(Department for Culture, Media and Sport, 2002). More recently, the Scottish Government has produced its first ever National Physical Activity Implementation Plan, in conjunction with National Health Service (NHS) Scotland – 'A more active Scotland'. This follows from the national PA strategy of 2003, *Let's make Scotland more active* (Scottish Executive, 2003), which was implemented to attempt to reduce the decline in activity and provide objectives and a framework to increase PA. The new 10-year plan incorporates the key parts of the Toronto Charter for PA directly into the Scottish Government's agenda for the legacy of the Commonwealth Games in Glasgow in 2014.

How do we assess physical activity across the spectrum of policy, application, results and health?

The Active Healthy Kids Scotland Report Card is a meritorious example of a 'state of the nation' report on PA and health – this example being for Scottish children and adolescents. Active Healthy Kids Scotland published its first report card in 2013 in line with the Active Healthy Kids Canada Report Card and the international network of Active Healthy Kids Report Cards (Tremblay et al, 2015; see also the Active Healthy Kids Global Alliance, available at: www. activehealthykids.org). There are 10 health indicators that contribute to the overall grade: Overall PA and Health Behaviours and Outcomes (Sedentary Behaviour, Overall PA, Active Transport, Active and Outdoor Play, Organised Sport Participation, Diet, and Obesity) and Settings and Influences on PA and Health (Family and Peer Influence, Community and the Built Environment, and National Policy, Strategy and Investment). It is hoped that the report card will provide up-to-date information on the PA and health of Scottish children and adolescents, and can be used by: the government to develop policy and inform investment; researchers/academics to share with students and shape grant applications; teachers, coaches, health professionals, charitable organisations to inform their work; and funding bodies to help shape funding strategy and decisions. An equivalent report card for these aspects in adults or at the population level would certainly provide critical and up-to-date information on PA and health in the chosen population.

How do we measure PA?

There are a number of ways to assess PA that vary in cost, accuracy and feasibility. Vanhees et al (2005) nicely summarise the methods into three categories:

- *Criterion methods*, such as doubly labelled water, indirect calorimetry and direct observation, which are accurate, valid and useful for small population samples. These methods are expensive, require expertise for analysis and are limited to the laboratory setting.
- *Objective methods*, such as pedometers, accelerometers and heart-rate monitors. These are lightweight and portable devices that provide a detailed, objective recording over an extended period of time. They measure the intensity but not the gradient of exercise or specific activity (total daily PA).
- *Subjective methods*, such as self-report questionnaires, interview-assisted questionnaires, proxy-report questionnaires and diaries, are useful for population-level research (eg epidemiological studies), and some have been validated with other measurements. The detail collected depends on participants' memory and interpretation, which can sometimes lead to an overestimation of PA (Troiano et al, 2008).

A number of factors determine the optimal measure to use, including the size of the sample to be measured, the required outcomes and the required measures. There are various questionnaire data that have been validated against other measurements. The Scottish Physical Activity Screening Questionnaire (Scot-PASQ) was developed by NHS Health Scotland for use in an NHS PA pilot (for details, see: http://www.paha.org.uk/Resource/scottish-physical-activity-screening-question-scot-pasq).

Physical activity guidelines

Given the importance of PA to health, many governments around the world have made recommendations. In the most recent UK guidelines (Department of Health, Physical Activity, Health Improvement and Protection, 2011), the Chief Medical Officer recommended the following:

- Adults (aged 19–64 years): adults should aim to be active daily. Activity should add up to 150 minutes of moderate-intensity activity per week and should be done in bouts of 10 minutes or more (eg 30 minutes × five days). The same benefits can be achieved through 75 minutes of vigorous-intensity activity throughout the week or a combination of moderate and vigorous. Adults should also take part in PA to improve muscle strength on two days of the week. Furthermore, all adults should minimise the amount of time spent sitting for extended periods.

• Children (aged 5–18 years): children and young people should take part in at least 60 minutes of moderate- to vigorous-intensity PA each day. The recommendations suggest taking part in vigorous-intensity activities, including those that strengthen muscle and bone, at least three days per week. All children and young people should reduce/minimise the amount of time they spend sitting for extended periods.

• Older Adults (aged 65+): the guidelines for older adults recommend taking part in any type of PA to provide health benefits, including the maintenance of physical and cognitive function. Older adults should be active daily and their activity should add up to 150 minutes of moderate-intensity activity (also in bouts of 10 minutes or more). For those who are already active, 75 minutes of vigorous-intensity activity or a combination of moderate- and vigorous-intensity activity should be undertaken. Similar to the adult recommendations, older adults are recommended to undertake PA to improve strength on at least two days of the week and should reduce the amount of time sitting for extended periods. Older adults at risk of falling should incorporate PA to improve balance and coordination at least two days of the week.

These guidelines build on the previous recommendations published in 2008. The 2011 guidelines begin to address sedentary behaviour and in addition to increasing PA, they promote a reduction in sitting time. Reducing sedentary time, such as TV viewing, computer use, motorised transport and sitting for leisure time, has been advised since sedentary behaviour is negatively associated with obesity, insulin resistance, type 2 diabetes, some cancers, cardiovascular disease and all-cause mortality (Tremblay et al, 2010). The recommended volume of exercise (150 minutes of moderate-intensity exercise) has been reported to be beneficial for health (O'Donovan et al, 2010; Warburton et al, 2010), although the guidelines do point out that higher volumes of activity ($\geq$ 150 minutes per week) are associated with additional health benefits (eg Australian PA guidelines recommend up to 300 minutes per week of moderate-intensity activity). The guidelines also highlight that benefits of vigorous-intensity exercise are similar or more than those observed for moderate-intensity activity (O'Donovan et al, 2010; Warburton et al, 2010). The importance of muscle-strengthening exercises is important to build muscle strength and power, as well as to improve or maintain functional ability, bone formation and reduction in bone loss. This is especially important for older adults, but is beneficial for all adults. There is also evidence suggesting that there is a beneficial effect of strength training on glucose metabolism and blood pressure (Braith and Stewart, 2006).

Examples of successful public health and community interventions to increase physical activity

This section will touch on a number of successful interventions to increase PA in the community. These by no means encompass all the excellent research and community projects that are being undertaken, but they give a little insight into some of the factors and organisations contributing to encouraging communities and individuals to be more physically active.

The Daily Mile

Although the majority of this book chapter has focused on adults, the Daily Mile is an initiative to improve health and well-being in children. The Daily Mile began at St Ninian's Primary School in Stirling, pioneered by the then Head Teacher Elaine Wyllie. Each day, the pupils run, jog or walk outside for 15 minutes. The average distance covered is approximately one mile. The aim of the Daily Mile is to improve the physical, emotional and social health and well-being of the children. Anecdotal evidence suggests that the Daily Mile improves fitness levels, reduces obesity, improves concentration in class, improves social interactions with peers and teachers, and improves well-being – and that the children enjoy it! The Daily Mile is simple, non-competitive and fully inclusive, so each child can improve and succeed. The Daily Mile has been encouraged by the Scottish government, and has been rolled out in large parts of the UK, with thousands of children and many schools taking part in the Daily Mile. Our research group (DM WHEEL, University of Stirling) is currently undertaking a large research project investigating the Daily Mile in the local area and wider as opportunities arise. Results are expected by late 2016.

Football Fans in Training

An excellent example of a public health intervention involving lifestyle intervention was started in Scotland and has now expanded out into Europe. The Football Fans in Training (FFIT) programme is a 12-week, gender-sensitised, weight management and PA programme delivered, initially, to groups of men – at first, at Scottish Premier League Football Clubs (Hunt et al, 2014). The aim of the intervention was to encourage individuals to make lifestyle choices and changes to reduce their risk of ill health by losing weight, becoming more physically active and consuming a healthier diet. After 12 weeks, participants lost body mass, reduced waist circumference and BMI, improved dietary intake, and increased their self-esteem, mental health, physical health and quality of life. The programme also had a retention rate of 90% – a key point in its ongoing success. The programme has recently been rolled out to 15 football clubs in Europe (Van Nassau et al, 2016).

There have been a number of key research projects investigating health promotion for socially disadvantaged groups, such as homeless individuals and hard-to-reach populations. The following is by no means a complete list, but it highlights a number of successful interventions for the readership:

- Everton Football Club's Football in the Community (FitC) recruited men living in homeless shelters and/or recovering from substance misuse. Their 12-week programme consisted of two-hour football sessions twice weekly, together with education about healthy living. The results suggest that programmes can improve psychosocial health and well-being but there are many challenges in engaging these individuals in PA and health behaviours, and adherence was poor (Curran et al, 2016).
- Street soccer/football has been investigated on a number of levels for benefits in homeless individuals who take part. Randers et al (2012) report improved physical fitness (reduced body mass (fat percentage), cholesterol, improved diastolic blood pressure [BP]) after 12 weeks of street soccer training. This group of researchers further measured bone marker profile and balance and found improvements after 12 weeks of training with 75% attendance (Helge et al, 2014).
- We have recently presented similar findings of improved metabolic health after participation in a community-based exercise intervention in women from previously disadvantaged backgrounds in South African townships. Our research involved initiating and maintaining a community-based exercise intervention, demonstrating that the

programme was both feasible and effective in the South African township setting (Brooks et al, 2014). The exercise programme continues to run today, led by community members who have been trained to facilitate the programme.

- In a number of reported studies, homeless women (Wilson, 2005) and men (Quine et al, 2004) both practise health-promoting behaviours within the constraints of their situations, but scored lowest on PA and nutrition. These are areas for awareness and improvement for these population groups.
- In addition to research studies that are investigating the benefits of PA, there are many groups throughout the UK that are working to implement and encourage the government's guidelines and frameworks for increasing PA. Further details can be found on the government's website but include Active Scotland (available at: www. activescotland.org.uk), Paths for All (available at: www.pathsforall. org.uk), Healthy Living (available at: www.takelifeon.co.uk), promoting PA at work (available at: www.healthyworkinglives.com) and associated equivalents across the UK.

Summary

It is evident that PA in the community is essential for health and well-being. Although we understand the benefits of PA and exercise, the numbers of those taking part in PA is low, and here we highlight the importance of working together to promote PA for health, including government, health practitioners, exercise physiologists, behavioural psychologists, community groups and so on. The benefits to health and well-being span throughout the lifespan and healthspan, and are for everyone. This chapter has highlighted the importance of PA and exercise for health and well-being, given current government guidelines for how much PA should be undertaken, and provided some examples of research and community projects currently under way in the community.

References

Abubakari, A.R., Lauder, W., Jones, M.C., Kirk, A., Agyemang, C. and Bhopal, R.S. (2009) 'Prevalence and time trends in diabetes and physical inactivity among adult West African populations: the epidemic has arrived', *Public Health*, 123(9): 602–14.

Ainsworth, B.E., Haskell, W.L., Whitt, M.C., Irwin, M.L., Swartz, A.M., Strath, S.J., O'Brien, W.L., Bassett, D.R., Schmitz, K.H., Emplaincourt, P.O., Jacobs, D.R. and Leon, A.S. (2000) 'Compendium of physical activities: an update of activity codes and MET intensities', *Med Sci Sports Exerc*, 32(9 Suppl): S498–504.

Ainsworth, B.E., Haskell, W.L., Herrmann, S.D., Meckes, N., Bassett, D.R., Tudor-Locke, C., Greer, J.L., Vezina, J., Whitt-Glover, M.C. and Leon, A.S. (2011) '2011 compendium of physical activities: a second update of codes and MET values', *Med Sci Sports Exerc*, 43(8): 1575–81.

Archer, E. and Blair, S.N. (2011) 'Physical activity and the prevention of cardiovascular disease: from evolution to epidemiology', *Prog Cardiovasc Disease*, 53(6): 387–96.

Beaglehole, R., Bonita, R., Alleyne, G., Horton, R., Li, L., Lincoln, P., Mbanya, J.C., McKee, M., Moodie, R., Nishtar, S., Piot, P., Reddy, K.S., Stuckler, D. and Lancet NCD Action Group (2011) 'UN High-Level Meeting on Non-Communicable Diseases: addressing four questions', *Lancet*, 378(9789): 449–55.

Blair, S.N. (1988) *Exercise within a healthy lifestyle* (edited by R. Dishman), Champaign, IL: Human Kinetics.

Blair, S.N. and Brodney, S. (1999) 'Effects of physical inactivity and obesity on morbidity and mortality: current evidence and research issues', *Med Sci Sports Exerc*, 31(11 Suppl): S646–62.

Braith, R.W. and Stewart, K.J. (2006) 'Resistance exercise training: its role in the prevention of cardiovascular disease', *Circulation*, 113(22): 2642–50.

Brooks, N,, Bowes, J., Gava, L., January, N., Esterhuizen, A. and Myburgh, K.H. (2014) 'Twelve weeks of community exercise improves health parameters in women living in a semi-rural township in South Africa', *FASEB J*, 28: 884.25.

Bull, F.C., Bellew, B., Schöppe, S. and Bauman, A.E. (2004) 'Developments in national physical activity policy: an international review and recommendations towards better practice', *J Sci Med Sport*, 7(1 Suppl): 93–104.

Byers, T., Nestle, M., McTiernan, A., Doyle, C., Currie-Williams, A., Gansler, T., Thun, M. and American Cancer Society 2001 Nutrition and Physical Activity Guidelines Advisory Committee (2002) 'American Cancer Society guidelines on nutrition and physical activity for cancer prevention: reducing the risk of cancer with healthy food choices and physical activity', *CA: A Cancer Journal for Clinicians*, 52(2): 92–119.

Caspersen, C.J., Powell, K.E. and Christenson, G.M. (1985) 'Physical activity, exercise, and physical fitness: definitions and distinctions for health-related research', *Public Health Reports (Washington, D.C.: 1974)*, 100(2): 126–31.

Courneya, K.S. and Friedenreich, C.M. (1999) 'Physical exercise and quality of life following cancer diagnosis: a literature review', *Ann Behav Med*, 21(2): 171–9.

Curran, K., Drust, B., Murphy, R., Pringle, A. and Richardson, D. (2016) 'The challenge and impact of engaging hard-to-reach populations in regular physical activity and health behaviours: an examination of an English Premier League "Football in the Community" men's health programme', *Public Health*, 135: 14–22.

Danaei, G., Ding, E.L., Mozaffarian, D., Taylor, B., Rehm, J., Murray, C.J.L. and Ezzati, M. (2009) 'The preventable causes of death in the United States: comparative risk assessment of dietary, lifestyle, and metabolic risk factors', *PLoS Medicine*, 6(4): e1000058.

De Backer, G., Ambrosioni, E., Borch-Johnsen, K., Brotons, C., Cifkova, R., Dallongeville, J., Ebrahim, S., Faergeman, O., Graham, I., Mancia, G., Cats, V., Orth-Gomér, K., Perk, J., Pyörälä, K., Rodicio, J., Sans, S., Sansoy, V., Sechtem, U., Silber, S., Thomsen, T., Wood, D. and Practice GES of CC (2003) 'European guidelines on cardiovascular disease prevention in clinical practice: third joint task force of European and other societies on cardiovascular disease prevention in clinical practice (constituted by representatives of eight societies and by invit)', *European J Cardiovasc Prev Rehab: Official J Eur Soc Cardiology*, 10(4): S1–S10.

Department for Culture, Media and Sport (2002) *Game plan: A strategy for delivering government's sport and physical activity objectives*, London.

Department of Health, Physical Activity, Health Improvement and Protection (2011) *Start active, stay active: A report on physical activity from the four home countries' Chief Medical Officers*. Available at: https://www.gov.uk/government/uploads/system/uploads/attachment_data/file/216370/dh_128210.pdf

Ding, D., Lawson, K.D., Kolbe-Alexander, T.L., Finkelstein, E.A., Katzmarzyk, P.T., van Mechelen, W., Pratt, M. and Lancet Physical Activity Series 2 Executive Committee. (2016) 'The economic burden of physical inactivity: a global analysis of major non-communicable diseases', *Lancet*, 388(10051): 1311-24.

Eriksson, J.G. (1999) 'Exercise and the treatment of type 2 diabetes mellitus. An update', *Sports Med*, 27(6): 381–91.

Fagard, R.H. (2001) 'Exercise characteristics and the blood pressure response to dynamic physical training', *Med Sci Sports Exerc*, 33(6 Suppl): S484-94.

Fletcher, G., Balady, G., Blair, S., Blumenthal, J., Caspersen, C,, Chaitman, B., Epstein, S., Froelicher, E.S., Froelicher, V., Pina, I. and Pollock, M. (1996) 'Statement on exercise: benefits and recommendations for physical activity programs for all Americans. A statement for health professionals by the Committee on Exercise and Cardiac Rehabilitation of the Council on Clinical Cardiology, American Heart Association', *Circulation*, 94(4): 857–862.

Global Advocacy Council for Physical Activity and International Society for Physical Activity and Health (2010) 'The Toronto Charter for Physical Activity: a global call to action'. Available at: http://www.paha.org.uk/Resource/toronto-charter-for-physical-activity-a-global-call-for-action

Hallal, P.C., Andersen, L.B., Bull, F.C., Guthold, R., Haskell, W., Ekelund, U. and Lancet Physical Activity Series Working Group. (2012) 'Global physical activity levels: surveillance progress, pitfalls, and prospects', *Lancet*, 380(9838): 247–57.

Helge, E.W., Randers, M.B., Hornstrup, T., Nielsen, J.J., Blackwell, J., Jackman, S.R. and Krustrup, P. (2014) 'Street football is a feasible health-enhancing activity for homeless men: biochemical bone marker profile and balance improved', *Scand J Med Sci Sports*, 24(Suppl 1): 122–9.

Hunt, K., Wyke, S., Gray, C.M., Anderson, A.S., Brady, A., Bunn, C., Donnan, P.T., Fenwick, E., Grieve, E., Leishman, J., Miller, E., Mutrie, N., Rauchhaus, P., White, A. and Treweek, S. (2014) 'A gender-sensitised weight loss and healthy living programme for overweight and obese men delivered by Scottish Premier League football clubs (FFIT): a pragmatic randomised controlled trial', *Lancet*, 383(9924): 1211–21.

Kavanagh, T., Mertens, D.J., Hamm, L.F., Beyene, J., Kennedy, J., Corey, P. and Shephard, R.J. (2002) 'Prediction of long-term prognosis in 12169 men referred for cardiac rehabilitation', *Circulation*, 106(6): 666–71.

Kohl, H.W. and Hootman, J.M. (2012) 'Reflections before moving forward', *J Phys Act Health*, 9(1): 1–2.

LaMonte, M.J., Blair, S.N. and Church, T.S. (2005) 'Physical activity and diabetes prevention', *J Appl Physiol*, 99(3): 1205–13.

Lee, I,-M., Shiroma, E.J., Lobelo, F., Puska, P., Blair, S.N., Katzmarzyk, P.T. and Lancet Physical Activity Series Working Group (2012) 'Effect of physical inactivity on major non-communicable diseases worldwide: an analysis of burden of disease and life expectancy', *Lancet*, 380(9838): 219–29.

McAuley, P.A. and Blair, S.N. (2011) 'Obesity paradoxes', *J Sports Sci*, 29(8): 773–82.

Morris, J.N., Heady, J.A., Raffle, P.A., Roberts, C.G. and Parks, J.W. (1953a) 'Coronary heart-disease and physical activity of work', *Lancet*, 265(6796): 1111–20.

Morris, J.N., Heady, J.A., Raffle, P.A., Roberts, C.G. and Parks, J.W. (1953b) 'Coronary heart-disease and physical activity of work', *Lancet*, 265(6795): 1053–7.

Ng, S.W., Norton, E.C. and Popkin, B.M. (2009) 'Why have physical activity levels declined among Chinese adults? Findings from the 1991–2006 China Health and Nutrition Surveys', *Social Sci Med*, 68(7): 1305–14.

O'Donovan, G., Blazevich, A.J., Boreham, C., Cooper, A.R., Crank, H., Ekelund, U., Fox, K.R., Gately, P., Giles-Corti, B., Gill, J.M.R., Hamer, M., McDermott, I., Murphy, M., Mutrie, N., Reilly, J.J., Saxton, J.M. and Stamatakis, E. (2010) 'The ABC of physical activity for health: a consensus statement from the British Association of Sport and Exercise Sciences', *J Sport Sci*, 28(6): 573–91.

Petrella, R.J. (1998) 'How effective is exercise training for the treatment of hypertension?', *Clin J Sport Med*, 8(3): 224–31.

Quine, S., Kendig, H., Russell, C. and Touchard, D. (2004) 'Health promotion for socially disadvantaged groups: the case of homeless older men in Australia', *Health Promot Int*, 19(2): 157–65.

Randers, M.B., Petersen, J., Andersen, L.J., Krustrup, B.R., Hornstrup, T., Nielsen, J.J., Nordentoft, M. and Krustrup, P. (2012) 'Short-term street soccer improves fitness and cardiovascular health status of homeless men', *Eur J Appl Physiol*, 112(6): 2097–106.

Reis, R.S,, Salvo, D., Ogilvie, D., Lambert, E.V., Goenka, S., Brownson, R.C. and Lancet Physical Activity Series 2 Executive Committee (2016) 'Scaling up physical activity interventions worldwide: stepping up to larger and smarter approaches to get people moving', *Lancet*, 388(10051):1337-48.

Scottish Executive (2003) *Let's make Scotland more active: A strategy for physical activity*, Edinburgh.

Seidell, J.C., Visscher, T.L. and Hoogeveen, R.T. (1999) 'Overweight and obesity in the mortality rate data: current evidence and research issues', *Med Sci Sports Exerc*, 31(11 Suppl): S597–601.

Tremblay, M.S., Colley, R.C., Saunders, T.J., Healy, G.N. and Owen, N. (2010) 'Physiological and health implications of a sedentary lifestyle', *Appl Physiol Nutr Metab*, 35(6): 725–40.

Tremblay, M.S., Gonzalezm, S.A., Katzmarzyk, P.T., Onywera, V.O., Reilly, J.J., Tomkinson, G. and Active Healthy Kids Global Alliance (2015) 'Physical activity report cards: Active Healthy Kids Global Alliance and The Lancet Physical Activity Observatory', *J Phys Act Health*, 12(3): 297–8.

Troiano, R,P,, Berrigan, D., Dodd, K.W., Mâsse, L.C., Tilert, T. and McDowell, M. (2008) 'Physical activity in the United States measured by accelerometer', *Med Sci Sports Exerc*, 40(1): 181–8.

UN (United Nations) (2011) *Political declaration of the high-level meeting of the General Assembly on the prevention and control of non-communicable diseases*, New York, NY.

Vanhees, L., Lefevre, J., Philippaerts, R., Martens, M., Huygens, W., Troosters, T. and Beunen, G. (2005) 'How to assess physical activity? How to assess physical fitness?', *Eur J Cardiovasc Prev Rehab*, 12(2): 102–14.

van Nassau, F., van der Ploeg, H.P., Abrahamsen, F., Andersen, E., Anderson, A.S., Bosmans, J.E., Bunn, C., Chalmers, M., Clissmann, C., Gill, J.M.R., Gray, C.M., Hunt, K., Jelsma, J.G.M., La Guardia, J.G., Lemyre, P.N., Loudon, D.W., Macaulay, L., Maxwell, D.J., McConnachie, A., Martin, A., Mourselas, N., Mutrie, N., Nijhuis-van der Sanden, R., O'Brien, K., Pereira, H.V., Philpott, M., Roberts, G.C., Rooksby, J., Rost, M., Røynesdal, Ø., Sattar, N., Silva, M.N., Sorensen, M., Teixeira, P.J., Treweek, S., van Achterberg, T., van de Glind, I., van Mechelen, W. and Wyke, S. (2016) 'Study protocol of European Fans in Training (EuroFIT): a four-country randomised controlled trial of a lifestyle program for men delivered in elite football clubs', *BMC Public Health*, 16: 598.

Warburton, D.E., Charlesworth, S., Ivey, A., Nettlefold, L. and Bredin, S.S. (2010) 'A systematic review of the evidence for Canada's physical activity guidelines for adults', *Int J Behavior Nutr Phys Act*, 7: 39.

WHO (World Health Organization) (2000) *Obesity: Preventing and managing the global epidemic. Report of a WHO consultation*, Geneva: WHO.

WHO (2004) 'Diet and physical activity: a public health priority'. Available at: http://www.who.int/dietphysicalactivity/strategy/eb11344/strategy_english_web.pdf

WHO (2009) *Mortality and burden of disease estimates for WHO member states in 2004*, Geneva: WHO.

Wilson, M. (2005) 'Health-promoting behaviors of sheltered homeless women', *Fam Comm Health*, 28(1): 51–63.

EIGHT

Health and well-being in the digital society

Nathan Critchlow

Introduction

This chapter provides a narrative review of evidence that links increased use of technology to negative health and well-being. While the chapter touches on several issues, it particularly focuses on two case studies of influencing alcohol use in young people. The chapter begins by reviewing internet use. Second, it considers how growing engagement with technology has influenced sedentary behaviour and, third, how it can influence mental well-being. Fourth, the chapter considers how the content created by other internet users may encourage or reinforce health risk behaviours, presenting the first alcohol case study. Finally, it considers the influence of digital marketing on behaviour, thus presenting the second alcohol case study.

The digital society and internet use

The half-century either side of the millennium has been characterised by a digital revolution, driven by increasing advancements in technology and accessibility to online spaces (Halfpenny and Procter, 2015). This revolution has also been driven by the increased social importance that we subscribe to online environments, and the ways in which technology has infiltrated our lives. This online revolution is characterised by the many not the few. For example, half of the estimated 3 billion internet users worldwide (Kende, 2015) are now members of social networking website Facebook (Facebook, 2015). Indeed, if Facebook was considered a country, it would have a population greater than any other in our physical world (Stenovic, 2015). In the UK specifically, internet use continues to steadily increase (Office for National Statistics, 2015). Frequency of use, the amount of time spent online and many online behaviours are also negatively correlated with age (OFCOM,

2015a, 2015b). This suggests that it is young people, who remain in a state of mental and social development, whose health may be most influenced by our digital society.

Technological developments have also fundamentally changed how we engage with media. Throughout the 20th century, traditional media channels saw audiences as passive observers with little power to influence content (Jenkins, 2006). Digital media, however, has instead created a culture where users have many opportunities to participate, predominantly through social networking and media-sharing websites designed specifically for this purpose (Kaplan and Haenlein, 2010). Highlighting this growth of user involvement, it is estimated that 500 million Tweets are sent every day (Oreskovic, 2015), over 300 hours of video footage are uploaded to YouTube every minute (Statistics Brain, 2015a) and over 410 million multimedia messages are sent daily via SnapChat (Statistics Brain, 2015b). A further negative correlation with age again suggests that it is young adults who take an active role in content creation (OFCOM, 2015a, 2015b).

Influence on sedentary behaviour

One facet of well-being influenced by increased technology use is our physical health. This is because many online tasks have little need for movement, and thus increase sedentary behaviour. This is important as decreased physical activity is associated with many negative outcomes, most notably, obesity (Trembley et al, 2011; Biswas et al, 2015). Understanding the drivers of obesity is important as it results in an estimated £15.8 billion cost to the UK economy each year (Morgan and Dent, 2010). For young people, the concerns about sedentary activity mainly focus on how new media entertainment, such as playing video games, can be achieved with little movement, thus leading to the term 'screenagers' (Biddle et al, 2010: 44). For adults, concerns have also been raised about how the increased use of technology in professional settings now means that large proportions of the population spend most of their working day sitting down (Buckley et al, 2015).

The suggestion that sedentary lifestyles may be influenced by technology is supported by evidence (Biddle et al, 2010). The Health Behaviour in School Aged Children Survey (HBSC), for example, indicates that the proportion of 11–15 year olds in England, Scotland and Wales who use computers for gaming, emails, homework or general browsing for two or more hours on weekdays is higher than the average across the other 40 countries surveyed (Townsend et al, 2015). With regards to workplace activity, the Health Survey for England indicates that over half of men (59%) and women (54%) spend five or more hours sitting or standing at work each day (Townsend et al, 2015). Research further suggests that the sedentary behaviour brought about by technology has a negative influence on physical health, including obesity (Vandleanotte et al, 2009), body mass (Arora et al, 2013), impaired vision (Bener et al, 2011), venous thromboembolism (Healy et al, 2010) and musculoskeletal pain (Costigan et al, 2013). A study of 11,931 adolescents in Europe further found that the prevalence of poor lifestyle reporting (eg sleeping patterns, nutrition and physical activity) was higher in participants who also reported maladaptive or pathological levels of internet use, thus suggesting a dose–response relationship with physical health risk (Durkee et al, 2016).

Influence on mental health

Another facet of well-being influenced by the digital society is mental health. For example, research suggests that individuals can become addicted to internet use itself, or specific online activities such as pornography, cyber-relationships and gaming (Young et al, 2000; Widyanto and Griffiths, 2006; Petry and O'Brien, 2013; Brand et al, 2014). It is also suggested that such Web-based addictions can generate serious concomitant harms, including poor academic performance (Gentile et al, 2011) and job loss (Young, 2004). Research has also demonstrated that the internet provides a platform in which mental health issues may be initiated or exacerbated (Huang, 2010; Harwood et al, 2014). This includes negative mental health outcomes as a result of sedentary behaviour (Hamer et al, 2010) or specific online activities, such as social media use, influencing low self-esteem, depression and symptoms of psychiatric disorders (Rosen et al, 2013; Richards et al, 2015; Cavazos-Rehg et al, 2016). It is further noted that mental health can be worsened by other interpersonal factors, such as cyber-bullying, which can cause depression, anxiety and suicidal tendencies (Daine et al, 2013).

Interpersonal influence on health and well-being: the first alcohol case study

The suggestion that online content influences interpersonal socialisation is supported by decades of research into observational learning and media influence (Bryant and Oliver, 2009). Social learning theory, for example, suggests that behavioural schemas are vicariously modelled on, and reinforced by, observing the outcomes experienced by others, including those in the media (O'Rorke, 2006). Cultivation theory further suggests that perceptions of behaviour can be influenced by the themes and ideological messages presented in the media (Gerbner, 1998). Further perspectives also suggest that media characters may act as '*super peers*' who provide prototypes of behaviour that may not be available in immediate social environments (Brown et al, 2005). This provides a means of understanding how negative behaviour may develop even when there is no immediate family history. Finally, the uses and gratification theory suggests that audiences may even seek out media content in a goal-oriented manner to reinforce existing cognitions of behaviour (Ruggiero, 2000).

There is a variety of research to support that this theoretical influence is realised in real-world behaviour. This includes associations between online engagement and offline health risk behaviours, such as legal high use (Norman et al, 2014), smoking (Van Hoof et al, 2014), sexual risk (Kletteke et al, 2014), violent behaviour (Linkletter et al, 2010), physical injury (Avery et al, 2016) and multiple health risks (Moreno et al, 2007). Evidence also suggests links between online engagement and other learnt aspects of dysfunctional socialisation, including links between video games and aggression (APA, 2015), distorted perceptions of body image (Tiggemman and Slater, 2013) and cyber-bullying (Hardaker, 2010).

One frequently referenced relationship is the influence of digital content on alcohol knowledge, attitudes and behaviour in young people (Moreno and Whitehill, 2013). The viral 'Neknominate' game, in which participants encouraged each other to partake in a risky drinking challenge, provides a high-profile example (Wombacher et al, 2016). Understanding the drivers of alcohol use is important as excessive consumption is linked with increased mortality, morbidity and a range of social harms (World Health Organization, 2014), with the annual accumulated social and economic costs in England estimated to be £21 billion (Public Health England, 2014).

Content analysis research supports the theory that messages encouraging alcohol use feature across a range of new media, including social networking websites (Griffiths and Casswell, 2010), Twitter (Cavazos-Rehg et al, 2014), YouTube (Primack et al, 2015) and smartphone applications (Weaver et al, 2013). Such messages also appear to represent a normal part of young people's online experiences and receive considerable levels of engagement and positive appraisal (Beullens and Schepers, 2013; Primack et al, 2015). The narratives within such content are also reported to promote alcohol use both explicitly, by showing or encouraging drinking (Moreno et al, 2010), and implicitly, by featuring contexts and cultures associated with consumption (eg nightclubs) (Atkinson et al, 2014). There are also suggestions that content frames consumption, and the associated consequences, in a positive manner (Cavazos-Rehg et al, 2014; Primack et al, 2015). Even when negative outcomes are featured, they are still suggested to be a desirable part of telling an enjoyable drinking story (Atkinson et al, 2014). It is also suggested that such content may target and appeal to young people by frequently depicting those around the legal purchasing age (Fournier and Clarke, 2011), adopting designs popular in these age groups (eg games) (Weaver et al, 2013), referring to popular culture (Atkinson et al, 2014) and having no effective processes to restrict underage exposure (Mart et al, 2009).

Audience research, based on surveys and experimental designs, provides further evidence that young people are exposed a range of content that promotes alcohol use, including encouraged risky alcohol consumption on popular social media websites (Westgate et al, 2014; Canbrera-Nguyen et al, 2016). This research also suggests that this exposure is associated with a range of drinking behaviours (Stoddard et al, 2012; Miller et al, 2014), alcohol-related harm (Ridout et al, 2012) and social cognitions that predispose consumption (Thompson and Romo, 2016). Qualitative research, based on interviews and focus groups, also further suggests that these alcohol-related messages play an instrumental role in establishing and confirming peer appraisal and social values, reinforcing friendship group belonging, providing life markers that facilitate social exchanges, and establishing or maintaining a drinking identity (Atkinson et al, 2014; Lyons et al, 2014).

The influence of commercial digital marketing: the second alcohol case study

Critics have long questioned the influence that commercial marketing has on young people's knowledge, attitudes and behaviours (Bakan, 2012). Since the turn of the century, rising internet use and technology developments have further fuelled interest in how commercial marketing goals can be fulfilled through digital media (Chaffey and Ellis-Chadwick, 2012). In comparison to other media channels, digital advertising is not only the fastest growing, but also receives the greatest proportion of expenditure (OFCOM, 2015c). Advertising expenditure, however, only provides a snapshot of understanding, and one likely to underestimate the true volume of marketing. A social media page, for example, can be created for little or no expenditure. The lower cost of promotion, compared to traditional media, also means that a greater volume of marketing can be created for equal, or even less, outlay (Chaffey and Ellis-Chadwick, 2012). Expenditure also fails to account for user-generated and co-created content (eg fans pages), which can extend the life and reach of a marketing message (Arnhold, 2010).

Research supports the theory that digital marketing is being used to promote a range of health risk behaviours, including the consumption of unhealthy food (Kelly et al, 2015) and gambling (Gainsbury et al, 2015), with the latter also greatly enhanced by the ability of technology to make gambling almost omnipresent in terms accessibility (eg mobile applications). One commodity that has attracted particular research attention, however, is how the alcohol industry is using digital channels to market their products, and the implications that this has for consumption and underage drinking (Bonner and Gilmore, 2012). That digital media allows marketing to be targeted at specific audiences and locations, that content can be virally spread or accessed at any time and in almost any context, and that age restrictions are difficult to effectively apply when online has led some to claim that digital alcohol marketing may be more powerful and less controllable than marketing using traditional media (Hastings and Sheron, 2013).

Content research identifies three themes about how the alcohol industry has embraced new media, and how such activity may influence risky consumption or underage drinking. The first, relating to presence and style, suggests that digital alcohol marketing is global and extensive in audience and volume, and that it represents an important feature in 360-degree marketing strategies (Chester et al, 2010). It is also suggested that the industry uses a variety of channels and styles, invests significant resources towards associating their products with popular cultures or identities, and creates real-time conversations that blur the boundaries between marketing and peer-created content (Nicholls, 2012; Atkinson et al, 2014; Moraes et al, 2014). The second theme suggests that marketing may reach young people due to ineffective age verification (Winpenny et al, 2013; Barry et al, 2015) and also appeal to them directly through style and design, as well as indirectly by associating with contexts and themes that may resonate with young people (Nicholls, 2012; Atkinson et al, 2014; Carah et al, 2015). The final theme suggests that marketing may also promote risky drinking by: (1) undermining regulations; (2) relating alcohol to contexts synonymous with risky drinking (Carah et al, 2015); (3) the inadequate promotion of responsible drinking (Nicholls, 2012; Atkinson et al, 2014); and (4) allowing user-generated branding to promote messages otherwise prohibited in marketing (Brooks, 2010).

Survey research provides further empirical evidence that young adults are aware of, and participating with, digital alcohol marketing, and this exposure is associated with consumption and risky drinking (Critchlow et al, 2016; De Bruijn et al, 2016). Survey research has further shown that exposure to digital alcohol marketing is also associated with changes in alcohol-related social cognitions in young people, for example outcome expectancies (de Bruijn et al, 2012). This helps to move the debate away from whether marketing influence consumption and onto how this influence occurs. These findings are also further supplemented by experimental research which suggests that digital marketing does not just encourage consumption, but also that the marketing messages supersede the effect of co-presented messages that attempt to promote responsible drinking (Alhabash et al, 2015).

Interviews and focus groups further suggest that young people are exposed to a range of digital alcohol marketing, particularly on social networking websites (Atkinson et al, 2014; Lyons et al, 2014). Young people further suggest that marketing is often blurred with peer-created content, which both makes it difficult to recognise what is marketing and potentially strengthens the impact that it has (Lyons et al, 2014; Weaver et al, 2016). Qualitative research further demonstrates that: (1) alcohol marketing is considered a ubiquitous and normal part of social media use; (2) young people are content to use global and local marketing discourses as a means of narrating their social and cultural identities; and (3) the power of financial or social reward is a strong influence on their engagement with such marketing (Atkinson et al, 2014; Lyons et al, 2014; Moares et al, 2014; Purves et al, 2014). Notably, young people also consistently see themselves as media-savvy users who are not vulnerable to the effects of marketing, a finding that contrasts with survey research which suggests that exposure is associated with consumption. Finally, the ambiguous mix of commercial marketing, user-created promotion and messages about responsible consumption leaves young people confused about the attractions and dangers of alcohol, and leads them to question the fairness about the marketing they see online (Lyons et al, 2014; Purves et al, 2014).

Conclusion

This narrative review is underpinned by five conclusions. The first is that extensive internet use, particularly in young people, highlights the importance of identifying and addressing determinants of health and well-being in our digital society. The second is that internet use, by virtue of its nature, is increasing sedentary behaviour that leads to a range of acute and chronic physical and mental outcomes. The third is that the digital society is influencing mental health, both by initiating new addictive behaviours and also by providing an environment in which existing issues can be exacerbated. The fourth is that the content observed online appears to have a powerful influence on socialisation and learned behaviour, including a range of health risk behaviours. Finally, digital technology provides a further environment in which commercial marketing can reach and influence young people, including highly prevalent and persuasive marketing for products that provide a gateway to a range of individual, social and economics harms (eg alcohol).

References

Alhabash, S., McAlister, A.R., Quilliam, E.T., Richards, J.I. and Lou, C. (2015) 'Alcohol's getting a bit more social: when alcohol marketing messages on Facebook increase young adults' intentions to imbibe', *Mass Communication and Society*, 18(3): 350–75.

American Psychological Association Task Force on Violent Media (2015) 'Technical report on the review of the violent video game literature', APA. Available at: http://www.apa.org/pi/families/review-video-games.pdf

Arnhold, U. (2010) *User generated branding: Integrating user generated content into brand management*, Bremen: Springer Gabler Research.

Arora, T., Lam, K-B. H., Yao, G.L., Thomas, N. and Teheri, S. (2013) 'Exploring the complex pathways among specific types of technology, self-report sleep duration and body mass index', *International Journal of Obesity*, 37: 1253–60.

Atkinson, A.M., Ross, K.M., Begley, E. and Sumnall, H. (2014) *Constructing alcohol identities: The role of social network sites (SNS) in young peoples' drinking cultures*, Alcohol insight number 119, London: Alcohol Research UK.

Avery, A., Rae, L., Summit, J. and Kahn, S.A. (2016) 'The fire challenge: a case of report and analysis of self-inflicted flame injury posted on social media', *Journal of Burn Care and Research*, 37(2): 161–5.

Bakan, J. (2012) *Childhood under siege: How big business targets your children*, New York, NY: Free Press.

Barry, A.E., Bates, A.M., Olysanya, O., Vinal, C., Martin, E., Peoples, J., Jackson, Z.A., Billinger, S.A., Yusuf, A., Cauley, D.A. and Montano, J.R. (2015) 'Alcohol marketing on Twitter and Instagram: evidence of directly advertising to youth and adolescents', *Alcohol and Alcoholism*, 51(4): 487–92.

Bener, A., Al-Mahdi, H.S., Al-Nufal, M., Vanhhani, P.J. and Tewfid, I. (2011) 'Obesity and low vision as a result of excessive Internet use and television viewing', *International Journal of Food Sciences and Nutrition*, 62(1): 60–2.

Beullens, K. and Schepers, A. (2013) 'Display of alcohol use on Facebook: a content analysis', *Cyberpsychology: Behavior and Social Networking*, 16(7): 497–503.

Biddle, S., Cavill, N., Ekelund, U, Gorely, T., Griffiths, M.D. and Jago, R. (2010) *Sedentary behaviour and obesity: Review of the current scientific evidence*, London: Department of Health.

Biswas, A., Oh, P.I., Faulkner, G.E., Bajaj, R.R., Silver, M.A., Mitchell, M.S. and Alter, D.A. (2015) 'Sedentary time and its association with risk for disease incidence, mortality and hospitalisation in adults', *Annals of Internal Medicine*, 162: 123–32.

Bonner, A. and Gilmore, I. (2012) 'The UK responsibility deal and its implications for effective alcohol policy in the UK and internationally', *Addiction*, 107(12): 2063–5.

Brand, M., Laier, C. and Young, K.S. (2014) 'Internet addiction: coping styles, experiences and treatment implications', *Frontiers in Psychology*, 5(11): 1–14.

Brooks, O. (2010) *'Routes to magic': The alcoholic beverage industry's use of new media in alcohol marketing*, Stirling: Institute for Social Marketing, University of Stirling.

Brown, J.D., Halpern, C.T. and L'Engle, K.L. (2005) 'Mass media as a sexual super peer for early maturing girls', *Journal of Adolescent Health*, 36: 420–7.

Bryant, J. and Oliver, M.B. (2009) *Media effects: Advances in theory and research*, London: Routledge & Sons.

Buckley, J.P., Hedge, A., Yates, T., Copeland, R.J., Loosemore, M., Hamer, M., Bradley, and Dunstan, D.W. (2015) 'The sedentary office: a growing case for change towards better health and productivity: Expert statement commissioned by Public Health England and the Active Working Community Interest Company', *British Journal of Sports Medicine*, 49: 1357–62.

Canbrera-Nguyen, E.P., Cavozos-Rehg, P., Krauss, M., Bierut, L.J. and Moreno, M.A. (2016) 'Young adults' exposure to alcohol and marijuana related content on Twitter', *Journal of Studies on Alcohol and Drugs*, 77(2): 349–53.

Carah, N., Brodmerkel, S. and Shaul, M. (2015) *Breaching the code: Alcohol, Facebook and self-regulation*, Canberra: Foundation for Alcohol Research and Education.

Cavavos-Rehg, P.A., Krauss, M.J., Sowles, S.J. and Bierut, L.J. (2014) '"Hey everyone, I'm drunk." An evaluation of drinking-related Twitter chatter', *Journal of Studies on Alcohol and Drugs*, 76(4): 635–43.

Cavazos-Rehg, P.A., Krauss, M.K., Sowles, S., Connolly, S., Rosas, C., Bharadwaj, M. and Bierut, L.J. (2016) 'A content analysis of depression-related tweets', *Computers in Human Behaviour*, 54: 351–357.

Chaffey, D. and Ellis-Chadwick, F. (2012) *Digital marketing: Strategy, implementation and practice*, New York, NY: Pearson PLC.

Chester, J., Montgomery, K. and Dorfman, L. (2010) *Alcohol marketing in the digital age*, Berkley, CA: Berkley Media Studies Group.

Costigan, S.A., Barnett, L., Plotnikoff, R.C. and Lubans, D.R. (2013) 'The health indicators associated with screen-based sedentary behaviour among adolescent girls: a systematic review', *Journal of Adolescent Health*, 53: 382–92.

Critchlow, N., Moodie, C., Bauld, L., Bonner, A. and Hastings, G. (2016) 'Awareness of, and participation with, digital alcohol marketing, and the association with frequency of high episodic drinking among young adults', *Drugs: Education, Prevention and Policy*, 23(4): 328–36.

Daine, K., Hawton, K., Singaravelu, V., Stewart, A., Simkin, S. and Montgomery, P. (2013) 'The power of the Web: a systematic review of studies of the influence of the Internet on self-harm and suicide in young people', *PLoS One*, 8(10): e77555.

de Bruijn, A., Tanghe, J., Beccaria, F., Bujalski, M., Celata, C., Gosselt, J., Schreckenberg, D. and Slowdonik, L. (2012) *Report on the impact of European alcohol marketing exposure on youth alcohol expectancies and youth drinking*, Deliverable 2.3 and 3.7, Work Package 4, Europe: AMPHORA Project.

de Bruijn, A., Tanghe, J., de Leew, R., Engels, R., Anderson, P., Beccaria, F., Bukalski, M., Celata, C., Gosselt, J., Schrenkenberg, D., Slowdonik, L., Wothge, J. and van Dalen, W. (2016) 'European longitudinal study on the relationship between adolescents' alcohol marketing exposure and alcohol use', *Addiction*, 11(10): 1774–83.

Durkee, T., Carli, V., Floderus, B., Wasserman, Sarchiapone, M., Apter, A., Balazs, J.A., Bobes, J., Brunner, R., Corcoran, P., Cosman, D., Haring, C., Hoven, C.W., Kaess, M., Kahnm J.P., Nemes, B., Postuvan, V., Saiz, P.A., Varnik, P. and Wasserman, D. (2016) 'Pathological Internet use and risk-behaviours among European adolescents', *International Journal of Environmental Research and Public Health*, 13(3): 1–17.

Facebook (2015) 'Facebook Q2 2015 results'. Available at: http://files.shareholder.com/downloads/AMDA-NJ5DZ/0x0x842064/619A417E-5E3E-496C-B125-987FA25A0570/FB_Q215EarningsSlides.pdf

Fournier, A.K. and Clarke, S.W. (2011) 'Do college students use Facebook to communicate about alcohol? An analysis of student profile pages', *Cyberpsychology: Journal of Psychosocial Research on Cyberspace*, 5(2).

Gainsbury, S.M., Russell, A., Hing, N., Wood, R., Lubman, D. and Blaszczynski, A. (2015) 'How the Internet is changing gambling: findings from an Australian prevalence survey', *Journal of Gambling Studies*, 31(1): 1–15.

Gentile, D.A., Choo, H., Liau, A., Sim, T., Li, D., Fung, D. and Khoo, A. (2011) 'Pathological video game use among youths: a two-year longitudinal study', *Pediatrics*, 127(2): 319–29.

Gerbner, G. (1998) 'Cultivation analysis: an overview', *Mass Communication & Society*, 1(3/4): 175–94.

Griffiths, R. and Casswell, S. (2010) 'Intoxigenic digital spaces? Youth, social networking sites and alcohol marketing', *Drug and Alcohol Review*, 29(5): 525–30.

Halfpenny, P. and Proctor, R. (2015) *Innovations in digital research methods*, London: Sage Publications.

Hamer, M., Stamatakis, E. and Mishra, G.D. (2010) 'Television and screen-based activity and mental wellbeing in adults', *American Journal of Preventative Medicine*, 38(4): 375–80.

Hardaker, C. (2010) 'Trolling in asynchronous computer mediated communications: from user discussions to academic definitions', *Journal of Politeness Research*, 6(2): 215–42.

Harwood, J., Dooley, J.J., Scott, A.J. and Joiner, R. (2014) 'Constantly connected: the effects of smart devices on mental health', *Computers in Human Behaviour*, 34: 267–72.

Hastings, G. and Sheron, N. (2013) 'Alcohol marketing: grooming the next generation', *British Medical Journal*, 346, f1227.

Healy, B., Levin, E., Perrin, K., Weatherall, M. and Beasley, R. (2010) 'Prolonged work and computer related seated immobility and risk of venous thromboembolism', *Journal of the Royal Society of Medicine*, 103: 447–64.

Huang, C. (2010) 'Internet use and psychological well-being: a meta-analysis', *Cyberpsychology, Behaviour and Social Networking*, 13(3): 241–9.

Jenkins, H. (2006) *Convergence culture: Where old and new media collide*, New York, NY: New York University Press.

Kaplan, A.M. and Haenlein, M. (2010) 'Users of the world, unite! The challenges and opportunities of social media', *Business Horizons*, 53(1): 59–68.

Kelly, B., Vandevijvere, S., Freeman, B. and Jenkins, G. (2015) 'New media but same old tricks: food marketing to children in the digital age', *Current Obesity Reports*, 4(1): 37–45.

Kende, M. (2015) *Internet society: Global Internet Report 2015*, Geneva: Internet Society.

Kletteke, B., Hallford, D.J. and Mellor, D.J. (2014) 'Sexting prevalence and correlates: a systematic literature review', *Clinical Psychology Review*, 34(1): 44–53.

Linkletter, M., Gordon, K. and Dooley, J. (2010) 'The choking game and YouTube: a dangerous combination', *Clinical Pediatrics*, 49(3): 274–9.

Lyons, A., McCreanor, T., Hutton, F., Goodwin, I., Barnes, H.M., Griffin, C., Kerryellen, V., O'Carroll, A.D., Niland, P. and Samu, L. (2014) *Flaunting it on Facebook: Young adults, drinking cultures and the cult of celebrity*, Wellington: Massey University School of Psychology.

Mart, S., Mergendoller, J. and Simon, M. (2009) 'Alcohol promotion on Facebook', *The Journal of Global Drug Policy and Practice*, 3(18): 1–8.

Miller, J., Prichard, I., Hutchinson, A. and Wilson, C. (2014) 'The relationship between exposure to alcohol-related content on Facebook and predictors of alcohol consumption among female emerging adults', *Cyberpsychology, Behavior and Social Networking*, 17(2): 735–41.

Moraes, C., Michaelidou, N. and Meneses, R.W. (2014) 'The use of Facebook to promote drinking among young people', *Journal of Marketing Management*, 30(13/14): 1377–401.

Moreno, M.A. and Whitehill, J.M. (2013) 'Influence of social media on consumption in adolescents and young adults', *Alcohol Research: Current Reviews*, 36(1): 91–100.

Moreno, M.A., Parks, M. and Richardson, L.P. (2007) 'What are adolescents showing the world about their health risk behaviours on MySpace?', *Medscape General Medicine*, 9(4): 9–15.

Moreno, M.A., Briner, L.R., Williams, A., Brockman, L., Walker, L. and Christakis, D.A. (2010). A content analysis of displayed alcohol references on a social networking website, *Journal of Adolescent Health*, 47(2), 168-175.

Morgan, L. and Dent, M. (2010) *The economic burden of obesity*, Oxford: National Obesity Observatory.

Nicholls, J. (2012) 'Everyday, everywhere: alcohol marketing and social media – current trends', *Alcohol and Alcoholism*, 47(4): 486–93.

Norman, J., Grace, S. and Lloyd, C. (2014) 'Legal high groups on the Internet: the creation of new organised deviant groups?', *Drugs: Education, Prevention and Policy,* 21(1): 14–23.

OFCOM (Office of Communications) (2015a) *Adults' media use and attitudes report, 2015,* London: OFCOM.

OFCOM (2015b) *Children and parents: Media use and attitudes report, 2015,* London: OFCOM.

OFCOM (2015c) *The communications market 2015,* London: OFCOM.

Office for National Statistics (2015) *Statistical bulletin: Internet users, 2015,* London: Office for National Statistics.

Oreskovic, A. (2015) 'Here's another area where Twitter appears to have stalled: tweets per day', *Business Insider UK.* Available at: http://uk.businessinsider.com/twitter-tweets-per-day-appears-to-have-stalled-2015-6?r=US&IR=T

O'Rorke, K. (2006) 'Social learning theory and mass communication', *ABEBA Journal,* 25(2): 72–4.

Petry, N.M. and O'Brien, C.P. (2013) 'Internet gaming disorder and the DSM-5', *Addiction,* 108: 1186–7.

Primack, B.A., Colditz, J.B., Pang, K.C. and Jackson, K.M. (2015) 'Portrayal of alcohol intoxication on YouTube', *Alcoholism: Clinical and Experimental Research,* 39(3): 496–503.

Public Health England (2014) *Alcohol treatment in England, 2013–2014,* London: Public Health England.

Purves, R.I, Stead, M. and Eadie, D. (2014) *What are you meant to do when you see it everywhere? Young people, alcohol packaging and digital media,* London: Alcohol Research UK.

Richards, D., Caldwell, P.H.Y. and Go, H. (2015) 'Impact of social media on the health of children and young people', *Journal of Paediatrics and Child Health,* 51: 1152–7.

Ridout, B., Campbell, A. and Ellis, L. (2012) "'Off your Face(book)": alcohol in online social identity construction and its relation to problem drinking in university students', *Drug and Alcohol Review,* 31(1): 20–6.

Rosen, L.D., Whaling, K., Rab, S., Carrier, L.M. and Cheever, N.A. (2013) 'Is Facebook creating "iDisorders"? The link between clinical symptoms of psychiatrics disorders and technology use, attitudes and anxiety', *Computers in Human Behaviour,* 29: 1243–54.

Ruggiero, T. (2000) 'Uses and gratifications theory in the 21st century', *Mass Communications & Society,* 3(1): 3–73.

Statistics Brain (2015a) 'YouTube statistics', *Statistics Brain.* Available at: http://www.statisticbrain.com/youtube-statistics/

Statistics Brain (2015b) 'Snapchat company statistics', *Statistics Brain*. Available at: http://www.statisticbrain.com/snapchat-company-statistics/

Stenovec, T. (2015) 'Facebook is now bigger than the largest country on Earth', *Huffington Post*. Available at: http://www.huffingtonpost.com/2015/01/28/facebook-biggest-country_n_6565428.html

Stoddard, S.A., Bauermeister, J.E., Gordon-Messer, D., Johns, M. and Zimmerman, M.A. (2012) 'Permissive norms and young adults' alcohol and marijuana use: the role of online communities', *Journal of Studies on Alcohol and Drugs*, 73(6): 968–75.

Thompson, C.M. and Romo, L.K. (2016) 'College students' drinking and posting about alcohol: forwarding a model of motivation, behaviors, and consequences', *Journal of Health Communication*, 21(6): 688–95.

Tiggemann, M. and Slater, A. (2013) 'NetGirls: the Internet, Facebook and body image concern in adolescents girls', *International Journal of Eating Disorders*, 46(6): 630–3.

Townsend, N., Wickramasinghe, K., Williams, J., Bhatnager, P. and Rayner, M. (2015) *Physical activity statistics 2015*, London: British Heart Foundation.

Tremblay, M.S., LeBlanc, A., Kho, M.E., Saunders, T.J., Larouche, R., Colley, R.C., Goldfield, G. and Grober, S.C. (2011) 'Systematic review of sedentary behaviour and health indicators in school-aged children and youth', *International Journal of Behavioural Nutrition and Physical Activity*, 8(98): 1–22.

Vandelanotte, C., Sugiyama, T., Gardiner, P. and Owen, N. (2009) 'Association of leisure-time Internet and computer use with overweight and obesity, physical activity and sedentary behaviours: cross-sectional study', *Journal of Medical Internet Research*, 11(3): e28.

Van Hoof, J.J., Bekkers, J. and Van Vuuren, M. (2014) '"Son, you're smoking on Facebook!" College students' disclosure on social networking sites as indicators of real-life risk behaviours', *Computers in Human Behaviour*, 34: 249–57.

Weaver, E.R., Horyniak, D.R., Jenkinson, R., Dietze, P. and Lim, M.S.C. (2013) '"Let's get wasted" and other apps: characteristics, acceptability and use of alcohol-related smartphone application', *JMIR MHealth and UHealth*, 1(1): e9.

Weaver, E.R.N., Wright, C.J.C. and Dietze, P.M. (2016) '"A drink that makes you feel happier, relaxed and loving": Young people's perceptions of alcohol advertising on Facebook', *Alcohol and Alcoholism*, 51(4), 481–86.

Westgate, E.C., Neighbors, C., Heppner, H., Jahn, S. and Lindgren, K.P. (2014) '"I will take a shot for every 'like' I get on this status": posting alcohol-related Facebook content is linked to drinking outcomes', *Journal of Studies on Alcohol and Drugs*, 75(3): 390–8.

Widyanto, L. and Griffiths, M. (2006) 'Internet addiction: a critical review', *International Journal of Mental Health Addiction*, 4(1): 31–51.

Winpenny, E.M., Marteau, T.M. and Nolte, E. (2013) 'Exposure of children and adolescents to alcohol marketing and social media websites', *Alcohol and Alcoholism*, 49(2): 154–9.

Wombacher, K., Reno, J.E. and Veil, S.R. (2016) 'NekNominate: social norms, social media and binge drinking', *Health Communication*. Available at: http://www.tandfonline.com/doi/full/10.1080/10410 236.2016.1146567

World Health Organization (2014) *Global status report on alcohol and health 2014*, Geneva: World Health Organization.

Young, K.S. (2004) 'Internet addiction: a new clinical phenomenon and its consequences', *American Behaviour Scientist*, 48(4): 402–15.

Young, K.S., Pistner, M., O'Mara, J. and Buchanan, J. (2000) 'Cyber-disorders: the mental health concern for the new millennium', *Cyberpsychology and Behaviour*, 3(5): 475–9.

Part Three
Social and community networks

At this time of austerity, economic planning and significant reductions in funding for local authorities, the need to promote volunteering and support an inclusive society are central to a healthy and flourishing community. Volunteers contribute to the promotion of *social capital* and are mostly associated with third sector and faith-based organisations. They not only fill in the gaps in services provided by statutory agencies, but also support vulnerable people and help in transforming people and communities through relationship building, contributing to the health and well-being of others as well as themselves. This is an important community response to the problematic lifestyle issues noted in Part Two. Support for people with learning disabilities is good example of where community organisation and 'circles of support' provide physical and emotional support to an underfunded group of vulnerable people at risk of social exclusion. The development of both statutory and third sector programmes of support should be aimed at the real, identified needs of the target group. The last two chapters in this part provide introductions to 'realist' research into 'what works, for whom, where and when'.

NINE

Building an inclusive community through social capital: the role of volunteering in reaching those on the edge of community

Claire Bonham

This chapter focuses specifically on one group of people who are bringing those on the edge of community into their social networks – volunteers. It will use the lens of social capital to look specifically at how volunteering can build inclusive communities. A recent NFP Synergy publication notes that 'volunteering, at its core, remains transformational. It transforms both the giver and the receiver' (Saxton et al, 2015: 3). It is this contention that volunteering has a transformational effect on both the individuals involved (volunteers and beneficiaries) and society as a whole that this chapter explores.

Social capital is a multifaceted concept, and is a useful way of thinking about civil society: the space between government institutions and the market. Broadly speaking, social capital starts from the viewpoint that relationships matter: social networks are a way of creating cohesive communities that have shared norms and values, and facilitating cooperation within and between groups. Social science research has tended to favour either the civic tradition (Putnam, 2000) or the instrumental tradition (Bourdieu, 1983; Coleman, 1994) when speaking about changes and trends in society. These different approaches can best be described as: a *civic good*, how our social interactions build trust and reciprocity in the community; or an *instrumental good*, which brings individual-level goods such as improved health, access to jobs and so on through social interactions.

These two ways of understanding social capital are often set in opposition to each other, but this chapter will argue that it is possible to see a correlation between both a civic and an instrumental measure of social capital as civic engagements can directly produce instrumental capital when channelled in the right way, thus building *both* a *public good* (civic tradition) and a *private good* (instrumental tradition). It will argue that both can build communities and enhance existing levels of social capital by bringing those on the edge of our communities into the social networks enjoyed by those who already have strong community ties.

This will be illustrated through looking at volunteer-involving community programmes run by the Salvation Army in the UK that demonstrate the transformative power of volunteering in building social capital. This chapter will only be able to offer a broad-brush overview of the impact of volunteer-involving programmes on building social capital, and data on volunteer-involving programmes are mainly based on the author's observations and conversations with volunteers. This is clearly limited in scope, so the chapter concludes with recommendations for further research.

The emergence of volunteering research

Volunteering has been of interest to policymakers for a long time and charities, civil society and communities rely on volunteers in order to function effectively. The 2010 Coalition government prioritised strengthening civil society through encouraging social action, devolving power to local communities and opening up public services to numerous providers, including the voluntary sector.[1] There has been a significant rise of volunteer-involving initiatives that provide vital services for those on the edge of community through organisations working to offset the impact of cuts to housing, welfare and other public services, with a huge increase in services such as food banks (Curtis, 2013).

Volunteering is also a growing area of interest for social scientists but there are few studies into how volunteering can build social capital. Alongside social science research into areas such as well-being (see Centre for Wellbeing and elsewhere in this book [Chapter Eleven]), there is increasing academic research, policy and government interest around the benefits of volunteering (Davis Smith, 2007). Studies are mostly input-based and use evidence such as the number of hours people are volunteering and the frequency of volunteering to measure the market value of volunteering to a particular society (Brown, 1999; Putnam, 2000; Li et al, 2003; Mayer, 2003; Foster, 2013; Fujiwara et al, 2013; Haldene, 2014). However, research into what those volunteers are doing and, more importantly, how the act of volunteering can create change in communities is limited. Thus, it seems timely to explore how volunteering can transform our communities and increase social capital.

What is social capital?

The concept of social capital originates from the early 20th century, but in the last 30 years, it has gained momentum within the social sciences by those interested in the way that strong networks of people and neighbourhoods can aid the development of a community or civil society. It is, in essence, the *productive* value of social connections, where the notion of production is not simply about the production of goods and services, but also about the production of well-being in terms of both public and private goods.

Bourdieu has taken an instrumental approach to social capital, using a Marxist analysis of capital as an economic resource to explain how power and resources are maintained in an unequal society. For Bourdieu, social capital is 'the aggregate of the actual or potential resources which are linked to possession of a durable network of more or less institutionalized relationships of mutual acquaintance and recognition' (Bourdieu, 1983: 249). In other words, social capital is about a person's access to resources through their social networks – it is not what you know, but who you know – and about how you can use the social network you have in order to leverage more resources to improve your economic situation. Bourdieu argued that this leads to a centralising of unequal access to power and resources by the social, economic and cultural elite.

Sociologist Coleman (1994) also sees social capital as a resource for individuals, and believes it is defined by its function. He argues that some social institutions are more suited to producing social capital than others – through processes such as trustworthiness, reciprocity and information channels – and that social capital is not 'owned' by anyone, but exists within social relationships and networks. Social capital is not just class-based, but can cut across different types of institutions, for example, families, religious groups and community groups.

Both Bourdieu and Coleman focus on social capital as a private good, where networks of people, mutual trust and reciprocity are good things, but they are framed in terms of enhancing one's personal advancement or good. Robert Putnam, on the other hand, focused his work on the public good, and it is his work on social capital that has most resonance with the work of social scientists looking to understand how communities work together (Putnam, 2000).

Putnam started from a political science perspective in wanting to understand the quality of civic engagement in a democratic society. He suggested that social networks are made up of both horizontal elements, or people with equivalent power or status, and *vertical* elements, or networks that contain people of different status that produce power relations and hierarchies of dependence (Scrivens, 2013: 14). Norms of trust and reciprocity are key to developing a strong sense of civic engagement, and active participation in local community associations, for example, churches, neighbourhood associations and sports clubs, foster these relations. For Putnam (2000: 19):

> social capital refers to connections among individuals – social networks and the norms of reciprocity and trustworthiness that arise from them ...'social capital' calls attention to the fact that civic virtue is most powerful when embedded in a sense network of reciprocal social relations. A society of many virtuous but isolated individuals is not necessarily rich in social capital.

Bonding, bridging and linking social capital

Within the concept of social capital, Putnam makes a distinction between *bonding* and *bridging* social capital. Bonding social capital can be characterised as exclusive, or networks that are inward-looking and tend to reinforce exclusive identities and homogenous groups. Examples of bonding capital would be 'old-boys' networks', country clubs or support groups for a particular ethnicity or group of people, for example, disabled people or single parents. Bridging capital, on the other hand, is inclusive or outward looking, and seeks to build social networks across different social strata, e.g. the civil rights movement or ecumenical religious organisations (Putnam, 2000: 22).

Neither bonding nor bridging forms of social capital are wholly positive or negative; rather, they have different functions. Instead of either/or categories to which all social networks can be assigned, these different types of social capital form a continuum along a 'more–less' axis, and can change over time. This is context-specific as we all have multiple identities at the same time, for example, as a wife, daughter, part of an ethnic group, supporter of a particular football team and so on; thus, relationships can be both bonding and bridging.

Woolcock (2001: 13–14) identified another form of social capital: *linking* capital. This emphasises social networks that reach out to people who would not otherwise come into contact with each other, including those who are outside our existing communities, enabling them to leverage a wider set of resources than are available within their community. It is this idea of people who are often excluded from our communities coming together in the same social space that will be demonstrated by the Salvation Army community programm outlined in the following.

Building social capital: Salvation Army community programmes

There are gaps in the existing literature on social capital to explain how volunteer-involving interventions that reach out to those on the edge of community can *change the nature of these social networks and relationships* – either in quality of relationships or quantity of members of a particular social network. This section turns attention to specific examples of how social capital is increased in both a civic and instrumental capacity through volunteering.

The Salvation Army has developed high levels of trust or social capital locally in many situations; the first benefit of this is that it attracts a diverse range of volunteers to assist with its programmes. Whatever social strata volunteers come from, they are generally civic-minded citizens interested in improving their communities and have seen the work of the Salvation Army in other contexts, that is to say, they choose to volunteer because of the social capital that the Salvation Army has built in their existing social networks. One volunteer, Mike, explained why he chose to volunteer with the Salvation Army in the local charity shop:

> "I did thirty years as a fire-fighter ... and when you get those big jobs, the Salvation Army canteen van turns up. They were always there, and I just decided that one day when I retire I was going to come to the Salvation Army and give something back." (Interview, 25 February 2016)

Neil, a volunteer with the Salvation Army community programme in Croydon, had a career in finance before volunteering as a befriender. He said: "*I have always admired the work the Salvation Army does in the community so I thought if I could contribute to the work at the Croydon Corps in any small way, it would be something very worthwhile*" (interview, 26 February 2016). At the heart of these communities, the social capital in terms of trust and reciprocity is high for the Salvation Army; therefore, when people want to volunteer or do something positive to build their community's social capital, the Salvation Army is often the first port of call. This demonstrates bridging social capital, or, to put it another way:

ـ

·ing has a powerful role in creating and sustaining
·apital, precisely because it is one of the few ways
ow people from other backgrounds and other
·d to do so outside of the monetary economy.
., 2015: 83)

ـ ɔalvation Army is a church first and foremost, and Putnam (2000: 22) notes that 'churchgoers are substantially more likely to be involved in … organisations, to vote and participate politically in other ways, and to have deeper informal social connections'.[1] Thus, both volunteers who have chosen the Salvation Army and those who give their time because they see it as part of their Christian service are highly motivated and come from a variety of social networks – many of whom would not necessarily come into contact regularly – but who are all committed to building the social capital of their local community.

However, the real sense of *linking* social capital comes when these volunteers interact with clients of the Salvation Army's community programmes. Volunteers work with a huge variety of people at the edge of community – from those experiencing homelessness or battling addictions to those with physical and learning disabilities, and from older people who are socially isolated to the long-term unemployed. Volunteers are uniquely placed to build relationships with clients as they are not in a position of authority and are not paid to work with people, but come alongside individuals out of a sense of unconditional care. Furthermore, clients are often encouraged to become volunteers and are, therefore, able to build relationships across diverse sectors of the community. Evidence suggests that voluntary organisations that involve a more diverse membership, across different social groups, ethnicities and nationalities, produce significantly higher levels of trust than those generated within more homogeneous groups (Aldridge et al, 2002: 43).

The Salvation Army's local expressions have also built significant social capital by developing high levels of trust and reciprocity with those on the edge of the community. This gives a huge benefit when it comes to engaging those who are hardest to reach – the Salvation Army often gets people in through its doors where other agencies cannot. This should interest local government policymakers who find it difficult to encourage those on the edge of community to access statutory services if their social capital is low. For those with chaotic lives, who are often wary of police and staff of statutory agencies, attending an appointment at a certain time with caseworkers who are paid to be there rather than necessarily being interested in you (this is how it may feel to the recipient) can be daunting. However, allowing people to access these services at the Bridge Centre and Croydon Community Centre drop-ins demonstrates that the Salvation Army's social capital is allowing them to reach those at the edge of community, linking them to resources and equipping them with both skills and relationships that allow the individuals to build up their instrumental social capital.

The Bridge Centre – Blackpool

The Salvation Army Bridge Centre in Blackpool serves homeless and vulnerable people resident in the Blackpool area. The centre runs a daily programme of activities and services supporting clients experiencing financial, emotional or personal hardship, including those affected by homelessness, abuse, poor mental health and alcohol/ substance misuse. Volunteers work alongside staff to support clients at the project between the hours of 9am and 3pm at the centre, which is based within the Salvation Army Corps building. They run daily education programmes delivered by qualified tutors, for which clients have to enrol. The subjects offered are designed to improve clients' life skills, social interaction, personal growth and aspirations; topics include budgeting, healthy eating, computer skills and first aid. Some of these courses are accredited, and a free breakfast and lunch is provided to all attendees as an incentive. The Bridge is then open in the afternoons as a drop-in centre for anyone who needs help, the majority of whom are socially excluded in some way. In 2014, they had 7,815 service users attend their drop-in (Blackpool Citadel, 2016).

Due to the high levels of trust and reciprocity that the Salvation Army has built up in the area, the Bridge Project is able to reach those on the edge of the community who are often not reached by mainstream services, such as the National Health Service (NHS), Job Centre and so on. As noted earlier, social capital can work vertically as well as horizontally; in this instance, it can link individuals on the margins in a hierarchical network with other individuals, organisations or institutions with greater available resources. The team at the Bridge work with a range of local authority and statutory service providers to build up a portfolio of services for their clients, including NHS nurses, the Housing Options Team from Blackpool Council, Horizons (Addiction Dependency Services) and a partnership with Lancashire Police to reduce street drinking. Volunteers at the Bridge Centre also offer help with benefits – offering computers to access the forms and support in completing them.

Croydon Community Centre

The Salvation Army Citadel in Croydon runs a community programme that works with different groups on the edge of community through a series of drop-in centres. On a Monday, they run a drop-in for the homeless, regularly receiving over 50 clients per day. On Tuesdays and Thursdays, they run games and craft clubs in the morning, a lunch club, followed by a social activity, for example, indoor bowls, quizzes and karaoke, aimed at both people with learning disabilities and elderly people suffering from social isolation. Initially, the morning activities were aimed at people with learning disabilities and the afternoon session was aimed at older people, with both being able to attend the lunch club. However, in an interesting example of linking social capital, the team discovered that the different groups enjoyed spending time together and all the sessions are now open to both, thereby enabling them to come into contact with people outside their usual social networks. The Croydon community programme is supported by over 30 volunteers from a wide range of backgrounds, including one volunteer who has Down's syndrome and has previously been a service user there. She now volunteers in the kitchen several days a week, and her experience has resulted in her also volunteering in a Croydon charity shop.

On a Monday, there is a wide range of statutory agencies that attend the homeless drop-in centre, again demonstrating the power of social capital in brokering relationships between those on the edge of the community and statutory and community-based organisations. As of March 2016, those agencies include: Crisis, the local NHS health centre, the Job Centre, Turning Point (drug and alcohol service) and Thames Reach (a London-wide homelessness charity).

Building instrumental social capital

So, how does this help individuals build their instrumental social capital? There are several ways in which this can be measured, and there are three ways in particular that are helpful in this context: (1) educational and skills attainment, leading to higher levels of aspiration; (2) lower levels of negative behaviour; and (3) better health and well-being through reducing isolation and depression.

By building people's education and skills, both through formal programmes leading to a qualification and through 'life skills' courses at the Bridge, for example, budgeting and computer skills, individuals are in a better position to access social networks that may otherwise be unavailable. Most importantly, though, those who are able to gain these qualifications or skills are coming into contact with tutors and volunteers delivering this training, thus building their social network to include people in a different socio-economic group who may be able to link them with employment opportunities and encourage them to adjust their aspirations. Larger and more diverse networks will allow clients to access a diversity of learning experiences and broaden their horizons of what they may be able to achieve. In the longer term, this may well lead to increased opportunities for finding employment as the social relationships that make up an individual's social capital can be highly cost-effective mechanisms for facilitating this. The type of social capital identified earlier as bridging capital is particularly important here as studies have demonstrated that more unemployed people find employment through friends and personal contacts than through any other single route (6, 1997; Petersen et al, 2000).

Second, by being involved in projects such as the Bridge, clients can be exposed to different norms and values that do not reinforce negative or destructive behaviours. If you are able to increase your social network to include people who have a different set of accepted norms and behaviours, this can lead to the production of different norms, values and standards of behaviour. For example, at the Croydon Community Centre drop-in on Mondays, over 100 people were coming each week, and the team noticed certain behavioural issues. By asking clients to sign up to a charter and pay £1 a day to access the service, they have seen attendance drop to a more manageable number and a marked improvement in behaviour. This is because clients have now invested in a transactional relationship with the services and know that they are expected to behave in a certain way, and that if they do not honour their agreement, then they will not be allowed to stay in the centre.

Third, building social capital can improve health by reducing social isolation and loneliness. Social isolation is likely to disproportionately affect those who are already disadvantaged in some way – people who are unemployed or on low incomes, the elderly, and those with physical or mental disabilities. Research has shown that wider social relationships, and the society around people, may have an effect on health through their impact on: individuals' perceptions of their social status; stress; the strength of social affiliations (weaker social affiliations are associated with poorer health); 'daily hassles'; and more general feelings of safety and fear (Wilkinson, 2002).

Improved confidence and feeling that they may have something of worth to contribute to their community often leads to clients wanting to 'give something back' and use their newly increased social capital to benefit society. In this author's observation of many Salvation Army community programmes, one common theme emerges, and that is the number of ex-clients who now volunteer for the community programmes from which they have benefited. One volunteer in a Salvation Army charity shop explained: *"because I've been helped with being homeless I wanted to give something back for what I've been given"* (interview, 25 February 2016). At the Bridge Centre in Blackpool, they have six volunteers who were previously clients, all who have taken at least a six-month break before volunteering in order to ensure that they will be able to work with clients without putting anyone at risk. For many, this will be a key point on their way to employment as volunteering gives them experience of a regular commitment, responsibilities and accepted behaviours. Subjective well-being and mental health (eg increased confidence in relationships and developing personal skills) can be seen as benefits from volunteering (Scrivens, 2013: 32).

When those on the edge of community volunteer, it both provides the volunteer with instrumental capital in terms of the social networks and resources that they can now leverage, and also raises the social capital of our communities by producing elevated levels of trust and civic engagement that extend beyond the direct value of work carried out by volunteers. These have been described as being 'multiplier effects' of volunteering on social capital (Mayer, 2003: 4). The Community Life Survey found that the number of people in the least deprived areas that regularly volunteer was 36%, compared to 19% of those living in deprived areas (Cabinet Office, 2013). Recent research from Time Bank (2013) found that 'people classified as being at risk of social inclusion … were less likely to regularly participate in volunteering'. Therefore, enabling people who have previously used a service to then become volunteers builds both an individual's *instrumental* capital and the general *civic capital* of a local community.

Conclusion

This chapter has used social capital as a lens through which to view the work of volunteer-involving community programmes seeking to reach those on the edge of our communities. By looking at two Salvation Army expressions of community engagement, it has demonstrated that rather than viewing social capital as producing *either* a public good or private good, volunteer-involving initiatives show that it is possible that one can kind of social capital can *generate* another. It has also demonstrated that social capital does not have to lead to greater inequality as those with high levels of social relationships who volunteer are providing bridging and linking capital, and are therefore able to build deeper relational networks with people who would not otherwise come into contact. There is evidence to suggest that more diverse, heterogeneous groups have higher levels of trust and cohesion, and thus the work that volunteers do is capable of transforming society through building inclusive communities.

There is clearly a need for in-depth studies into the way in which volunteering develops instrumental capital, particularly when ex-clients then volunteer themselves. One way in which this could be measured is through the emerging focus on well-being, in particular, how volunteering can have a positive effect on a person's well-being, especially when one is going through difficult or chaotic life circumstances. There is some research that uses the Wellbeing Valuation to estimate the increase in well-being associated with goods or services, one of which is volunteering (Fujiwara et al, 2013; Kamerãde, 2015). It is not clear what the causes and effects of well-being are for people who volunteer – it is possible that those who choose to volunteer already have a greater sense of well-being, which means that they may benefit less than someone who has a lower sense of well-being (Dolan et al, 2011: 11).

In a time when health and social care is in crisis, will volunteering become increasingly politicised and seen as a solution to budget cuts? If so, will that detract from the 'added value' that volunteers provide in working to build social capital across their communities? It is clear that we are embarking on a new journey in delivering interventions that meet the needs of those on the edge of our communities, and that volunteering is one way in which we are able to draw communities together. In order to understand and develop the unrealised potential of volunteering in building both civic and instrumental social capital, we need to do far more than simply measure the numbers, time and contribution of our volunteers to the economy.

The 2016 vote to leave the European Union (EU), the 2016 US presidential election and the resurgence of nationalist parties across Europe suggest that our communities are becoming increasingly divided between those who feel connected to the opportunities of globalisation and those who feel left behind. This raises many questions about the future of our communities where many feel excluded. Will these divisions across different socio-economic groups affect the bridging capital that can be created through volunteering opportunities such as those discussed earlier? The examples of Salvation Army projects enhancing the social capital of both volunteers and recipients are being replicated by numerous charities, social enterprises and other initiatives across the country, and it is high time that their endeavours were the subject of detailed academic research. Now, more than ever, we should explore how social capital can be utilised to unite rather than divide.

Note

[1.] A recent nfpSynergy survey showed that regular worshippers are the most likely of all groups to volunteer –39% compared with 19% of non-worshippers (Saxton et al, 2015: 32).

References

6, P. (1997) *Escaping poverty: From safety nets to networks of opportunity*, London: Demos.

Aldridge, S., Halpern, D. and Fitzpatrick, S. (2002) 'Social capital: a discussion paper', Performance and Innovation Unit. Available at: http://www.thinklocalactpersonal.org.uk/_library/BCC/Social_Capital_PIU_Discussion_Paper.pdf

Blackpool Citadel (2016) 'Bridge project', The Salvation Army Blackpool Citadel Corps. Available at: http://www.blackpoolcitadel.co.uk/bridge-project.html (accessed 29 March 2016).

Bonner, A. and Luscombe, C. (2008) *The seeds of exclusion*, London: The Salvation Army.

Bourdieu, P. (1983) 'Forms of capital', in J.C. Richards (ed) *Handbook of theory and research for the sociology of education*, New York, NY: Greenwood Press.

Brown, E. (1999) 'Assessing the value of volunteer activity', *Nonprofit and Voluntary Sector Quarterly*, March: 3–17.

Cabinet Office (2013) *Giving of time and money: Findings from the 2012–13 Community Life Survey*, London: Cabinet Office.

Cabinet Office (2014) *Community Life Survey: England 2013–2014*, London: Cabinet Office.

Coleman, J.C. (1994) *Foundations of social theory*, Cambridge, MA: Harvard University Press.

Curtis, A. (2013) *Volunteering for stronger communities research project year one report: Summary and key findings*, London: Institute for Volunteer Research.

Davis Smith, J. (2007) 'Beyond social capital: what next for voluntary action research?', in J. Davis Smith and M. Locke (eds) *Volunteering and the test of time*, London: Institute for Volunteering Research, p 117.

Dolan, P., Layard, R. and Metcalfe, R. (2011) *Measuring subjective well-being for public policy*, London: Office for National Statistics.

Foster, R. (2013) *Household satellite accounts – valuing voluntary activity in the UK*, London: Office for National Statistics.

Fujiwara, D., Oroyemi, P. and McKinnon, E. (2013) *Wellbeing and civil society: Estimating the value of volunteering using subjective wellbeing data*, London: Department for Work and Pensions.

Haldene, A.G. (2014) *In giving, how much do we receive? The social value of volunteering*, Pro Bono Economics lecture to the Society of Business Economists, London: Bank of England.

Kamerãde, D. (2015) 'Volunteering, subjective wellbeing and mental health: what we know and what we don't know', State of Social Capital in Britain conference paper, Understanding Society.

Li, Y., Savage, M. and Pickles, A. (2003) 'Social capital and social exclusion in England and Wales (1972–1999)', *The British Journal of Sociology*, 54(4): 497–526.

Mayer, P. (2003) *The wider economic value of social capital and volunteering in South Australia*, Adelaide: Government of South Australia.

Petersen, T., Saporta, I. and Seidel, M. (2000) 'Offering a job: meritocracy and social networks', *American Journal of Sociology*, November: 763–816.

Putnam, R. (2000) *Bowling alone: The collapse and revival of the American community*, New York, NY: Simon & Schuster.

Saxton, J., Harrison, T. and Guild, M. (2015) *How volunteering turns donations of time and talent into human gold*, London: NFP Synergy.

Scrivens, K.S. (2013) 'Four interpretations of social capital: an agenda for measurement', OECD Statistics Working Papers. Available at: http://dx.doi.org/10.1787/5jzbcx010wmt-en

Time Bank (2013) 'Time Bank key facts'. Available at: http://timebank.org.uk/key-facts (accessed 28 March 2016).

Wilkinson, R. (2002) 'Liberty, fraternity, equality', *International Journal of Epidemiology*, January: 538–43.

Woolcock, M. (2001) 'The place of social capital in understanding social and economic outcomes', *Isuma: Canadian Journal of Policy Research*, 2(1): 1–17.

TEN

Support for people with learning disabilities: promoting an inclusive community

Barbara McIntosh

Introduction

One-and-a-half million people with learning disabilities (LDs) live in the UK. For 30 years, Britain has moved away from institutional care to small-scale domestic-size homes based on person-centred support that seeks the views of the person. For many people with LDs, there is a gap between UK policy and reality, made worse by recent cuts in public spending. Nevertheless, progress has been achieved and we have come a long way from the institutions so valued by the Victorians. New approaches are needed to address cuts in services, the increasing complexity of the needs of people and increasing levels of loneliness, bullying and hate crimes.

What is a learning disability?

There is no world consensus on the definition of the term 'learning disability', now generally preferred in the UK, replacing terms such as 'learning difficulty', 'mental handicap' and 'mental retardation,. Some countries use the term 'intellectual disability' (Emerson and Heslop, 2010: 1–4). The Department of Health (2001) describes LD as a significantly reduced ability to understand new or complex information and to learn new skills.

LDs occur when the brain's development is affected, either before birth, during birth or in childhood. Causal factors include:

- maternal illness during pregnancy;
- the inheritance of certain genes;
- genetic changes during pregnancy;

- difficulties at birth causing oxygen deprivation and brain damage; and
- illness, such as meningitis, or injury in early childhood.

There are thus many causes but often no identified cause.
Some conditions associated with LD include:

- Down's syndrome;
- Fragile X syndrome;
- Prader Willi Syndrome;
- cerebral palsy;
- autism;
- epilepsy; and
- Foetal Alcohol Syndrome.

How does a learning disability present?

The presence of an LD can be recognised at birth or in early childhood. An LD can be mild, moderate or severe. Some people with an LD can communicate easily and look after themselves but take longer to learn new skills, while others may not be able to communicate in a conventional way. People with LDs can grow up to be quite independent, but others need help with everyday tasks, such as getting dressed, and need support throughout life.

The diagnosis of profound and multiple learning disability (PMLD) is used when a person has more than one disability, with the most significant being an LD. People in this group may also have a sensory or physical disability, complex health needs, or mental health difficulties. People with PMLD need carers to help them with all aspects of life (Live Well, 2015a).

A brief history

Policies to protect and promote the rights of people with LDs have emerged in response to changes in social attitudes and political views, as well as to institutional/individual abuse situations. Starting with the Victorian asylums and the passing of the Mental Incapacity Act in 1913, thousands of people in the UK were deemed to be 'feeble-minded' or 'morally defective'. Many lived in large rural Victorian asylums, in wards with little privacy and with little or no contact with family. Men and women were separated to prevent pregnancies. The asylums were a Victorian phenomenon aiming to create a humane, safe environment away from crowded urban areas. In the long term, they did not achieve these aims. Victorian hospitals were influenced by the Eugenics movement, seeing the increase in the number of disabled people as a problem to society (Atherton, 2003). While some employment and support was available within asylums, many people reported mistreatment, inhumane care, no private space and a lack of education opportunities.

The Second World War and post-war period significantly altered views on the rights of people with LDs across Europe. In Germany, people with LDs did not conform to the concept of a master race in the eyes of the Nazis. The Holocaust Memorial Museum in New York estimates that despite public protests, about 200,000 disabled people were murdered between 1936 and 1945. The Nazis euthanasia programme saw the systematic killing of people who were deemed unworthy of life (Burleigh, 1994). Post-war legislation emerged in response to the deaths of thousands of people with LDs in Germany and Austria during the Second World War.

Despite this, it was 1970 before laws mandated the education of children with LDs (Open University, 2016). For most of the 20th century, people were segregated from the rest of society. The influence of Irving Goffman's (1961) book *Asylums* in the early 1960s, post-war reforms following the Holocaust, the Human Rights Act, widely publicised abuse within UK institutions and more informed compassionate views all led the hospitals to be closed. It took 45 years to achieve.

The promotion of people's rights as citizens and their right to an ordinary life has been and remains a core theme in the delivery of services. The Disability Discrimination Act 1995, 'Valuing people' (Department of Health, 2001), the 2007 United Nations Convention on the Rights of Persons with Disabilities and the Human Rights Act 1998 challenged discrimination and set out principles to promote the value of individuals. The rights to decent housing, employment, education, health care and access to individual budgets were addressed. These policies hold up the principles of an inclusive society, promoting equality and the importance of good-quality support. The closure of long-stay hospitals and large government institutions has now been achieved in the UK, with the exception of some treatment and assessment units. Britain's LD services are generally seen as progressive, providing good practice examples to other countries and having policy and legislative frameworks to promote community living. The challenge is how to preserve these improvements with severe pressure to cut costs and with local authorities reducing spending. The developing role of the Care Quality Commission (CQC) has contributed to improving standards and competence in services.

The decrease in involvement and leadership from the Department of Health has been partially in response to the recession of 2008, which reduced staffing at a national level to cover LDs. There has been a devolution of responsibility to local government and, in parallel, a severe reduction in funding due to significant reductions in the revenue budget from central government. One disadvantage is the variation in spending and quality from one area to another.

Challenges

Prevalence

In order to plan for the future and identify resources, it is important to know the numbers of people involved now and in the future. Of the 1.5 million people in the UK who have an LD, it is thought that up to 350,000 people have severe LDs. This figure is increasing but is an estimate (Emerson and Hatton, 2008). There is no accurate figure for the national prevalence of LDs in the UK.

Using information on the population of children with LDs in the UK, we can predict our future adult population. The latest information (from January 2006) indicates that of 8.2 million pupils, 171,740 (2.1%) had an identified primary special educational need (SEN) associated with a moderate LD, 30,440 (0.4%) had an identified primary SEN associated with a severe LD and 8,330 (0.1%) had an identified primary SEN associated with a PMLD. In total, 210,510 pupils (2.6%) were identified as having a primary SEN associated with LDs but the authors of this report point out that these statistics are also a significant underestimate of the true figures.

Emerson and Hatton looked at demographic factors that will influence the future size and composition of the English population (eg changes in birth rate, migration and mortality) and possible changes in the incidence and prevalence of LDs. From their previous work, they identify three factors likely to lead to an increase in the age-specific prevalence rates for adults with LD over the next two decades:

1. an increase in the proportion of younger English adults who belong to South Asian minority ethnic communities (where evidence suggests that there may be a two- to threefold increase in the prevalence of more severe learning LDs in children and young adults);

2. increased survival rates among young people with severe and complex disabilities; and
3. reduced mortality among older adults with LDs.

Health inequalities

People with LDS have poorer health than the general population. These health inequalities often start early in life. The inequalities are made worse by people having difficulties communicating and identifying their symptoms of poor health, which can lead to delayed treatment. There is wide variation in the service that people receive across the UK, and people can face difficulties in accessing timely, appropriate and effective health care. The impact of these health inequalities is serious. As well as having a poorer quality of life, people with LDs die at a younger age than their non-disabled peers (Live Well, 2015b).

The Confidential Inquiry into Premature Deaths of People with LDs (CIPOLD) found that, on average, men with LDs died 13 years younger than men in the general population and women 20 years younger. CIPOLD data also show that people with LDs are three times as likely as people in the general population to have a death classified as potentially avoidable through the provision of good-quality health care (Heslop et al, 2013). This suggests that if we improve the quality of health care, we can improve mortality outcomes.

Employment

Having a job gives us an identity, an income and status. People with LDs have consistently had low levels of employment but show an interest in being part of the labour force. Just over 60% ranked employment as a priority (McIntosh and Whittaker, 1998). Despite this, our national statistics are poor – 7.1% employed in the UK in 2012 (Emerson et al, 2012) compared to Canada, where 25% are employed (Canadian Association for Community Living, 2010). Rates of employment have fallen from 6.8% in 2013/14 to 6% in 2014/15, primarily due to the recession and the withdrawal of funds from supported employment initiatives (BASE, no date).

The Organisation for Economic Co-operation and Development (OECD) report 'Transforming disability into ability' (OECD, 2003: 11–12) notes that despite member countries being wealthy, none stand out as having very successful initiatives to promote the employment of disabled people. The report recommends that disability should not be allied with the assumption of inability to work. A mutual commitment from employers and the disabled person is needed to integrate the disabled into the workforce.

Key principles to achieve higher levels of employment for people with LDs include:

- *Supported employment.* Supported employment offers a job coach or mentor with on-the-job support given to the disabled person. Denmark offers up to 20 hours per week of personal assistance, the highest in the OECD. This model can also help adapt the job to suit the person's strengths and abilities. Fellow employees can be offered enhanced rates of pay to support their disabled colleague.
- *Sheltered employment,* for example, Remploy, has existed for many years and provides settings where all employees are disabled. The model is valued by some but has less good outcomes in achieving the social inclusion of disabled people. Making the transition to regular employment is not achieved by many, with Norway achieving the highest rate of 30% moving to ordinary jobs.
- *Quotas* set by the government to urge employers to hire disabled people are used in France, Germany, Italy, Poland and Spain (OECD, 2003: 111–13).
- *Subsidised employment,* where employers receive government funding for each disabled employee, reducing over time, is well developed in Sweden, Denmark, France and Norway (OECD, 2003).
- *Removing financial disincentives to work* so that salaries are higher than welfare benefits.
- *Access to work* in the UK offers a job advisor for training and funds to help with employers' extra costs, for example, specialist equipment.

Funding for job coaches and mentors in the workplace is needed, and the Business Disability Forum can offer advice and support. The Foundation for People with Learning Disabilities 'In Business' project ran for six years. People with LDs were supported to set up their own businesses, building on their interests and talents. The project saw businesses including recycling, dog walking, baking services and furniture removal develop. The impact of having a job raises people's self-esteem, helps address depression and isolation, and gives people an income. Those in employment see it as improving the quality of their lives (Changing Days Programme, 1996).

Mental health

For people with LDs, the prevalence rate of a diagnosable mental health disorder is 36%, compared with 8% of those who do not have a disability. People with LDs are also 33 times more likely to be on the autistic spectrum and are much more likely than others to have emotional and conduct disorders (Mental Health Foundation, 2011).

Children and young people with LDs are much more likely than others to live in poverty, to have few friends and to have additional long-term health problems, such as epilepsy and sensory impairments. All these factors are associated with mental health problems:

- The prevalence of dementia is much higher among older adults with LDs compared to the general population (21.6% versus 5.7% aged 65+) (Cooper, 1997).
- People with Down's syndrome are at high risk of developing dementia, with an age of onset 30–40 years younger than the general population (Holland et al, 1998).
- Prevalence rates for schizophrenia in people with LDs are approximately three times greater than for the general population (3% versus 1%) (Doody et al, 1998).
- Reported prevalence rates for anxiety and depression among people with LDs vary widely but are generally reported to be at least as prevalent as the general population and higher among people with Down's syndrome (Collacott et al, 1998).
- Challenging behaviours (aggression, destruction, self-injury and others) are shown by 10–15% of people with LDs, with age-specific prevalence peaking between the ages of 20 and 49 (Emerson et al, 2012).

Much more attention is needed to help people manage their mental health problems, and diagnose people's mental health problems when they have little or no verbal communication.

Early intervention and prevention can be achieved by working with children who have developmental disorders. Paula Barrett of the University of Queensland works with the Pathway to Resilience Trust, which works to implement Fun Friends and Friends for Life. These programmes focus on preventing and treating anxiety and depression, as well as on suicide prevention (Barrett, 2010).

Improving decision-making by people with learning disabilities

The Mental Capacity Act 2005 is designed to protect and restore power to vulnerable people who lack capacity, and to help them take part as much as possible in decisions that affect them. It aims to promote and strengthen supported decision-making. There are five core principles to the Act:

- *Principle 1: A presumption of capacity* – every adult has the right to make his or her own decisions and must be assumed to have capacity to do so unless it is proven otherwise.
- *Principle 2: Individuals being supported to make their own decisions* – people must be given all appropriate help to make a decision before anyone concludes that they cannot make that decision.
- *Principle 3: Unwise decisions* – individuals must be able to make what might be seen as unwise decisions.
- *Principle 4: Best interests* – anything done for or on behalf of people who lack capacity must be in their best interests.
- *Principle 5: Less restrictive option* – anything done in the best interests of people who lack capacity should be the option that is least restrictive of their basic human rights.

The culture of co-production and joint decision-making in implementing the Act has proved popular with people who have LDs.

Housing

Residential care for people with LDs has reduced, with a move towards supported housing/supported living. The aim is to provide housing and support that gives people more autonomy, personal support and independence with their own tenancy. This approach allows access to better funding opportunities for local authorities. Supported housing allows people to use personal budgets, which give a more tailor-made package of support.

Many people need support to become a part of their community. Staff need the right supervision and training to help people build friendships and participate in community events. People with LDs report that being involved in decision-making about their life and feeling that they are part of their community are two factors that result in higher levels of happiness, lower levels of depression and greater self-esteem (Strong and Hall, 2011).

The model of support

Many positives were gained by a shift away from the medical model to a social care model with personalised support, focusing on people's abilities and helping people to make choices. Negotiating health care in the community requires staff to advocate for better health care and is dependent on community medical staff with knowledge about LDs and associated health problems. Support staff can find it difficult to cope with the complex health problems of those with an LD. General practitioners (GPs) may not have had experience of LDs and the quality of primary care can be inconsistent. GPs are now encouraged to offer people with LDs annual health-care checks in order to change to a preventive and early intervention approach.

The model of care for people who no longer live with their families is increasingly supported living, which can mean living alone or with a small number of people in ordinary housing. Support staff are recruited and support each person in their own home according to the level of need. This approach offers more freedom, autonomy and independence.

Abuse

People with LDs experience higher rates of abuse than non-disabled people. Hate crimes, bullying and other forms of mistreatment, including financial, emotional, physical and sexual abuse, are not uncommon and need cross-agency community approaches to tackle. People can feel vulnerable, leading them to remain indoors and feeling isolated from neighbours and community. In a study undertaken by Reiter et al (2007), most physical abuse was reported as occurring in the local neighbourhood and McCormack et al (2005) identified the most common location of abuse as being the family home, followed by day services and public places.

Recently, we have seen growing concerns regarding hate crimes experienced by people with LDs, with one study suggesting that almost nine out of every 10 people with LDs have been harassed or bullied, that two thirds are bullied at least once a month and that just under one third are bullied on a daily or weekly basis. In a more recent study (Gravell, 2012), 67 people with LDs were interviewed and the most frequent types of incidents reported were name-calling or verbal abuse (27%), attacks on property, uninvited entry, burglary or destroying possessions (23%), borrowing or stealing money or being made to buy things (20%), and physical abuse, threats or assaults (18%) (Looking into Abuse, 2013).

Awareness programmes run in schools have had a positive impact. By hearing about people's experiences and meeting people with LDs, pupils develop supportive, compassionate attitudes to those with LDs.

Winterbourne View and institutional abuse

Policies were already in place in 2012 when BBC Panorama reported on Winterbourne View, a private hospital in Bristol. Recommendations followed and policies, alongside greater public awareness, in-depth staff training and adherence to CQC guidelines, are all used to reduce abuse.

Financial constraint

Emerson and Hatton's (2008) analysis shows an increase in the population of people with complex needs over the next 15 years, helping us to plan and develop services, although new money for service development is scarce. The cost of implementing the National Living Wage for front-line support workers is challenging services to find funds. The setting of a National Living Wage is positive for staff who are on low wages but local authorities are struggling to find the funds.

The future

New approaches to care and support are needed. No one solution will meet all needs. Innovations might include harnessing the skills and talents of volunteers in the community, who could offer mentoring, advocacy and social relationships to people with LDs. Dutch approaches to disability include free housing offered to students who live alongside disabled people and offer several hours of support, access to community and friendship for people who may have been isolated due to their disability (Humanitas Tandem, 2011).

Circles of Support have been used by a number of people in the UK. Cuts in social care funding, the wish to have a more humane approach, frustration with the long wait times for services and a feeling that public services can be bureaucratic and impersonal have brought this approach to people's attention. These Circles of Support bring unpaid people together to work collectively to hear the views of the disabled person, achieve their goals and work on positive changes desired by the individual. It is a model driven by active citizenship and can include paid professionals.

Circles of Support are well suited to periods of change in a person's life, such as a young person wanting to leave home or move from college to an adult way of life. In this case, Circle of Support members listen to the person and work to help achieve the person's choices, such as a finding a place to live, finding the right support to maximise independence, getting a job, finding a friendship network or participating in local activities. If the disabled person does not communicate with conventional speech, effort is made to identify the person's 'yes' and 'no' signals or nonverbal signs of agreement or disagreement. The disabled person's preferences can be collected by people who know them well. Circles of Support promote a culture that focuses on the person's strengths, uniqueness and abilities rather than on the disability, and tap into the knowledge and enterprise of community members to help the disabled person thrive (Circles UK, no date).

Public monies cannot meet need just now and tapping into funds from private industries and companies, especially those with a social responsibility arm to their organisation, will add valued resources. The growth of the voluntary sector has been partially driven by the contracting out of local authority services. Voluntary organisations can tap into funding from other charities (such as the Big Lottery) that statutory services cannot access, and this has become an important stream of revenue.

Increasingly, technology is helping disabled people with their communication and independence. Several LD providers have invested in technology, introducing such things as fingerprint door entry, which provides security, freeing concerns about losing front door keys while allowing people to come and go independently without a support worker. Sleep pads that monitor a person's epilepsy during the night and alert staff when there is a problem can enable a person to live more independently but have staff on hand when needed (Young Epilepsy, 2012). The use of smart phones with apps such as Skype and Face Time can help in sustaining friendship, addressing isolation through contact with others and receiving medical information from health-care staff, which all contribute to improved quality of life. Using a mobile phone with a location-tracking device can increase freedom and security for the person with an LD.

Conclusion

Services for people with LDs will continue to move forward while facing debilitating funding cuts. New collaborations across organisations, harnessing the talents of ordinary citizens, shifting to prevention (particularly in mental health) and seeking funds from new sources will all be required to meet increasing need. Resources and funding should be offered according to the person's needs and not based on where they live. Finally, new generations of children and adults will need to be influenced by policies and education so that more inclusive and enabling attitudes are common and the marginalisation and mistreatment seen in the past is not repeated.

References

Atherton, H. (2003) 'Getting it right together', Unit 3 – A history of learning disabilities, University of Hull. Available at: www.lx.iriss. org.uk

Barrett, P. (2010) 'Friends for Life'. Available at: www.pathwayshrc. com.au

BASE (British Association of Supported Employment) (no date) 'Home/information for commissioners/key facts and data'. Available at: www.base-uk.org

Burleigh, M. (1994) *'Death and deliverance': Euthanasia in Germany 1900–1945*, Cambridge: Cambridge University Press.

Canadian Association for Community Living (2010) 'Position statement on employment', June. Available at: www.cacl.ca

Changing Days Programme (1996) (ed) Alison Wethheimer, King's Fund Publishing, 35–47.

Circles UK (no date) 'About Circles'. Available at: www.Circles-UK. org.uk

Collacott, R.A., Cooper, S.A., Branford, B. and McGrother, C. (1998) 'Behaviour phenotype for Down's syndrome', *The British Journal of Psychiatry*, 172(1) 85–9.

Cooper, S,A. (1997) 'Epidemiology of psychiatric disorders in elderly compared with younger adults with learning disabilities', *The British Journal of Psychiatry*, 170(4): 375–80.

Department of Health (2001) 'Valuing people: a new strategy for learning disability for the 21st century'. Available at: www.gov. uk/government/publications/valuing-people-a-new-strategy-for-Learning-Disability-for-the-21st-Century

Doody, G.A., Johnstone, E.C., Sanderson, T.L., Owens, D.G. and Muir, W.J. (1998) '"Pfropfschizophrenie" revisited. Schizophrenia in people with mild learning disability', *The British Journal of Psychiatry*, 173(2): 145–53.

Emerson, E. and Hatton, C. (2008) 'People with learning disabilities in England', Centre for Disability Research, Lancaster University, UK. Available at: www.lancaster.ac.uk

Emerson, E. and Heslop, P. (2010) 'A working definition of learning disabilities', Improving Health and Lives, Learning Disabilities Observatory. Available at: https://www.researchgate.net/publication/265306674_A_working_definition_of_Learning_Disabilities

Emerson, E., Hatton, C., Robertson, J., Baines, S., Christie, A. and Glover, G. (2012) 'People with learning disabilities in England 2012', Improving Health and Lives, Learning Disability Observatory. Available at: www.glh.org.uk/pdfs/PWDAR2011.pdf

Goffman, E. (1961) *Asylums: Essays on the social situation of mental patients and other inmates* (Vol 277) New York: Anchor Books, Random House.

Gravell, C. (2012) *Loneliness + cruelty. People with learning disabilities and their experience of harassment, abuse, and related crime in the community*, London: Lemos and Crane.

Heslop, P., Blair, P., Fleming, P., Hoghton, M., Marriott, A. and Russ, L. (2013) 'Confidential inquiry into premature deaths of people with learning disabilities' (CIPOLD), Final Report. Available at: http://www.bristol.ac.uk/cipold/fullfinalreport.pdf

Holland, A.J., Hon, J., Huppert, F.A., Stevens, F. and Watson, P. (1998) 'Population-based study of the prevalence and presentation of dementia in adults with Down's syndrome'. *The British Journal of Psychiatry*, 172(6): 493–8.

Humanitas Tandem (2011) 'A Netherlands befriending project'. Available at: www.mandbf.org

Live Well (2015a) 'What is a learning disability?', NHS Choices. Available at: www.nhs.uk

Live Well (2015b) '"Learning disabilities": annual health checks', NHS Choices. Available at: www.nhs.uk

Looking into Abuse (2013) 'Research by people with learning disabilities', University of Glamorgan, Rhondda Cynon Taff People First and New Pathways. Available at: http://udid.research.southwales.ac.uk/media/files/documents/2013-03-05/Final_report.pdf

McCormack, B., Kavanagh, D., Caffrey, S. and Power, A. (2005) 'Investigating sexual abuse: findings of a 15-year longitudinal study', *Journal of Applied Research into Intellectual Disabilities*, 18: 217–27.

McIntosh, B. and Whittaker, A. (eds) (1998) 'Days of change: a practical guide to developing day opportunities for people with learning difficulties', The Kings Fund.

Mental Capacity Act (2005) Section 1, Clauses 2–6. Available at: www.legislation.gov.uk/ukpga/2005

Mental Health Foundation (2011) 'People with learning disabilities in England 2011', https:www.mentalhealth.org.uk/learning-disabilities/help-information/learning-disability-statistics-/187699

OECD (Organisation for Economic Co-operation and Development) (2003) 'Transforming disability into ability: policies to promote work and income for disabled people', OECD.

Open University (2016) 'Timeline of learning disability history'. Available at: www.open.ac.uk

Reiter, S. Bryen, D. and Shachar, Y. (2007) 'Adolescents with intellectual disabilities as victims of crimes', *Journal of Intellectual Disability Research*, 11: 1–17.

Strong, S. and Hall, C. (20o1) 'Feeling Settled project: guide prepared for NDTI'. Available at: www.ndti.org.uk/.../Feeling_Settled_Final_Report_February_2011. pdf 26-31

Young Epilepsy (2012) 'Seizure bed alarms'. Available at: www.youngepilepsy.org.uk

ELEVEN

Community well-being programmes: reviewing 'what works'

Anne-Marie Bagnall

Introduction

This chapter will explore the challenges inherent in choosing the most appropriate methodologies to determine what works to improve the well-being of communities. Well-being is arguably a nebulous concept to define in the individual context, but when we think about the well-being of communities, additional concepts, such as the way a community functions, how that impacts on the well-being of individuals and what influences both of these outcomes, create interesting challenges for researchers. Contextual influences, such as housing, access to local services, social inclusion and local democratic processes, can be both part of the change being evaluated and the outcomes being assessed. Moreover, many community-led programmes, while potentially highly effective in their local context, have not been published or evaluated with the same techniques or rigour as professionally-led interventions.

This chapter will report on how the multidisciplinary What Works: Wellbeing Centre's[1] Communities Evidence Programme has decided to approach these challenges: from extensive consultation with a wide range of stakeholders to define the issues, to the development of a working Theory of Change, to innovative search strategies, leading to the inclusion and critique of evidence from many different traditions and contexts. The aim of the Centre is to produce findings that are relevant and useful to both local and national stakeholders.

What Works: Wellbeing Centre

The What Works: Wellbeing Centre is part of a network of What Works centres in the UK, which also include the National Institute for Health and Care Excellence (NICE), the Centre for Ageing Better and the Early Intervention Foundation. With initial funding from Public Health England and the Economic and Social Research Council, the What Works: Wellbeing Centre comprises four collaborative evidence programmes: Communities; Culture and Sport; Work and Learning; and a cross-cutting stream. The four evidence programmes are overseen by a central 'Hub', which manages and approves work delivery plans for each of the four programmes, and took the lead on developing a collaborative 'methods' guide for conducting systematic reviews for the Centre, with input from methodological experts from each of the four evidence programmes (Snape et al, 2016).

The What Works: Wellbeing Centre's Communities Evidence Programme is led by a consortium of 10 partners, both academic and non-academic. These are: the University of Liverpool, Leeds Beckett University, Sheffield University, Durham University, Happy City, Locality, the New Economics Foundation, Goldsmiths College (University of London), the Centre for Local Economic Strategies (CLES) and Social Life. Their work is overseen by an advisory board that includes academic and policy experts on epidemiology, health inequalities, town planning, local government and community policy. They also have access to a wider network of stakeholders from other academic, governmental and non-governmental (third sector) organisations, who have contributed knowledge by taking part in surveys and attending workshops in the first six-month phase of the Centre's development.

The initial three-year set-up period of the Centre comprised three phases: a six-month collaborative development phase, during which the topics to be researched were decided in consultation with stakeholders; a two-year evidence review phase, during which systematic reviews are being carried out on the topics of interest; and another six-month collaborative phase, where the findings of the systematic reviews will be 'road-tested' and given a reality check by further consultation with stakeholders who will be using the findings. At the end of this, a 'roadmap' will be prepared, which will present the findings from the systematic review in a way that is accessible to stakeholders and policymakers.

What is well-being?

The What Works: Wellbeing Centre uses the definition of well-being developed by the Office for National Statistics (2013):

Wellbeing, put simply, is about 'how we are doing' as individuals, communities and as a nation and how sustainable this is for the future. We define wellbeing as having 10 broad dimensions which have been shown to matter most to people in the UK as identified through a national debate. The dimensions are: the natural environment, personal well-being, our relationships, health, what we do, where we live, personal finance, the economy, education and skills and governance. Personal wellbeing is a particularly important dimension which we define as how satisfied we are with our lives, our sense that what we do in life is worthwhile, our day to day emotional experiences (happiness and anxiety) and our wider mental wellbeing. (https://whatworkswellbeing.org/about/what-is-wellbeing/)

As part of the collaborative development phase for the Communities Evidence Programme, an online survey of local government, voluntary and community sector stakeholders was carried out (Communities Evidence Programme, 2015). One of the aims of the survey was to develop a current working definition of 'well-being' and 'community well-being'.

In total, 317 people responded to the online survey from across the UK. The most popular definition of 'well-being' was: 'functioning well in life, for example having a strong sense of meaning and feeling connected to other people'. The most popular understanding of 'community well-being' was: 'strong networks of relationships and support between people in a community, both in close relationships and friendships, and between neighbours'. Another popular definition was: 'people feeling able to take action to improve things in, and influence decisions about, their community'.

What is community?

Community is perhaps a slightly less contested concept than well-being, but there are differences between communities of place and communities of interest. The What Works: Wellbeing Centre's Communities Evidence Programme is using the same definition as NICE (2016):

A community is a group of people who have common characteristics or interests. Communities can be defined by: geographical location, race, ethnicity, age, occupation, a shared interest or affinity (such as religion and faith) or other common bonds, such as health need or disadvantage.

What is community well-being?

Community well-being is more than just an aggregate of individuals' well-being within a defined population or geographic area. Pre-existing community conditions (including features of the environment, socio-economic factors, relationships with others and power and control) impact upon individual well-being, and individual well-being impacts upon community conditions, in ways that are likely to be complex and context-specific (Lee and Kim, 2015). Improving community and social capital has been linked to improved health outcomes (CSDH, 2008; Marmot et al, 2010) but socio-economic inequalities, in turn, affect the quality of community conditions and social relationships (Friedli, 2009), and the relationships between them are complex and not always obvious (Seaman and Edgar, 2015).

Three of the early outputs of the What Works: Wellbeing Centre's Communities Evidence Programme are a working Theory of Change on Building Community Well-being (South et al, 2017), which will be updated in the light of emerging findings from the systematic review programme, a scoping review of indicators of community well-being and related concepts (Bagnall et al, 2017), and a conceptual review of community-level phenomena that may influence community well-being (such as trust, sense of belonging and connection, and shared objectives) (Atkinson et al, 2017).

Early findings of the scoping review of indicators found many synonyms in use for community well-being (Bagnall et al, 2017). These included: social capital; local well-being; asset-based approaches; social outcomes; resilience; neighbourhood satisfaction; neighbourliness; community capital; community cohesion; national success; city liveability; and community prosperity. Therefore, the What Works: Wellbeing Centre's Communities Evidence Programme has initially taken a broad inclusive approach to the concept of community well-being.

What do we know about what works for community well-being?

A recent report from Public Health England and NHS England (2015) identified a 'family' of community-centred approaches to improve health and well-being, which can be grouped into four main themes:

- Strengthening communities: where approaches involve building on community capacities to take action on health and the social determinants of health.
- Collaborations and partnerships: where approaches involve communities and local services working together at any stage of the planning cycle, from identifying needs through to implementation and evaluation.
- Volunteer and peer approaches: where approaches focus on enhancing individuals' capabilities to provide advice, information and support, or to organise activities around health and well-being in their or other communities.
- Access to community resources: where approaches connect people to community resources, practical help, group activities and volunteering opportunities to meet health needs and increase social participation.

The report (Public Health England and NHS England, 2015), which was underpinned by a rapid scoping review of 128 relevant reviews (of which 32 were systematic reviews) (Bagnall et al, 2015a), found 'reasonably strong evidence on the positive impact of social participation, taking part in volunteering, and community engagement with a range of benefits reported including better physical and emotional health, increased wellbeing, self-confidence, self-esteem, and social relationships'.

One of the largest reviews included was a systematic review of the effectiveness of community engagement for improving health and reducing health inequalities, which included 315 studies (O'Mara-Eves et al, 2013). The conclusions of this review were that:

> Overall, community engagement interventions are effective in improving health behaviours, health consequences, participant self-efficacy and perceived social support for disadvantaged groups. There are some variations in the observed effectiveness, suggesting that community engagement in public health is more likely to require a 'fit for purpose' rather than 'one size fits all' approach. (O'Mara-Eves et al, 2013: 68, xvii)

The Public Health England and NHS England (2015) report identified evidence gaps, including a publication bias towards professionally led interventions, as many small, successful community-led interventions, have not undertaken formal evaluations and therefore not published reports either as 'grey literature' or in peer-reviewed academic journals. Equally, the dynamic nature of participatory methods and the long-term nature of the outcomes produced are not always reflected in published academic papers, as changes are often seen long after the formal evaluative stage of a project has ended. The report concluded that:

> At a collective level, confident and connected communities provide the social fabric that is necessary for people to flourish. An equitable health system involves people in determining the big questions about health and care and actively removes barriers to social inclusion. That is why individual and community empowerment have to be core to efforts to improve the population's health and reduce health inequalities. (Public Health England and NHS England, 2015: 36)

The recently updated NICE guidance on community engagement (NICE, 2016), underpinned by five systematic reviews (Brunton et al, 2014, 2015; Bagnall et al, 2015b; Harden et al, 2015; Stokes et al, 2015), a cost-effectiveness review (Optimity Advisors, 2015) and primary qualitative research (Bagnall et al, 2016), made the following recommendations:

- Ensure local communities, community and voluntary sector organisations, and statutory services *work together* to plan, design, develop, deliver and evaluate health and well-being initiatives.
- Recognise that building relationships, trust, commitment, leadership and capacity across local communities and statutory organisations needs *time*.
- Support and promote sustainable community engagement by encouraging local communities to get involved in *all stages* of a health and well-being initiative.
- Ensure decision-making groups include members of the local community who reflect the *diversity* of that community.
- *Feed back* the results of engagement to the local communities concerned, as well as other partners.
- *Support the development of collaborations and partnerships* to encourage local communities to take part in initiatives to improve their health and well-being, and to reduce health inequalities.
- Base collaborations and partnerships on local needs and priorities.

- Effective approaches are:
  - An asset-based approach – to build on the strengths and capabilities of local communities.
  - Community development – to give local communities at risk of poor health support to help identify their needs and tackle the root causes. This support comes from statutory organisations.
  - Community-based participatory research – to provide collaborations and partnerships with background knowledge and insights into the nature of the community that they are working with.
  - Area-based initiatives – to work with local communities to improve local health and education and to support urban regeneration and development to tackle social or economic disadvantage.
  - Co-production methods – to ensure statutory organisations and the community can participate on an equal basis to design and deliver health and well-being initiatives.
- Consider offering *training and mentoring support* to community members. Also consider providing formal recognition of their contribution and other opportunities for development. This could include, for example, accredited training.
- Address *health inequalities* by ensuring additional efforts are made to involve local communities at risk of poor health. This includes people who are vulnerable, marginalised, isolated or living in deprived areas.
- Work with local communities and community and voluntary organisations to identify barriers to involvement and decide which types of communication would get people interested and involved.
- Provide the support people need to get involved (NICE, 2016).

Implications of health and social inequalities for the evidence base

Types of studies

Traditionally, systematic reviews of effectiveness restrict inclusion to randomised controlled trials (RCTs) and clinical or so-called 'hard' outcomes. The recent systematic mapping review of current and emerging policy and practice in UK community engagement (Bagnall et al, 2015b) included 316 articles, of which 227 (72%) were research or evaluation studies. Only 15 (7%) of these were RCTs; most were mixed-methods evaluations or qualitative studies. The systematic review of effectiveness (Brunton et al, 2014), which was also conducted to underpin the NICE guidance on community engagement and was an update of the 2013 systematic review by O'Mara-Eves et al, included only 28 RCTs, 22 of which were from the US and most of which focused on individual behaviour change, such as healthy eating or physical activity. By contrast, the UK-based mapping review (Bagnall et al, 2015b) found that the health and well-being issues addressed most frequently by UK community engagement initiatives were community-level or well-being outcomes, specifically:

- social capital or social cohesion ($n = 129$; 41%);
- community well-being ($n = 110$; 35%), for example, community resilience (Cinderby et al, 2014) and empowerment (Hothi et al, 2007);
- personal well-being ($n = 82$; 26%), for example, positive mental health (Tunariu et al, 2011; IRISS, 2012) and quality of life (Nazroo and Matthews, 2012);
- general health – personal ($n = 99$; 31%), for example, weight management (Jennings et al, 2013) and healthy lifestyle promotion (Robinson et al, 2010); and
- general health – community ($n = 95$; 30%), for example, setting up group activities (Woodall et al, 2013) and reducing health inequalities (Race for Health, 2010).

Types of participants

It is well documented that people who consent to take part in RCTs are not wholly representative of the intended population sample. They tend to be predominantly male (as females of childbearing age are excluded from many RCTs) and middle-aged (Kennedy-Martin et al, 2015). RCTs require commitment from participants, who consent to undergo clinical or psychometric tests at both baseline and at least one follow-up point. If the informed consent process is carried out correctly, this would involve at least three attendances at the clinical setting. This almost automatically rules out certain groups of people, in addition to the groups already excluded by basic RCT requirements, such as: those who are homeless or insecurely housed; Gypsies, Romanies and Irish Travellers; refugees and asylum seekers; and people with mental health issues and/or substance use disorders that cause problems with memory and organisation. Many RCTs also require participants to be competent to consent, thus indirectly ruling out people with learning disabilities, severe mental health disorders and (often) those who do not speak the language of the host country. By contrast, the UK mapping review of community engagement practice (Bagnall et al, 2015b) found that community engagement initiatives in the UK actively seek to engage some of the most marginalised, disadvantaged or excluded population groups.

Publication bias

The noted tendency for evidence on professionally led interventions to be evaluated and published, while community-led interventions 'operate under the radar of formal evaluations' (Savage et al, 2010) presents challenges for systematic reviewers. Searching for 'grey' literature in the form of organisational reports may not be enough to identify the full range of community-led health and well-being initiatives taking place, and review teams are likely to have to go further than this in their searching efforts. The systematic mapping review of current and emerging UK policy and practice in community engagement (Bagnall et al, 2015b) set up a register of interest and put out a call for evidence to existing networks of contacts in local government, community and voluntary sector organisations to complement the NICE call for evidence that goes to registered stakeholders. The review team also searched websites of relevant organisations and carried out qualitative case studies in six projects, two of which had not published a formal evaluation report (Bagnall et al, 2016). In the mapping review, more than a quarter (26%) of included initiatives were found through website searches and the calls for evidence, rather than through traditional database and citation searching.

Well-being inequalities

The evidence base on well-being inequalities, compared to health inequalities, is relatively sparse but is expected to follow a similar pattern (Quick, 2015); as for health, interventions to improve overall well-being in a population may increase well-being inequalities if these are not an explicit focus. Research into differences in well-being between population groups has found that:

- Lower-income and/or education groups have lower average well-being than higher-income and education groups (Stoll et al, 2012; Eurofound, 2013; Helliwell et al, 2015).
- Studies from the UK and US have found that many minority ethnic groups have lower well-being than the rest of the population. This

holds even after controlling for other factors, such as income or education (Stevenson and Rao, 2014).

- Different age groups seem to have different levels of well-being, with the lowest life satisfaction occurring between about 35 and 50 years, and higher levels of well-being at younger and older ages.
- Men have higher well-being in some countries, and women in others, with some countries showing no difference at all (Quick, 2015).

When considering policies or interventions, rather than simply asking 'Does this policy improve well-being?', we should be asking 'Whose well-being will this policy improve?' (Quick, 2015).

Implications for systematic review methods

Considerations of equity should be explicit in every part of a systematic review protocol (Welch et al, 2015, Snape et al, 2016), including the search strategy and study selection criteria. Study designs should not be restricted to RCTs or even quantitative designs. For example, there is much to be learned from process evaluations (which are usually qualitative in design, though often attached to RCTs), which are particularly important when evaluating complex interventions (Moore et al, 2015). The NICE public health methods guide (NICE, 2012) acknowledged the role of non-randomised study designs in systematic reviews of public health interventions, and the What Works: Wellbeing Centre's methods guide takes this a step further by including qualitative study designs as sources of outcome data, as well as process data (Snape et al, 2016).

There are several 'good practice' guides to combining qualitative and quantitative evidence in systematic reviews (Gough et al, 2012; Thomas et al, 2004; Dixon-Woods et al, 2005); the most prevalent approach has been to synthesise the qualitative evidence to develop review questions or potential moderators or mediators of effect to test out in a meta-analysis of the 'hard' quantitative data (Thomas and Harden, 2008). This can be described as a 'sequential' approach to mixed-methods systematic reviews. However, there is also a less used 'convergent' approach that treats the qualitative data as outcome data (where appropriate), as well as process data, and so combines quantitative and qualitative data for the same outcome. An example of this approach can be seen in a systematic review of peer interventions in prison settings (South et al, 2014).

Our inclusive approach

Following the findings of a recent case-study report (Bagnall et al, 2016), which concluded that a key theme related to successful community engagement was respect for community members' expertise, and emerging evidence on the value of involving community members at every stage (NESTA, 2012; South and Phillips, 2014), our approach to reviewing the evidence aims to engage and involve the end-user as much as possible in collaborating and co-producing a relevant and useful set of findings on what works for community well-being.

In the collaborative development phase, this took the form of carrying out 10 three-hour workshops with 224 stakeholders across the UK, carrying out a short online survey (317 respondents) and conducting 11 in-depth interviews with key senior stakeholders from central government, local government and the third sector in order to understand the opportunities and barriers to using well-being evidence, as well as carrying out three community sounding board exercises to ensure that the opinions of stakeholders with a professional interest resonated with members of the public in community settings (Communities Evidence Programme, 2015).

Within the systematic reviews, the What Works: Wellbeing Centre's methods guide advocates taking a broad, inclusive approach to evidence, not restricted to RCTs or quantitative study designs unless appropriate, while still being rigorous about validity assessment of every included study design and outcome (Snape et al, 2016).

Based on the results of the collaborative development phase (Communities Evidence Programme, 2015), we are carrying out systematic reviews in the following broad topic areas: housing; co-production; boosting social relations; and five ways to well-being. We will first carry out rapid scoping reviews to determine what is already known and where the evidence gaps lie within these topic areas, and then, following brief consultation with community stakeholders, undertake full systematic reviews of more focused questions within each of these broad topic areas. Both quantitative and qualitative study designs will be eligible for inclusion, depending on what is most appropriate for the review question.

Conclusion

In conclusion, finding out what works to improve community well-being must involve making every effort to include those who are excluded from society and from traditional research, and making their voice heard within the evidence base, with the aim of reducing inequalities in well-being, as well as improving overall community well-being.

Note
1. See: https://whatworkswellbeing.org/

References
Atkinson, S.J., Bagnall, A., Corcoran, R. and South, J. (2017) *Conceptual review of community wellbeing*, London: What Works Centre for Wellbeing.

Bagnall, A.M., Southby, K., Mitchell, B. and South, J. (2015a) 'Bibliography and map of community-centred interventions for health and wellbeing', Centre for Health Promotion Research, Leeds Beckett University, Leeds.

Bagnall, A., South, J., Trigwell, J., Kinsella, K., White, J. and Harden, A. (2015b) 'Community engagement – approaches to improve health. Map of the literature on current and emerging community engagement policy and practice in the UK', Centre for Health Promotion Research, Leeds Beckett University/Institute for Health and Human Development, University of East London, Leeds.

Bagnall, A., Kinsella, K., Trigwell, J., South, J., Sheridan, K. and Harden, A. (2016) 'Community engagement – approaches to improve health. Map of current UK practice based on a case study approach', Centre for Health Promotion Research, Leeds Beckett University/ Institute for Health and Human Development, University of East London.

Bagnall, A., South, J., Mitchell, B., Pilkington, G., Newton, R. and Di Martino, S. (2017) *Systematic scoping review of indicators of community wellbeing in the UK*, London: What Works Centre for Wellbeing.

Brunton, G., Caird, J., Stokes, G., Stansfield, C., Kneale, D., Richardson, M. and Thomas, J. (2014) *Community engagement for health via coalitions, collaborations and partnerships. A systematic review and meta-analysis*, London: EPPI-Centre.

Brunton, G., Caird, J., Kneale, D., Thomas, J. and Richardson, M. (2015) *Review 2: Community engagement for health via coalitions, collaborations and partnerships: A systematic review and meta-analysis*, London: EPPI-Centre, Social Science Research Unit, UCL Institute of Education, University College London.

Cinderby, S. (2014) 'Practical action to build community resilience: the good life initiative in New Earswick', Joseph Rowntree Foundation (JRF).

Communities Evidence Programme (2015) *Voice of the user report*, London: What Works Wellbeing Centre.

CSDH (Commission on Social Determinants of Health) (2008) *Closing the gap in a generation: Health equity through action on the social determinants of health. Final report of the Commission on Social Determinants of Health*, Geneva: World Health Organization.

Dixon-Woods, M., Agarwal, S., Jones, D., Young, B. and Sutton, A. (2005) 'Synthesising qualitative and quantitative evidence: a review of possible methods', *Journal of Health Services Research and Policy*, 10(1): 45–53.

Eurofound (2013) *Quality of Life Survey – Quality of life in Europe: Subjective well-being*, Luxembourg: Publications Office of the European Union.

Friedli, L. (2009) *Mental health, resilience and inequalities*, Denmark: World Health Organization Europe.

Gough, D., Oliver, S. and Thomas, J. (2012) *An introduction to systematic reviews*, London: Sage.

Harden, A., Sheridan, K., McKeown, A., Dan-Ogosi, I. and Bagnall, A.M. (2015) *Evidence review of barriers to, and facilitators of, community engagement approaches and practices in the UK*, London: Institute for Health and Human Development, University of East London.

Helliwell, J.F., Layard, R. and Sachs, J. (eds) (2015) *World happiness report 2015*, New York, NY: Sustainable Development Solutions Network.

Hothi, M., Bacon, N., Brophy, M. and Mulgan, G. (2007) *Neighbourliness + empowerment = wellbeing: Is there a formula for happy communities?*, London: The Young Foundation.

IRISS (Institute for Research and Innovation in Social Services) (2012) *Using an assets approach for positive mental health and wellbeing: An IRISS and East Dumbartonshire project*, Glasgow: Institute for Research and Innovation in Social Services.

Jennings, A., Barnes, S., Okereke, U. and Welch, A. (2013) 'Successful weight management and health behaviour change using a health trainer model', *Perspectives in Public Health*, 133: 221.

Kennedy-Martin, T., Curtis, S., Faries, D., Robinson, S. and Johnston, J. (2015) 'A literature review on the representativeness of randomized controlled trial samples and implications for the external validity of trial results', *Trials*, 16: 495.

Lee, S.J. and Kim, Y. (2015) 'Searching for the meaning of community wellbeing', in S.J. Lee, Y. Kim, and R. Phillips (eds) *Community well-being and community development*, New York: Springer, pp 9-23.

Marmot, M., Atkinson, T., Bell, J., Black, C., Broadfoot, P., Cumberlege, J., Diamond, I., Gilmore, I., Ham, C., Meacher, M. and Mulgan, G. (2010) *Fair society, healthy lives: The Marmot review: Strategic review of health inequalities in England post-2010*, London: The Marmot Review.

Moore, G.F., Audrey, S., Barker, M., Bond, L., Bonell, C., Hardeman, W., Moore, L., O'Cathain, A., Tinati, T., Wight, D. and Baird, J. (2015) 'Process evaluation of complex interventions: Medical Research Council guidance', *BMJ*, 350: h1258.

Nazroo, J. and Matthews, K. (2012) *The impact of volunteering on well-being in later life*, Cardiff: WRVS.

NESTA (formerly National Endowment for Science, Technology and the Arts) (2012) *The power of co-design and co-delivery*, London: The Innovation Unit.

NICE (National Institute for Health and Care Excellence) (2012) *Methods for the development of NICE public health guidance* (3rd edn), London: NICE. Available at: https://www.nice.org.uk/process/pmg4/chapter/introduction

NICE (2016) 'NICE guideline: community engagement: improving health and wellbeing and reducing health inequalities'. Available at: www.nice.org.uk/guidance/ng44

Office for National Statistics (2013) *Reflections on measuring national wellbeing*, London: Office for National Statistics.

O'Mara-Eves, A., Brunton, G., Mcdaid, D,. Oliver, S., Kavanagh, J., Jamal, F., Matosevic, T., Harden, A. and Thomas, J. (2013) 'Community engagement to reduce inequalities in health: a systematic review, meta-analysis and economic analysis', *Public Health Research*, 1(4): 1–525.

Optimity Advisors (2015) *Community engagement – approaches to improve health and reduce health inequalities: Précis of the economic chapter of the EPPI review (Component 1, Stream 3). Health economics 1*, London: Optimity Advisors.

Public Health England and NHS England (2015) *Community-centred approaches for health and wellbeing: Main report*, London: Public Health England, NHS England.

Quick, A. (2015) *Inequalities in wellbeing: Challenges and opportunities for research and policy*, London: New Economics Foundation.

Race For Health (2010) *In powerful health: How effective community engagement is challenging health inequalities and improving the lives of people from black and minority ethnic backgrounds*, Liverpool: Race for Health.

Robinson, M., Robertson, S., Mccullagh, J. and Hacking, S. (2010) 'Working towards men's health: findings from the Sefton Men's Health project', Centre for Men's Health, Leeds Beckett University, Leeds.

Savage, V., Cordes, C., Keenaghan-Clark, L. and O'Sullivan, C. (2010) 'Public services and civil society working together: promising ideas for effective local partnerships between state and citizen', The Young Foundation.

Seaman, P. and Edgar, F. (2015) *Exploring socio-cultural explanations of Glasgow's 'excess' mortality*, Glasgow: Glasgow Centre for Population Health.

Snape, D., Meads, C., Bagnall, A.M., Tregaskis, O. and Mansfield, L. (2016) *What Works Wellbeing: A guide to our evidence review methods*, London: What Works Wellbeing Centre.

South, J. and Phillips, G. (2014) 'Evaluating community engagement as part of the public health system', *J Epidemiol Community Health*, 68: 692–6.

South, J., Bagnall, A., Hulme, C., Woodall, J., Longo, R., Dixey, R., Kinsella, K., Raine, G., Vinall-Collier, K. and Wright, J. (2014) 'A systematic review of the effectiveness and cost-effectiveness of peer-based interventions to maintain and improve offender health in prison settings', *Health Serv Deliv Res*, 2(35): 1–217.

South, J., Abdallah, S., Bagnall, A., Curtis, S., Newton, R., Pennington A. and Corcoran, R. (2017) 'Building community wellbeing – an initial theory of change', Liverpool: University of Liverpool. Available at: https://whatworkswellbeing.files.wordpress.com/2017/05/theory-of-change-community-wellbeing-may-2017-what-works-centre-wellbeing.pdf

Stevenson, J. and Rao, M. (2014) 'Explaining levels of wellbeing in black and minority ethnic populations in England. Project report', University of East London, Institute for Health and Human Development.

Stokes, G., Richardson, M., Brunton, G., Khatwa, M. and Thomas, J. (2015) *Review 3: Community engagement for health via coalitions, collaborations and partnerships (on-line social media and social networks) – a systematic review and metaanalysis*, London: EPPI-Centre, Social Science Research Unit, UCL Institute of Education, University College London.

Stoll, L., Michaelson, J. and Seaford, C. (2012) *Well-being evidence for policy: A review*, London: New Economics Foundation. Available at: www.neweconomics.org/publications/well-beingevidence-for-policy-a-review

Thomas, J., Harden, A., Oakley, A., Oliver, S., Sutcliffe, K., Rees, R., Brunton, G. and Kavanagh, J. (2004) 'Integrating qualitative research with trials in systematic reviews', *BMJ*, 328(7446): 1010–2.

Tunariu, A., Boniwell, I., Yusef, D. and Jones, J. (2011) 'Well London DIY happiness project research evaluation report', Well London.

Welch, V., Petticrew, M., Petkovic, J., Moher, D., Waters, E., White, H., Tugwell, P. and PRISMA-Equity Bellagio Group (2015) 'Extending the PRISMA statement to equity-focused systematic reviews (PRISMA 2012): explanation and elaboration', *Int J Equity Health*, 14(1): 92.

Woodall, J., White, J. and South, J. (2013) 'Improving health and well-being through community health champions: a thematic evaluation of a programme in Yorkshire and Humber', *Perspectives in Public Health*, 133(2): 96–103.

TWELVE

Looking through a realist lens: services provided by faith-based and third sector organisations

Jean Hannah

Introduction

In recent years, perspectives, expectations and requirements of faith-based and third sector organisations (TSOs) as community support and social care providers have changed, with accompanying requirements for evidencing the impact of their programmes. This chapter aims to encourage faith-based organisations and TSOs to consider realist evaluation in helping to identify and evidence what it is about their programmes that offer benefit. It begins by considering the contexts of faith-based organisations and TSOs and those of people accessing their services, including those affected by multiple and deep exclusion. An introduction to realist evaluation is presented, followed by a realist-inspired evaluation examining what works, for whom, in what circumstances, how and why. This draws on the real-life experiences of two men who successfully addressed problematic alcohol use and its ramifications when accessing Salvation Army community programmes.

Context

Governmental Big Society reforms called on faith-based organisations and TSOs to develop and provide 'innovative, bottom-up services where expensive state provision has failed' (Office for Civil Society, 2010). The financial societal context was one of widespread challenges, with tendering required for services and contracts (Office for Civil Society, 2010). Successful bidding depends on evidence of impact, economic value and, on occasions, added value compared to competitors. While some programmes use reporting frameworks to meet organisational or statutory inspection bodies' requirements, others do not. Thus, it can be difficult for TSOs unfamiliar with such processes to examine what they are offering their client population and the associated outcomes. Simultaneously, the same TSOs are accustomed to working with people and situations overflowing with complexity, including those affected by problematic alcohol use.

'Tackling the UK's alcohol problem' (Siva, 2015) discusses the challenge of alcohol and its impact on individuals and health providers. Despite the health implications of problematic alcohol use, individuals may have limited benefit from health supports because of their 'failure to attend' – or perhaps because service provision does not consistently befit vulnerable people. Advantages in health providers working with TSOs are recognised – albeit that integration is perceived as currently inadequate (Brown, 2015). However, statutory providers may not always know where an individual sources help, including their daily supports from faith-based organisations or TSOs. These organisations may be core providers of nutrition, hygiene opportunities, clothing and companionship. They may enable benefit sanction avoidance, the maintenance of tenancies and financial stability, and the making and keeping of otherwise missed appointments. Such matters may lack priority or be forgotten by people with problematic alcohol use, especially those with the accompanying cognitive impairment found in alcohol-related brain damage.

The concept of faith-based organisations' or TSOs' pivotal role in the support of holistic health and well-being (see Chapter Three) may be unrecognised by some. However, their de-stigmatising approaches and support may open sticking doors to statutory health and social care provision. The *Lancet* identified individual and wider societal benefits of clearly structured engagement between faith-based groups and the public sector, with recommended activities to strengthen cross-sector partnerships (Duff and Buckingham, 2015). These included activities to measure and improve communication of the scope, scale, distinctiveness and results of faith-based groups' work in health care, to appreciate respective objectives, capacities, differences and limitations, and to increase investments and use efficient business styles in faith-based groups (Duff and Buckingham, 2015).

The Salvation Army, founded in 1865 by the Christian William Booth, has supported people experiencing difficulties, including due to alcohol, throughout its existence. Booth's vision is reflected in his 1912 last public address:

> While women weep, as they do now, I'll fight; while children go hungry, as they do now, I'll fight; while men go to prison, in and out, in and out, as they do now, I'll

fight; while there is a drunkard left, while there is a poor lost girl upon the streets, while there remains one dark soul without the light of God, I'll fight, I'll fight to the very end! (Smith, 1949: 123–24)

Today, these people could be viewed as affected by multiple or deep exclusion, stigma and alienation. The descriptions in the Salvation Army publication 'The seeds of exclusion 2009' (Bonner et al, 2009) of the experiences of people accessing their homelessness services concur with multiple-exclusion homelessness:

> ... if they have been 'homeless' (including experience of temporary/unsuitable accommodation as well as sleeping rough) and have also experienced one or more of the following ... 'institutional care' (prison, local authority care, psychiatric hospitals or wards); 'substance misuse' (drug problems, alcohol problems, abuse of solvents, glue or gas); or participation in 'street culture activities' (begging, street drinking, 'survival' shoplifting or sex work). (Fitzpatrick et al, 2011)

These individuals are likely to be among those more recently described as affected by severe and multiple disadvantage (Bramley et al, 2015), experiencing a greater sense of social isolation than other vulnerable low-income people. Due to their complex problems, they are also likely to experience weaker progress, in keeping with service provider reports elsewhere (Bramley et al, 2015).

Like other TSOs, the Salvation Army strives to evidence community programme impact, though may not routinely gather data, creating complexity in determining and measuring outcomes. Furthermore, lack of information available to statutory providers exacerbates the complexity of measuring individual, community, societal and economic programme benefits. However, realist evaluation approaches have been found helpful in a Salvation Army community programme in such a situation.

Looking through a realist lens

Use of a 'realist lens' is about looking at a programme, service or intervention from the philosophical stance of realists, discussed later in the chapter. Those involved in realist evaluation and synthesis informally refer to the 'hook line' of 'what works, for whom, in what circumstances and how or why'. When facing a raft of different evaluation approaches, this phrase makes sense. It addresses a desire to ensure that people are offered and receive services of benefit to them, and opportunities to demonstrate wise, effective and economical resource use. Realist evaluation and synthesis are well suited to TSO settings because they acknowledge the importance of complexity. This chapter aspires to encourage organisations to consider how the approaches might be used within their settings, in particular, to highlight added value compared to other providers and support the strengthening of cross-sector partnerships.

Terminology

Realist evaluation and synthesis encourage deepening, evolving knowledge and understanding and are of great value in the exploration of social programmes and their impacts. Realist evaluation is primary or novel research. Realist synthesis (or review) compiles evidence from sources including research journals, project initiation documents, 'grey literature' (Wong et al, 2016) and personal testimony (Pawson et al, 2005). Key definitions of realist evaluation and synthesis terms are found in Table 12.1, adapted and abbreviated from an article on community-based participatory research (Jagosh et al, 2015).

Social programmes are based upon theories that postulate: 'If we deliver a programme in this way or we manage services like so, then it will bring about some improved outcome' (Pawson, 2006b: 26). When developing programme theories, the quality, relevance and rigour of evidence used is important (Pawson, 2006b: 87–90). Nevertheless, evidence not reaching a desired standard of rigour or relevance can include 'nuggets' of information (Pawson, 2006a), resulting in a need to pause, revisit and revise programme theories. The theories help guide the questions and data (qualitative and/or quantitative) needed to test and determine their accuracy.

Retroductive thinking and reasoning in realist evaluation and synthesis is used to consider the influences on a programme's outcomes from all angles and beyond first perceptions (Blaikie, 2004). Retroduction can reveal multiple, interwoven contexts and mechanisms collectively impacting on these. Outcome patterns occur as mechanisms are triggered (or not) in a context through the introduction of the programme (Pawson, 2013: 34–46). Context–mechanism–outcome (CMO) configurations are built, adapted and refined, allowing, in turn, programme theories to more accurately reflect what works, for whom, in what circumstance, why and how. As emerging problems can outpace the speed of data availability, it is important to recognise the time limitations of programmes and anticipate that change will occur – with subsequent benefit from further theory testing and refinement (Pawson, 2013: 34–46).

Table 12.1: Realistic evaluation: definition of terms

Realist methodology*: 'Theory driven, interpretative approach uncovering underlying theories driving interventions and their multiple components, and illuminating contextual factors influencing mechanisms of change to produce outcomes'.
Programme or middle-range theory (Merton, 1968)*: Implicit or explicit explanatory theory sought initially then examined iteratively during the programme review explaining specific programme elements or how programme logic manifests in implementation.
Context–mechanism–outcome (CMO) configurations*:
practical problem-solving approach generating explanations about outcome causes
may reflect all or part of a programme, be embedded in another or configured in a series (ripple effect: the outcome of one CMO becomes the context for the next)
help generate and/or refine theory that becomes the final product of the review.
Context*:
often relates to programme 'backdrops', including location, culture, history, social networks and infrastructure
can change over time and in response to programme outcomes.
Mechanism(s)*:
intended or unintended resources created by an intervention and participants' responses (cognitive, emotional or motivational) to resources
can relate to participants' decisions to participate, internalise knowledge or change behaviour.
Outcome(s): intended, intermediate and unexpected impacts.

Source: Adapted and abbreviated (*) from Table 1 of Jagosh et al (2015).

The living history of realist evaluation and synthesis

Realist evaluation and synthesis are increasingly and inclusively used worldwide with accessible, enthusiastic experts keen to discuss different perspectives and approaches. This is possible through initiatives such as the RAMESES Project (see: http://www.ramesesproject.org). Experts and novices alike share views, experiences and recommendations about projects on the online forum.

Realist synthesis and evaluation were brought to the fore by Pawson and Tilley (1997) from foundations in Bhaskar's philosophy of critical realism. In recognition of 'enduring structures and generative mechanisms underlying and producing observable phenomena and events', Bhaskar (1989: 2) wrote:

> ... we will only be able to understand – and so change – the social world if we identify the structures at work that generate those events and discourses.... These structures are not spontaneously apparent in the observable pattern of events: they can only be identified through the practical and theoretical work of the social sciences.

One 'pillar' influencing realist thinking (Pawson, 2013: 3–12), described by Elster (2007), is the strength of social science in explaining why we think we know things that are not in fact the case. That 'knowledge' is important because knowledge owned by different participants within or about a programme can vary and impact on outcomes. Policymakers may launch an intervention that practitioners know will not work because of their knowledge of the complexity of the setting and their clients' lives. People delivering services may have setting contexts and complexities resulting in poor engagement with a new intervention likely to reap benefit. Programme priorities may not relate to client self-perceived needs, resulting in a mismatch between client and provider aspirations for outcomes. This was reflected in one person's view of a drug and alcohol programme: "*They think they get recovery, but they don't*" (personal communication).

Experiencing a realist-inspired evaluation of a Salvation Army community programme

This realist-inspired evaluation incorporates a video, some contextual background information and salutogenic theories of human health and well-being. Viewing a short video – 'Greenock drug and alcohol work – the Salvation Army' (available at: https://www.youtube.com/watch?v=cMgPj3CmwNI) – demonstrates the value of looking beyond traditional data sources. It contains interviews with clients, Chris and Willy, and Lesley, a Salvation Army drug and alcohol support worker. The video content (data) is examined through a realist lens to provoke thought about the work of a faith-based TSO and what realist evaluation can offer. In other realist evaluations, but not possible here, quantitative data might be used, such as numbers of people accessing services and achieving outcomes, including reduced alcohol intake, volunteering or employment.

Important contexts are those influencing outcomes. In this instance, the community programme is located in the Salvation Army's Scottish territory, a country known for its poor, inequitable health statistics (Burns, 2012, 2015). Burns's (2012, 2015) arguments for change are based upon Antonovsky's (1996) salutogenic origins of health theory – health relating to a person in their entirety. Antonovsky introduced the concepts of generalised resistance resources, which facilitate successful coping when exposed to life's stressors. He then looked for commonality within these resources, concluding that their sense of coherence enabled people to make sense of and understand experiences within their world in a manageable and meaningful way (Antonovsky, 1996).

A challenge for people with severe and multiple disadvantage (Bramley et al, 2015), including some accessing Salvation Army supports (Bonner et al, 2009), is lack of generalised resistance resources, including: strong, positive family relationships; educational and employment opportunities; and a secure home environment. Instead, they may have experienced abusive relationships, mental ill-health, substance misuse, engagement with prison services, homelessness and hopelessness. They risk alienation from family, friends, support networks (including health, housing, employment and benefit agencies) and society at large, with spiralling risk of mental ill-health and problematic substance use. Children of parents with problematic alcohol use were more likely to suffer multiple adverse experiences in childhood, accompanied by subsequent scope for intergenerational cycles of adult alcohol abuse and adverse childhood experiences (Usher et al, 2015). Thus, the Salvation Army community programme (the Scotland Drug and Alcohol Strategy) was launched in 2014 in an extremely complex societal-level context.

The Salvation Army review, *A time for recovery* (Scotland Drug and Alcohol Strategy Task Group, 2011), examined evidence on community-based services for people with problematic alcohol and drug use. In keeping with Salvation Army experiences elsewhere (Patterson et al, 2015), the review supported the adoption of the community reinforcement approach (Meyers et al, 2011) in Scotland. The approach aspires to enable an individual's context, or, to use Zinberg's (1984) words, set and setting, to be one with more positive opportunities and experiences available through avoiding alcohol and drugs than through using them. These can include social, family, work and leisure activities. Motivational interviewing is used with trials of sobriety and abstinence (sobriety sampling). Personal triggers for substance misuse are discussed and coping strategies developed, with skills development and incentives through leisure, vocational and social means. To support this work, drug and alcohol support workers were appointed in community programmes in Stirling, Aberdeen and Falkirk, in a programme that runs in parallel with the Salvation Army Greenock Floating Support Service, which successfully supports the capacity of people with experience of problematic alcohol use to maintain a housing tenancy.

Using realist thinking, the strands discussed so far are drawn into an initial programme theory:

> If the Salvation Army offers a Floating Support Service and a community programme of drug and alcohol support worker-led support for people with substance misuse in the ethos of the community reinforcement approach, then people living in local communities will develop and maintain a lifestyle more rewarding than one including substance misuse.

The overarching realist evaluation question centres upon what aspects of the community programme work to enable the development and maintenance of a lifestyle more rewarding than one dominated by substance misuse, in which people, in what circumstances and how or why. Realist evaluation offers the ability to begin at the outcome and work backwards. Thus, the outcome is that Chris's and Willy's lives are now more rewarding than when they were dependent upon alcohol: "*Things are going quite nicely for me at the moment.... I've got no major hiccoughs in my life that are going to make me want to go back to drink*" (Chris). They describe their lives as being transformed through engagement with the community programme and Floating Support Service. A synopsis configuration of Willy's CMOs is portrayed in Table 12.2.

Trust, self-esteem, feelings of belonging, purpose, fulfilment, and knowing reliable people to turn to at any time of need were instrumental to the outcomes here and incentivised ongoing engagement. They contributed to the enhancement of Willy's sense of coherence and generalised resistance resources (Antonovsky, 1996). Chris moved from a complex time in life to one with optimism for the future based on positive experiences through choosing to access and engage with freely available, accessible resources (see Table 12.3).

Table 12.2: Realist perspectives about Willy's context, mechanisms and outcomes

Willy's context	Mechanism	Outcome
Traumatic childhood Self-harmed and attempted suicide Problematic drug and alcohol use from young age Lacked confidence Unable to face other people, get involved in groups or work with others Past help from other agencies Context resources: community programme and Floating Support Service	Reasoning: supported by people he could rely on – trust Inclusion: opportunity and support to work in cafe Experiential reasoning: increased confidence associated with working in cafe, and increased confidence made him feel more able to interact with others	Alcohol- and drug-free Self-esteem increased: a lot of confidence Employment: working in cafe Relationships: able to work with other people and participate in groups Belonging: feeling of being in a family Trust: Someone to rely on, day in, day out, no matter what

Table 12.3: Realist perspectives about Chris's context, mechanisms and outcomes

Chris's context	Mechanism	Outcome
Traumatic personal events Developed problematic alcohol use Broken family relationships Unemployed Poor health Did not like leaving house Context resources: community programme and Floating Support Service	Reasoning: free support available Responding to incentives: opportunities provided were things he wanted to get involved in He chose to leave the house to take part	Alcohol-free Relationships: re-establishing family relationships Social capital: went out of house for positive purposes Education: undertook college courses Employment: hoping to return to work Optimism: life is good – nothing to make him want to go back to drink

The video offers additional contextual insight. Despite the initial waterfront shots, the community programme is not set in an affluent area. The church-style building has a large informal 'Welcome' sign. Although open to people of all belief constructs, Christian beliefs are presented: 'We do not lose heart ... our spirits are being renewed, 2 Corinthians 4:16'. The timing of new programmes is important, as is participant experience of similar programmes in the past, whether successful or not (Pawson, 2013: 3–12). Chris and Willy indicate past support from other agencies, though it appears that recent supports had most impact. To Chris, the timing of seeking and responding to offers of help is crucial: "*An' I do get frustrated that I know there's other*

*people out there.... They've got to be ready themself but ... it's like anything
– if you're not ready to accept anything, you won't accept the help"* (Chris).

The Floating Support Service, community programme and drug and
alcohol support worker offered added value through the integration of
formal services with general community-oriented activities. Overall,
there was a salutogenic opportunity incorporating generalised resistance
resources and sense of coherence, the former described by Antonovsky
(1990: 78) as 'Something that provided a person with a set of life
experiences involving feedback, sending messages like: Here is the
right track; you can handle things; you are of worth'.

Chris's and Willy's past coping strategies for traumatic events beyond
their ability to comprehend, manage and find meaning in, that is,
their sense of coherence, included alcohol. Their lives then changed
with achievements beyond their previous reach. Lesley described the
positive outcomes witnessed in people engaging with the community
programme: *"How do I measure success? By seeing a change in a life. By
seeing someone unloved, uncared for to becoming someone who is more confident
in themselves, who is able to make friendships and make relationships"* (Lesley).
Her words ring true with Antonovsky's: the transformation from being
unloved to recognising worth in self and to others.

The concept of added value

Realist evaluation provides opportunities for TSOs to demonstrate
complex contexts in which their clients are living and services are
provided, highlighting individual and organisational strengths and
outcomes. People other than Chris and Willy may remain in desperate
need, continuing to access community programme supports on a single,
sporadic or frequent basis. Welcoming engagement remains as people
'slip', returning to crisis, with self-prioritised supports continuing until
they begin to recognise that they are 'of worth', and the benefits of a
life without alcohol. In these instances, measurement of the value of
the recurrent Salvation Army's welcome and provision of basic support
may be reflected in rippling CMO configurations.

McCluskey's (2005) care-seeking stances aid understanding of the
complexity of people's presentations and reactions when seeking help,
from confident approaches for specific help to feeling beyond help in
crisis situations. Importantly, McCluskey (2011: 14) advises:

> The more experience a person has of an effective caregiver
> helping them to manage stressful situations, the more the
> person will be able to both seek appropriate help and

access memories of how they have been helped to manage in the past.

People with alcohol-related brain damage may or may not remember caregiver support that may influence future engagement. Although Chris and Willy do not describe their initial feelings when seeking help, they spoke of complex, troubled lives. They then built up memories of how they were helped and, through their empowering participation, encouraged others to do likewise: "*It's worked for me. Why can't other people come and give it a shot?*" (Chris).

This introductory realist-inspired evaluation has demonstrated that people with problematic alcohol use can develop and maintain a lifestyle more rewarding than one filled with substance misuse through accessing the Salvation Army Floating Support Service and community programme drug and alcohol support worker assistance in the ethos of the community reinforcement approach. Achievements arose through the development of trusting relationships, a sense of belonging, increased self-confidence and self-esteem, work and educational opportunities, and sobriety. Salutogenic inroads were made through Salvation Army supports and services for individuals and through the integration of people accessing services in the wider community. Although presented as a synopsis, this will have occurred in many intertwining stages, but against the backdrop on an individual level of having "*someone to rely on, day in, day out, no matter what*" (Willy).

Conclusion

The chapter aimed to introduce realist evaluation in order to encourage others to explore its potential benefits within their own contexts, with pointers to key authors and resources. For those in TSOs or faith-based organisations, the use of salutogenic theories and models in conjunction with a realist approach may be beneficial as they reflect on the support needs of many people affected by multiple and deep exclusion. While the brief evaluation provided does not claim to be an exemplar of the approach, it does provide a means of demonstrating how the voices of those accessing a community programme can be heard, with potential therefore for influence on shaping future programme provision. Realist evaluation is an expanding, supportive research field offering a refreshing honesty in expectations for all, and is ideally placed for use in complex social settings.

References

Antonovsky, A. (1990) 'A somewhat personal odyssey in studying the stress process', *Stress Medicine*, 6(2): 71–80.

Antonovsky, A. (1996) 'The salutogenic model as a theory to guide health promotion', *Health Promotion International*, 11(1): 11–18.

Bhaskar, R. (1989) *Reclaiming reality: A critical introduction to contemporary philosophy*, London: Verso.

Blaikie, N. (2004) 'Retroduction', in M.S. Lewis-Beck, A. Bryman and T.F. Liao (eds) *The SAGE encyclopedia of social science research methods*, Thousand Oaks, CA: Sage Publications, Inc., p 973.

Bonner, A., Luscombe, C., Van den Bree, M. and Taylor, P. (2009) 'The seeds of exclusion 2009', The Salvation Army, University of Kent, University of Cardiff.

Bramley, G., Fitzpatrick, S., Edwards, J., Ford, D., Johnsen, S., Sosenko, F. and Watkins, D. (2015) 'Hard edges: mapping severe and multiple disadvantage', The LankellyChase Foundation. Available at: http://lankellychase.org.uk/multiple-disadvantage/publications/hard-edges/

Brown, C. (2015) 'Better together', *Drink and Drugs News*, July/August: 12–13.

Burns, H. (2012) *Kilbrandon's vision. Healthier lives: Better futures. The tenth Kilbrandon lecture*, Edinburgh: Scottish Government.

Burns, H. (2015) 'Health inequalities – why so little progress?', *Public Health*, 129(7): 849–53.

Duff, J.F. and Buckingham, W.W. (2015) 'Strengthening of partnerships between the public sector and faith-based groups', *The Lancet*, 386(10005): 1786–94.

Elster, J. (2007) *Explaining social behaviour*, Cambridge: Cambridge University Press.

Fitzpatrick, S., Johnsen, S. and White, M. (2011) 'Multiple exclusion homelessness in the UK: key patterns and intersections', *Social Policy & Society*, 10(4): 501–12.

Jagosh, J., Bush, P.L., Salsberg, J., Macaulay, A.C., Greenhalgh, T., Wong, G., Cargo, M., Green, L.W., Herbert, C.P. and Pluye, P. (2015) 'A realist evaluation of community-based participatory research: partnership synergy, trust building and related ripple effects', *BMC Public Health*, 15: 725 doi: 10.1186/s12889-015-1949-1.

McCluskey, U. (2005) *To be met as a person: the dynamics of attachment in professional encounters*, London: Karnac Press.

McCluskey, U. (2011) 'The therapist as a fear-free caregiver: supporting change in the dynamic organisation of the self', *The Association for University & College Counselling Journal*, May: 12–17.

Merton, R.K. (1968) *Social theory and social structure*. New York, NY: The Free Press.

Meyers, R.J., Roozen, H.G. and Smith, J.E. (2011) 'The community reinforcement approach: an update of the evidence', *Alcohol Research & Health*, 33(4): 380–8.

Office for Civil Society (2010) *Building a stronger civil society. A strategy for voluntary and community groups, charities and social enterprises*, London: HM Government.

Patterson, T., Macleod, E., Egan, R., Cameron, C., Hobbs, L. and Gross, J. (2015) *Testing the bridge: an evaluation of the effectiveness of the Salvation Army's Bridge programme model of treatment*, Commissioned by the Salvation Army New Zealand, Fiji and Tonga Territory, Dunedin, New Zealand: Departments of Psychology, Psychological Medicine and Preventive & Social Medicine, University of Otago.

Pawson, R. (2006a) 'Digging for nuggets: how "bad" research can yield "good" evidence ', *International Journal of Social Research Methodology*, 9(2): 127–42.

Pawson, R. (2006b) *Evidence-based policy: A realist perspective*, London: Sage Publications Ltd.

Pawson, R. (2013) *The science of evaluation: A realist manifesto*, London: SAGE Publications Ltd.

Pawson, R. and Tilley, N. (1997) *Realistic evaluation*, London: Sage Publications, Inc.

Pawson, R., Greenhalgh, T., Harvey, G. and Walshe, K. (2005) 'Realist review – a new method of systematic review designed for complex policy interventions', *Journal of Health Services Research & Policy*, 10(Suppl 1): 21–34.

Scotland Drug and Alcohol Strategy Task Group (2011) *A time for recovery: A way forward for addiction services in Scotland*, The Salvation Army.

Siva, N. (2015) 'Tackling the UK's alcohol problems', *The Lancet*, 386(9989): 121–2.

Smith, J.E. (1949) *Booth, the beloved: Personal recollections of William Booth, founder of the Salvation Army*, Oxford: Oxford University Press.

Usher, A.M., McShane, K.E. and Dwyer, C. (2015) 'A realist review of family-based interventions for children of substance abusing parents', *Systems Review*, 4(1): 177.

Wong, G., Westhorp, G., Manzano, A., Greenhalgh, J., Jagosh, J. and Greenhalgh, T. (2016) 'RAMESES II reporting standards for realist evaluations', *BMC Medicine*, 14(1): 96. doi: 10.1186/s12916-016-0643-1.

Zinberg, N. (1984) *Drug, set, and setting: The basis for controlled intoxicant use*, New Haven, CT: Yale University Press.

Part Four
Employment and housing

Improvements in living conditions, the supply of food, working conditions and services such as education and health care have had a major impact on the health of people in the UK and other countries during recent years (see Chapters Two, Four and Twenty-three). Employment and housing can reduce social inequalities, with concomitant benefits to population health and community well-being. The employment needs of young people are reviewed in Chapter Thirteen, with specific focus on the role of social enterprises as an approach in helping people who have problems in gaining access to mainstream employment. Adequate accommodation, security and working conditions are essential for good health and well-being. Chapters Fourteen and Fifteen provide an insight into housing policy in England and Scotland, and the link between appropriate housing and health.

THIRTEEN

Social enterprise and the well-being of young people not in education, employment or training

Steve Coles

Introduction

What does social enterprise have to do with the well-being of young people who are not in education, employment or training (NEET)? Let us break the question down into smaller parts and ask further questions. What is NEET? How many young people in the UK are NEET? Why does it matter? What is well-being? What does it have to do with being NEET? What is social enterprise? What does social enterprise have to do with it all?

This chapter draws on research from academics, practitioners and policymakers, publicly available data, and my own experience of supporting more than 500 social enterprises over the last six years to measure, report and maximise their social impact. To begin, we need to understand what we mean by 'NEET', 'well-being' and 'social enterprise'.

NEET or 'NEETs' refer to young people aged 16 to 24 who are not in education, employment or training. Among them, there are two distinct subcategories: those who are actively seeking work (known as unemployed young people); and those who have not actively sought work recently and/or are unable to start work imminently (known as economically inactive young people) (ONS, 2016).

The UK government's Office for National Statistics (ONS) has been actively measuring and analysing 'well-being' since 2011,[1] although the field of research has been around a lot longer. Well-being is defined as:

> A positive, social and mental state; it is not just the absence
> of pain, discomfort and incapacity. It arises not only from
> the action of individuals, but from a host of collective goods
> and relationships with other people. It requires that basic

needs are met, that individuals have a sense of purpose, and that they feel able to achieve important personal goals and participate in society. It is enhanced by conditions that include supportive personal relationships, involvement in empowered communities, good health, financial security, rewarding employment and a healthy and attractive environment. (ONS, 2009: 6)

Even from this brief introduction, the areas of overlap between unemployment and well-being are already emerging. Professor Richard Layard (2011: 67) crisply makes the case as to 'why unemployment is such a disaster: it reduces income but it also reduces happiness directly by destroying the self-respect and social relationships created by work'. As such, young people who are NEET may well find themselves at the edges of community – isolated, outside of the usual social relationships created by work, financially disadvantaged, anxious or perhaps ostracised.

The definition of 'social enterprise' varies across countries and organisations. In the UK, the government defines social enterprise as 'a business with primarily social objectives whose surpluses are principally reinvested for that purpose in the business or in the community, rather than being driven by the need to maximise profit for shareholders and owners' (Department for Business, Innovation & Skills, 2011: 2). From my own experience as a social enterprise and social impact practitioner, I would define social enterprises as organisations that intentionally seek to increase well-being, whether of individuals, families, communities or society.

The prevalence and make-up of the NEET population

The following statistics about NEET young people are the latest available from the ONS at the time of writing. The August 2016 statistical release relates to the period April to June 2016, and shows that there were 843,000 young people aged from 16 to 24 in the UK who were NEET, down 78,000 from a year earlier. Expressed in percentages, the percentage of all young people in the UK who were NEET was 11.7%, down 0.9 percentage points from a year earlier. In the last five years, the peak was 16.9% of all 16 to 24 years olds being NEET in July to September 2011 (ONS, 2016). To better understand this long-lasting and seemingly intractable problem, which includes just over one in 10 young people, we need to investigate the statistics in more detail.

In the same period, 46% of all young people in the UK who were NEET were looking for work and available for work, and therefore classified as unemployed. The remaining 58% were either not looking for work and/or not available for work, and therefore classified as economically inactive (ONS, 2016). It is in the statistics for each subgroup that greater insight and potential concerns are to be found.

For April to June 2016, there were 390,000 NEET young people who were unemployed, down 41,000 from a year earlier. By gender, 230,000 of those were men and 159,000 were women; by age group, 30,000 of those were aged 16 to 17 (2.0% of the relevant population group) and 360,000 were aged 18 to 24 (6.3% of the relevant population group). For the same period, there were 453,000 NEET young people who were economically inactive, down 37,000 from a year earlier. By gender, this total included 179,000 men aged from 16 to 24 and 274,000 women; by age group, 33,000 were aged 16 to 17 (2.2% of the relevant population group) and 421,000 were aged 18 to 24 (7.3% of the relevant population group) (ONS, 2016).

Of particular note in these statistics is a significant gender difference between the two subcategories and the sharp increase in NEET rates in young people aged over 18. The number of unemployed young men is nearly half as many again as the number of unemployed young women, but in relation to economic inactivity, the difference is reversed, with 55% more young women being economically inactive compared to young men. The total NEET rate among 18 to 24 year olds is 13.6%, a figure greatly reduced when the age range is expanded to include 16 and 17 years olds (as the NEET rate for that group is only 4.3%).

Causes of NEET status

What might be the causes of becoming NEET? Research conducted in Scotland using the Scottish Longitudinal Study, which links anonymised individual records from the 1991, 2001 and 2011 Censuses and a wide range of data from a variety of sources, provides succinct details of the risk factors of becoming NEET:

- Educational qualification is the most important risk factor. No qualifications increased the risk of being NEET by six times for males and eight times for females (for those born in the 1980s).
- Other school factors are important, including time absent from school and number of exclusions.
- Two factors are important for females: being an unpaid carer for more than 20 hours per week and teenage pregnancy.

- Household factors are also important. Living in a social renting household, living in a family that is not headed by a married couple, living in a household with no employed adults and having a large number of siblings all increased the risk of becoming NEET.
- The local NEET rate is an important factor for both cohorts and genders, with the risk of NEET increasing with the local NEET rate (Social Research, 2015: 1–2).

We can also look back further into the lives of young people to see what happens to their well-being prior to the age of 16. Pioneering research undertaken by the New Economics Foundation (NEF) into well-being among young people in Nottingham exposed a worrying relationship between stages of education and levels of satisfaction (NEF, 2004). Young people were found to be far happier at primary school than at secondary school, and while there is a known 'transition' between school stages, this was not found to sufficiently account for such a severe drop in levels of satisfaction, both in terms of scale and abruptness. Between the 'senior primary' age (9–11 years old) and secondary school age (12–15), average school satisfaction scores fell from 3.62 out of 5 to 2.63, a 20% drop. Deeper questioning reveals further information. Percentages of school children strongly agreeing with the statement 'school is interesting' plummeted from 65% at primary school to 12% at secondary. Similarly, strong agreement with 'I enjoy school activities' fell from 65% to 18% and with 'I learn a lot at school' from 71% to 18% (NEF, 2004). At this point, we cannot draw a causal line between declining levels of well-being as schooling progresses and young people grow up and them becoming NEET post-16. However, in light of these findings, it is unsurprising that many young people have no desire to continue in formal education after the age of 16.

The need for new opportunities that are tangible, accessible and achievable for NEETs and all young people is also vital. According to Elkington and Hartigan (2008), it is lack of opportunities that leads to crime, violence and drug trafficking. While few NEETs may end up in such dismal circumstances, they also argue that, alongside those 'new opportunities', people want fun, art and technology in their lives, and that these are often lacking in inner-city areas, which is also where concentrations of NEETs are to be found.

Therefore, it seems that there are particular risk factors, if not direct causes, of becoming NEET. However, what are the consequences, particularly in relation to well-being?

Consequences of NEET status

In short, well-being and being NEET are related because a substantial weight of research demonstrates that unemployment has a negative effect on well-being (Argyle, 1999; Di Tella et al, 2003; Helliwell, 2003), with wellbeing levels of the unemployed being roughly half of the employed, including among young people (Clark and Oswald, 1994). This seems likely to be because paid work activities provide enjoyment (as, contrary to popular opinion, most people do not suffer employment in order to earn money, but obtain pleasure from even mundane jobs), as well as a daily structure, social contact, an opportunity to earn respect and an opportunity to find challenge and meaning (Diener and Seligman, 2004). We can see, therefore, how NEETs are at particular risk of becoming marginalised.

However, the consequences of being NEET go beyond the already significant economic, educational and social concerns. For example, low well-being resulting from being NEET may have a detrimental effect on social relationships, as well as mental and physical health (Diener and Seligman, 2004). The Scottish government's longitudinal research corroborates this, finding that being NEET is associated with a higher risk of both poor physical and mental health after 10 and 20 years. The research found that 'the risk for the NEET group was 1.6–2.5 times that for the non-NEET group, varying with different health outcomes' (Social Research, 2015). The same goes for mental health, with 'the risk of depression and anxiety prescription for the NEET group being over 50% higher than that for the non-NEET group' (Social Research, 2015).

Furthermore, 16- and 17-year-old NEETs may also be damaged for the long term. The job history of former NEETs now in their 40s shows that they are more prone to unemployment or to low-paid, low-skilled work (Turner, 2008). Specifically, it has been found that NEETs remain disadvantaged in their level of educational attainment. More than one in five of NEET young people in 2001 had no qualifications in 2011, compared with only one in 25 of non-NEETS. Furthermore, in relation to economic activity, there is also a 'scarring effect'. In comparison with their non-NEET peers, NEET young people in 2001 were 2.8 times as likely to be unemployed or economically inactive 10 years later. There is also an observable effect on the type of occupations that NEET young people take up: NEET young people in 2001 were 2.5 times as likely as their non-NEET peers to work in a low-status occupation in 2011, if they found work (Social Research, 2015). Clearly, the consequences of being NEET are significant and dire. Andrew Clark has studied these 'scarring effects' of unemployment in depth. Along with colleagues, he found that (for males at least) 'life satisfaction is greater for those who have suffered less than average unemployment in the past' (Clark et al, 2001). This should incentivise interventions that help NEET young people into work as it is likely to reduce the prevalence and magnitude of lower well-being in adult life.

Context: budgets and costs

Reflecting on their findings on the cumulative effect of being out of employment and education on later life chances, the Scottish government's report on NEETs concludes that 'this group is the most disadvantaged and in need of continuing support' (Social Research, 2015: 4). However, the wider economic and political context in which NEETs and future NEETs find themselves may have significant negative impacts on continuing support provision. To take one example, for which stark information is available, Cambridgeshire County Council, like many other councils and local authorities, faces significant, long-term challenges relating to funding and service delivery. An excerpt from one of their public consultation documents outlines the scale and duration of the difficulties ahead, particularly in relation to proposed changes to 'Enhanced and Preventative Services', the department responsible for providing a range of community-based and preventive services for vulnerable children and families:

> The funding position for the County Council is increasingly difficult; our funding is reducing at a time when our costs continue to rise significantly due to inflationary and demographic pressures. *There continues to be a high level of demand for services and rising demand for higher need services.* As an authority we need to find £41 million in savings in 2016/17 with more than £100 million over the next five years. Children, Families and Adults Services (CFA) have to make savings of £29.0m in 2016/17 and £85.6m across five years. *This is a 35% reduction by 2020 and means all services for children, families and adults will be affected.* For Enhanced and Preventative Services we are required to achieve £2,424,000 savings in total. (Cambridgeshire County Council, 2015: 4, emphases added)

While cutting budgets may be necessary, there is both a substantial personal cost to being NEET as well as a societal cost. According to recent research, NEETs will, on average, lose up to £50,000 in earnings over their working life compared to non-NEET peers and up to £225,000 over the same period compared to a non-NEET peer who has graduated from university (Impetus PEF, 2014). This is another example of the 'scarring effect' of a period of being NEET on a young person's future. In addition, if the 120,000 of 2014's 13 year olds at risk of becoming NEET are not prevented from doing so, they collectively stand to lose £6.4 billion. Furthermore, the lost taxes, additional public service costs and associated impacts, such as youth crime and poor health, will cost Britain in excess of £77 billion a year (Impetus PEF, 2014). University of York research gives a range for the possible costs attributable to the NEET population (aged 16–18), with total resource cost (including loss to the economy, welfare loss to the individual and the family, and the impact on the resources of or opportunity cost to society) estimated at between £22 billion and £77 billion. The 'unit resource cost' per NEET young person is estimated to be £104,312 (Coles et al, 2010). The costs to the young people themselves and to public finances are significant.

NEETs and entrepreneurship

However, there is reason for hope in the midst of this bleak situation. Campbell and Keck (2008) argue that NEET young people often display considerably creative and enterprising behaviour. Their activities may not always be legal or desirable, but they are nevertheless entrepreneurial, and there is potential for encouraging and guiding this enterprising behaviour towards appropriate expressions. Catching NEETs before their situation becomes critical is possible, although dependent upon 'recognition of the potential for internal change stemming from the emotional and psychological effects of being one's "own boss"' (Campbell and Keck, 2008: 128). Being able to achieve entrepreneurial ambitions and seize creative opportunities may help bring about that change. This brings us on to the topics of employment, entrepreneurship and social enterprise.

In the face of social ills, deprived communities, NEET young people and those at risk of being NEET, one of the most eloquent and challenging reasons to champion and redefine entrepreneurship is given by the Nobel Peace Prize winner Professor Mohammad Yunus, who claims that there is:

a blind spot in standard economic thinking: the assumption that 'entrepreneurship' is a rare quality. According to the textbooks, only a handful of people have the talent to spot business opportunities and the courage to risk their resources in developing those opportunities. On the contrary, my observations among the poorest people of the world suggest ... that entrepreneurial ability is practically universal. Almost everyone has the talent to recognise opportunities around them. And when they are given the tools to transform those opportunities into reality, almost everyone is eager to do so. (Yunus, 2007: 54)

Research among NEETs reveals that 69% believe entrepreneurship to be a good career move. For NEETs, being their own boss is about agency: the ability to determine personal goals and act upon them. In opening up opportunities for positive expressions of their entrepreneurial tendencies, entrepreneurship becomes not just about building a business, but about building up the spirit of the entrepreneur. For NEETs, entrepreneurship is about building or rebuilding self-esteem, and for them, enterprise and emancipation go hand-in-hand (Campbell and Keck, 2008). In my own research, I propose the concept of agency as a meeting point between well-being and entrepreneurship, with high levels of agency being associated with entrepreneurship and with higher well-being (Coles, 2008).

Research among people under the age of 30 suggests that the most important characteristic in a job is to have the opportunity to use initiative (Clark, 2001). For young adults, whether NEET or at risk of becoming NEET, self-employment and entrepreneurship may hold the opportunity to do just that. Indeed, according to the Royal Society for the encouragement of Arts, Manufactures and Commerce's (RSA's) research, in partnership with the bank Royal Bank of Scotland (RBS), it might do that and more:

> there is in fact another route for young people: entrepreneurship ... starting up in business is now very much a viable means for young people to earn a living. Indeed, new research by the Federation of Small Businesses shows that unemployed people are now more likely to find work through self-employment than within large firms. A record 14 percent of the workforce – the equivalent of around four million people – now work for themselves. But the benefits of youth enterprise are not limited to

young people. We all have a stake in helping our younger generation start up in business. These same entrepreneurs will be the employers of the future. They will also be the innovators, driving the creation of more and better quality products. This is not only a motor of growth, it is also a means of maintaining the economic diversity of our towns and cities. In short, youth enterprise is essential to building the kind of vibrant society and healthy economy. (RSA, 2013)

Of course, to get young people interested in entrepreneurship and to equip them for starting their own business, we will need engaging and innovative approaches to enterprise education and work experience. The following extract from a report called 'The way to work' explains the potential value and importance of enterprise education in helping all young people, including NEETs:

Teaching enterprise behaviours can play a key role in raising confidence and self-esteem, increasing attainment and helping young people classified as NEET back into education, work or training. However ... narrow understanding and applications are limiting its reach and efficacy in current practice. Our research underscores the need to de-stream enterprise from business studies in schools and higher education, and to inject enterprise more broadly into curricula.... Finally, it is important to reframe entrepreneurship – by debunking negative myths that make the concept off-putting to young people ... and providing young people with more accessible role models with whom they can better identify. Opening up the meaning of 'enterprise' as a more inclusive concept that signifies an attitude to life and a transferable skill set, rather than just something related to money, will be vital in widening the current narrow focus on self-employment. (Kahn et al, 2011: 43)

Returning to the RSA's wide-ranging research on self-employment and entrepreneurship, it was found that 'young people are more likely than other age groups to want to start a social enterprise' as they are more keen than other age groups to 'do something meaningful' and to 'make a difference' (RSA, 2013: 17). However, it should be tested whether this desire may be found in those with greater means, particularly financial means, to start a business as many young entrepreneurs that the RSA surveyed said that 'opportunity was the main driving force, rather than necessity' (RSA, 2013), in starting their own business. Those who are NEET may be driven more by necessity than opportunity. Therefore, while social enterprise might be an avenue for young people to actively pursue to gain a job, earn an income or fulfil deeper motivations, we might also ask what social enterprise can do to engage, encourage and support young NEETs to undertake a similar journey.

NEETs and social enterprise

Social enterprise is about 'changing the world through business. Social enterprises exist and trade not to maximise private profit, but to further their social and environmental aims' (Social Enterprise UK, 2015). There is no single or legal definition of social enterprises and they can take a number of structures and forms. What social enterprises do, where they are and whom they employ and benefit, however, is much clearer. According to Social Enterprise UK's State of Social Enterprise 2015 survey, social enterprises are:

- focused where they are most needed, with 31% working in the top 20% most deprived communities in the UK;
- inclusive and diverse, with 40% led by women, 31% having Black, Asian and Minority Ethnic (BAME directors and 40% with a director with a disability; and
- fair in relation to pay, with the average pay ratio between the chief executive officer (CEO) and the lowest-paid being 3.6:1 (compared to FTSE100 CEOs, for whom the ratio is 150:1) (Social Enterprise UK, 2015).

In the same research, it is evident what social enterprise has to do with unemployment, the unemployed and NEETs. In the 12 months prior to the State of Social Enterprise Survey 2015, 41% of social enterprises created jobs compared to 22% of all small- and medium-sized businesses, and of the jobs created, 59% of social enterprises employed at least one person who was disadvantaged in the labour market. Indeed, for 16% of social enterprises, at least half of all their employees are those who are disadvantaged in the labour market. Furthermore, 18% of all social enterprises surveyed said that 'education' was their principal trading activity, with 14% saying 'employment and skills' (Social Enterprise UK, 2015). It is clear, therefore, that there are social enterprises that intentionally seek to create employment, education and training opportunities for young people.

In Cambridge, Turtle Dove[2] creates work experience and training opportunities for women who are NEET or at risk of becoming NEET through working at events across the city, as well as hosting their own, usually intergenerational, community events. Across the UK, Catch22[3] is 'providing services that help vulnerable people turn their lives around' and now runs five independent alternative schools supporting 2,000 learners. Their apprenticeship programmes link to over 150 different employers. In London, K10[4] has created a range of innovative apprenticeships, enabling young people to train, develop and earn with major construction firms on large developments in their local area. In the last three years, K10 has created 450 apprenticeships in partnership with over 75 developers and contractors, and more than 30 local authorities and London boroughs. In Surrey, Eikon[5] works further 'upstream', working with 3,000 young people a year in schools and youth centres, offering support in areas such as parenting, conflict resolution, anger management and self-awareness, thus concentrating on the cause of the problem, not just the effects. While a charity in legal form, Eikon trades and earns most of its income through winning contracts from the local authority or selling its services directly to schools. As well as working across the country, Future First[6] is helping to create alumni communities in schools in the South-West, in Cornwall, Devon and Somerset. Another intervention 'upstream' from the problem of NEETs, the argument is that 'access to relevant and relatable role models is crucial for a young person's development', which also 'has a central part to play in increasing social mobility' (Future First, 2016). Across Scotland and the North-East, the award-winning Wise Group[7] has helped 30,000 people into work over the last 30 years. Their Talent Match North East programme specifically targets 18 to 24 year olds who are NEET, aiming to support 2,500 young people over five years to 2018. In Norwich, LEAP[8] gets NEETs into work by unlocking creativity, agency and accountability through coupling work experience in their catering social enterprise with one-to-one support and employment advice. These few examples are just a few of the social enterprises around the country changing the lives of NEET young people.

Conclusion

The problem of NEETs is clearly complex, costly and consequential. It affects young men and young women differently. However, by understanding the problem, the causes and consequences, and the ways in which well-being can be damaged or enhanced, we can detect existing solutions and devise new ones. Some of the existing solutions are found in organisations that intentionally seek to increase well-being – social enterprises – and they do so by being driven by social aims, focusing on areas of deprivation and adopting varied, localised, tailor-made approaches to the problem of NEETs, which often requires gender-specific, age-specific or location-specific solutions.

One facet might be encouraging young people to consider social entrepreneurship for themselves – unleashing their creativity, local knowledge, passion, sense of meaning and agency. Another facet might be supporting existing social enterprises to do more to better train, support, befriend, advise, include and realise the potential in young people. Enterprise education and pragmatic policies for supporting self-employment and the self-employed will need to play a part. Existing social enterprises also need to build capacity and grow in scale and impact. Social enterprises up and down the country are focused on ensuring that NEET young people have a sense of purpose, feel able to achieve important personal goals and participate in society, have supportive personal relationships and are involved in empowered communities, and find routes towards or opportunities for rewarding employment. Those are the building blocks of well-being and the keys to a full, flourishing life. This is what social enterprise has to do with the well-being of young people who are NEET.

Notes

[1.] For more, see: http://www.ons.gov.uk/peoplepopulationandcommunity/wellbeing
[2.] See: http://www.turtledovecambridge.com
[3.] See: http://www.catch-22.org.uk
[4.] See: https://www.k-10.co.uk
[5.] See: http://eikon.org.uk
[6.] See: http://futurefirst.org.uk
[7.] See: http://www.thewisegroup.co.uk
[8.] See: http://www.norwichleap.co.uk

References

Argyle, M. (1999) 'Causes and correlates of happiness', in D. Kahneman, E. Diener and N. Schwarz (eds) *Well-being: The foundations of hedonic psychology*, New York, NY: Russell Sage Foundation, pp 353–73.

Cambridgeshire County Council (2015) 'Formal consultation on the recommissioning of early help services (phase 2), children, families and adults services'. Downloaded from: http://www.cambridgeshire. gov.uk/download/downloads/id/4130/formal_consultation_on_ the_recommissioning_of_early_help_services.pdf [URL no longer available]

Campbell, T. and Keck, S.B. (2008) 'To be your own boss: enterprise and emancipation', in S. Keck and A. Buonfino (eds) *The future face of enterprise*, London: Demos, pp 127–37.

Clark A.E. (2001) 'What really matters in a job? Hedonic measurement using quit data', *Labour Economics*, 8(2): 223–42.

Clark, A.E. and Oswald, A.J. (1994) 'Unhappiness and unemployment', *The Economic Journal*, 104(424): 648–59.

Clark, A.E., Georgellis, Y. and Sanfey, P. (2001) 'Scarring: the psychological impact of past unemployment', *Economica*, 86: 221–41

Coles, B., Godfrey, C., Keung, A., Parrott, S. and Bradshaw, J. (2010) 'Estimating the life-time cost of NEET: 16–18 year olds not in education, employment or training', Department of Social Policy and Social Work and Department of Health Services, University of York.

Coles, S. (2008) *Does social entrepreneurship raise hope and optimism?*, London: Imperial College Business School.

Department for Business, Innovation and Skills (2011) 'A guide to legal forms for social enterprise'. Available at: https://www. gov.uk/government/uploads/system/uploads/attachment_data/ file/31677/11-1400-guide-legal-forms-for-social-enterprise.pdf

Diener, E. and Seligman, M.E.P. (2004) 'Beyond money: toward an economy of well-being', *Psychological Science in the Public Interest*, 5(1): 1–31.

Di Tella, R., MacCulloch, R.J. and Oswald, A.J. (2003) 'The macroeconomics of happiness', *The Review of Economics and Statistics*, 85(4): 809–27.

Elkington, J. and Hartigan, P. (2008) *The power of unreasonable people: How social entrepreneurs create markets that change the world*, Boston, MA: Harvard Business Press.

Future First (2016) 'Social mobility, careers advice & alumni networks'. Available at: http://files.futurefirst.org.uk/wp-content/uploads/ images/20170125092714/Future-First-Social-Mobility-Careers-Report.pdf

Helliwell, J.F. (2003) 'How's life? Combining individual and national variables to explain subjective well-being', *Economic Modelling*, 20(2): 331–60.

Impetus PEF (2014) 'Make NEETs History in 2014, London'. Available at: http://impetus-pef.org.uk/wp-content/uploads/2013/12/Make-NEETs-History-Report_ImpetusPEF_January-2014.pdf

Kahn, L., Abdo, M., Hewes, S., McNeil, B. and Norman, W. (2011) *The way to work*, London: The Youth of Today and The Young Foundation.

Layard, R. (2011) *Happiness: Lessons from a new science* (2nd edn), London: Penguin.

NEF (New Economics Foundation) (2004) 'The power and potential of well-being indicators: measuring young people's well-being in Nottingham', *The Power of Well-Being*, Report number 2.

ONS (Office for National Statistics) (2009) 'Working paper: Measuring societal wellbeing in the UK', Office for National Statistics.

ONS (2016) 'Young people not in education, employment or training (NEET), UK: Aug 2016, statistical bulletin', Office for National Statistics.

RSA (Royal Society for the encouragement of Arts, Manufactures and Commerce) (2013) 'A manifesto for youth enterprise', The RSA, London. Available at: https://www.thersa.org/discover/publications-and-articles/reports/a-manifesto-for-youth-enterprise-making-the-uk-a-better-place-to-start-up-a-business/

Social Enterprise UK (2015) 'Leading the world in social enterprise', State of Social Enterprise 2015, London. Available at: https://www.socialenterprise.org.uk/state-of-social-enterprise-report-2015

Social Research (2015) 'Consequences, risk factors, and geography of young people not in education, employment or training (NEET)', Scottish Government, January. Available at: http://dera.ioe.ac.uk/24628/1/00487865.pdf

Turner, D. (2008) 'Ministers' teenage problem improves', *The Financial Times*, 19 June. Available at: http://www.ft.com/cms/s/0/cf761e14-3e29-11dd-b16d-0000779fd2ac.html

Yunus, M. (2007) *Creating a world without poverty: Social business and the future of capitalism*, New York, NY: PublicAffairs.

FOURTEEN

Health and homelessness

Katy Hetherington and Neil Hamlet

Introduction

Homelessness is both a consequence and a cause of poverty and social and health inequality. It is also, in many cases, a 'late marker' of severe and complex disadvantage that can be identified across the life course of individuals (McDonagh, 2011). Poverty is a pervasive factor for those experiencing, and at risk of, homelessness, and with homelessness comes an increased risk of excess mortality. In Scotland, homeless people in Glasgow are 4.5 times more likely to die than their housed peers (Morrison, 2009). What, then, is the role of the National Health Service (NHS) and public services in preventing the severe health and social impacts of homelessness? This chapter reviews the opportunities to improve the health of homeless people and the challenge for the NHS, working with its partners, to play a full role in the prevention of homelessness. Through a better understanding of the diverse causes of homelessness and routes into and out of homelessness, public services can lead a collaborative approach to creating the right conditions for people to flourish. This can be summed up by the mnemonic we call 'the 5Rs', highlighting the individual and interdependent importance of 'Rafters', 'Relationships', 'Resources', 'Restoration' and, ultimately, 'Resilience' in the prevention and mitigation of homelessness. However, first, let us be reminded why homelessness is a public health and health equity issue.

Health and homelessness

Homeless people are not enjoying the right to the highest attainable standard of health, a right recognised within the European Convention on Economic, Social and Cultural Rights (Office of the High Commissioner for Human Rights, 2008). The right to health should be equally available, accessible, acceptable and of good quality to people experiencing homelessness. However, evidence demonstrates that homeless people experience poorer physical and mental health than the general population (Scottish Executive, 2005; St Mungo's, 2013; Homeless Link, 2014).

Homeless people have a much higher risk of death from a range of causes than the general population (Morrison, 2009). Many of the health conditions that homeless people develop in their 40s and 50s are more commonly seen in people decades older (Crisis, 2011). In 2013/14, the average age of death for a Crisis service user in Edinburgh was 36 years.

The most common health needs of homeless people relate to mental ill-health, alcohol abuse and illicit drug use, and dual diagnosis is frequent (Wright and Tompkins, 2006; Hwang and Burns, 2014). Violence, such as injuries, assaults and self-harm, is also a threat to the physical and psychological health of homeless people (Hwang, 2001; Fazel et al, 2014). Depression and suicides are higher among homeless people compared to the general population. Mental ill health is both a cause and a consequence of homelessness, as is alcohol and drug abuse (Edidin et al, 2012; Hwang and Burns, 2014). There is also a complex relationship between homelessness and offending, with an increase in the risk of homelessness for those who have spent time in prison and a lack of stable accommodation increasing the risk of (re) offending (Dore, 2005).

Homelessness adversely impacts children's health and well-being. Homeless children have higher rates of acute and chronic health problems than low-income children with homes (Council on Community Pediatrics, 2013). Children's development can be damaged and delayed by disruptions to important relationships and the failure to establish or maintain a familiar environment (Kirkman et al, 2010). Homelessness in childhood has been found to be part of most street homeless people's life histories, along with school or family problems, indicating the need to support families experiencing homelessness in order to avoid and break such patterns (Fitzpatrick et al, 2011; McDonagh, 2011). Homeless children are therefore a particularly vulnerable group, and unstable accommodation can result in difficulties for homeless families to access services (Rafferty, 2013).

In Scotland, there is currently a project to link homelessness data collected and reported to the Scottish Government by local authorities with NHS hospital data. This was first undertaken in Fife, where HL1 (a local authority statutory homelessness application data set) and local NHS hospital data were linked and analysed to identify the health-care experience of the local homeless population using routinely collected service data. It showed stark inequalities between the statutory homelessness population and the 'securely housed' general Fife population regarding the numbers of accident and emergency admissions, the age distribution of accident and emergency attendances, and also the number of multiple accident and emergency re-attendances (see Figure 14.1).

Figure 14.1: Accident and emergency attendance rate per 1,000 population: attendances at Queen Margaret Hospital and Victoria Hospital in Fife, Scotland

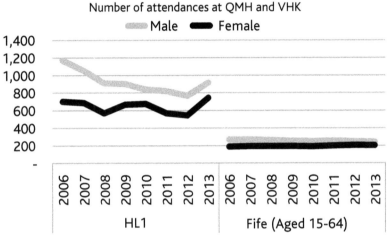

Notes: QMH = Queen Margaret Hospital; VHK = Victoria Hospital; HL1 = population who have made a formal application to Fife Council as homeless and can therefore be seen as experiencing 'insecure or no housing'; Fife = standard population of 'securely housed' Fife residents.

An all-Scotland data-linkage project reporting in 2017 will extend what has been done in Fife by linking all local authority homelessness data with a range of health data to quantify the use of health services over a 14-year period. It will categorically demonstrate the burden of the ill health and service costs of homelessness and how we need to reshape the provision of health care for the homeless population and reverse the inverse care law (Hart, 1971).

In summary, the research indicates that homeless households experience poorer physical and mental health, which can be exacerbated by continuing homelessness and insecure, poor living conditions. Mortality rates are higher, highlighting the extreme health inequalities experienced by this group. While a need therefore remains to mitigate the severe impact of homelessness on health and well-being, every opportunity must be taken to increase its prevention by better understanding the routes and key transition points into and out of homelessness.

Rafters – health is about housing; housing is about health

Scotland has a strong homelessness legislative framework, which has meant that from 2012, all people made homeless through no fault of their own have a right to settled accommodation. As well as the right to settled accommodation should a person become homeless, there is an emphasis on the prevention of homelessness through 'housing options' guidance to local authorities from the Scottish Government (2009). Recognition that the prevention of homelessness can save public finances is well known within the housing world, and with the data-linkage work being done with housing and health, there is the potential to demonstrate the cost of 'failure demand' within the health service (New Economics Foundation, 2008, cited in Department for Communities and Local Government, 2012a; Shelter, 2010). Local authorities have always had a specific requirement to prevent homelessness, recognising that such prevention will reduce pressure on other services, such as health, in the longer term.

The prevention of homelessness is also not new for the NHS in Scotland. National Health and Homelessness Standards were produced by the former Scottish Executive in 2005 (Scottish Executive, 2005). The Commission on Housing and Wellbeing (2015) restated the importance of good-quality, affordable housing in order for people to flourish throughout their lives. A number of recommendations were produced in the report and the response of the Scottish Government (2015a) welcomed the Commission's analysis that housing is fundamental for well-being, fairness and prosperity.

A house provides much more than shelter and safety; it is where, as a baby and in our early years, we can form and nurture relationships that can help or hinder us in life, and it provides us with links to the wider community in which we live, grow, work and age. The home is the bedrock salutogenic environment without which well-being cannot naturally grow and flourish.

Housing underpins the outcomes that the new Scottish Health and Social Care Partnerships must deliver to their local populations. Some partnerships, such as Glasgow City Council, have chosen to include homelessness within the remit of their Health and Social Care Partnership. This provides the opportunity to include homelessness services as part of front-line health and social care services. There remains an opportunity through integration to maximise the connections between housing, health and social care in order to ensure that those individuals and families affected by homelessness and at risk of homelessness are supported by all necessary agencies in novel and evidence-informed person-centred pathways.

Relationships

The provision of a homely setting from our earliest years is the environment within which we form meaningful relationships with our families and, indeed, ourselves. This takes us to the second 'R', which is 'Relationships'. It is such an environment that makes what we term a 'home'. The importance of bonding and responsive, predictable and caring relationships cannot be underestimated as these earliest experiences begin to hard-wire our developing brains for how we will navigate and relate our way into adult life (Bellis et al, 2014). Furthermore, it is the capacity to form, trust and keep relationships that impacts on the likelihood of later social difficulties that can spiral finally into a state of homelessness.

A deeper understanding of the psychodynamic roots of homelessness underpins approaches to both prevent homelessness and help those experiencing homelessness to rebuild those necessary relationships with self and others. There is increasing knowledge about the psychological and mental health problems that affect people experiencing homelessness, and in response to this, we have a growing awareness of the importance of providing psychologically informed services and environments (Breedvelt, 2016). There is also an evidence base around 'trauma-informed practice' that links closely to this theme. For the homeless, there are many histories of abuse, neglect and traumatic experiences in childhood (Fitzpatrick et al, 2011).

Similarly, the research around adverse childhood experiences and remove 'there is emerging' (Felitti et al, 1998). Adverse childhood experiences include direct experiences, such as abuse and neglect, as well as indirect experiences, such as living with a family member addicted to alcohol or drugs, in prison, or with a mental illness. Chronic stress from such experiences in the early years can affect development in childhood through to adulthood, leading to social, emotional and learning problems, health-harming behaviours and crimes, and, ultimately, an early death (Felitti et al, 1998). The work in Scotland to bring an increased focus to the prevention of homelessness, as well as psychologically informed service responses to homelessness, has therefore taken us right back to the critical early years of child development.

Distinguishing various routes into homelessness is helpful both for understanding its prevention and for service responses. For some people, homelessness may be a one-off occurrence due to a particular circumstance, which through an application to the local authority, can result in the housing need being met. Others may have more complex issues but can be supported into stable accommodation with the appropriate help. However, for those identified with the most complex issues or 'multiple exclusion homelessness' – a form of deep social exclusion including homelessness, mental health problems, drug and alcohol dependencies, street culture activities, and institutional experiences – homelessness can be the result of a number of issues that housing alone will not solve (Anna Evans Housing Consultancy, 2014). A large body of evidence has been building up on 'multiple exclusion homelessness' (Scottish Executive, 2007; McDonagh, 2011; Fitzpatrick, 2012). The complexity of issues faced by those experiencing 'multiple exclusion homelessness' raises important questions about how such complexity is best addressed by services and prevented in the future. The evidence that early childhood trauma can often be at the root of 'multiple exclusion homelessness' highlights the need to recognise this as an early sign of potential future homelessness, as well as poorer health in later life. It supports our argument that the ability to form positive and healthy relationships from the early years is a protective factor against future social difficulties that can lead to such forms of homelessness and social exclusion.

People who have a history of trauma may behave in a range of ways that mainstream services and staff can find challenging. Developing trusting relationships and managing emotions can be difficult for those who have experienced complex trauma in their lives. It is the relationship with care itself and, subsequently, how those providing care respond to how this manifests that can maintain the inverse care law. Supporting staff to understand the reasons for such behaviours through developing 'psychologically informed' environments can support a more constructive and creative approach (Department for Communities and Local Government, 2012b; Breedvelt, 2016). It is no surprise therefore to discover that a key success factor in many front-line services is the engagement of peer mentors, experts by experience and pathway navigators. Individuals who have personal experience of homelessness can be the best-placed volunteers or staff to truly engage with and help clients address their issues. The evidence for the success of 'Housing First' in Scotland points to the key role of such peer mentors in these pilot projects (Johnsen, 2014):

> For the moment, at least, the definitive marker of a PIE
> [Psychologically Informed Environment] is simply that, if

asked why the unit is run is such and such a way, the staff would give an answer couched in terms of the emotional and psychological needs of the service users, rather than giving some more logistical or practical rationale, such as convenience, costs or Health and Safety regulations. (Johnson and Haigh, 2010)

Therefore, an understanding of the importance of relationships (and past histories of damaged relationships) underpins both the required service response to the homeless client and also an approach to early intervention and preventive strategies for at-risk children and families.

Resources

Access to the resources that help us to live, learn, work, flourish and contribute to society is an essential part of living in a community and wider society. Poverty, often associated with homelessness, can be defined as a lack of access to resources, of which money is but one form. Lack of opportunity to access, or the ability to personally benefit from, resources such as education or employment, or, indeed, welfare benefits, is the third 'R' in the mnemonic. In order to access available societal resources, we need the building blocks of a secure home and trusting relationships from which we can benefit from education and other public services. The Adverse Childhood Experiences pathway proposes the links between early experiences and early death (Centers for Disease Control and Prevention, no date). Available money can also determine one's access to broader resources for life. Social inequity underpins the origins of homelessness. Therefore, it is action on social inequalities that is required if we are to prevent health inequalities (Dahlgren and Whitehead, 1991). Current understanding on the causes of health inequalities is shown in Figure 14.2.

A strategy to address homelessness as a significant health inequality will require action across all areas of the determinants of health inequalities: fundamental causes, environmental influences and individual experiences. Thus, the prevention and mitigation of homelessness requires an integrated approach that stretches from affordable social housing to investment in supporting parents and families, child development, education, employability, income maximisation, and social inclusion.

This is supported by a recent analysis, drawing on quantitative sources on experiences of homelessness in the UK, concluded that poverty, especially childhood poverty, was associated with later homelessness. It reported that '... homelessness is not randomely distributed across the population, but rather the odds of experiencing it are systematically structured around a set of identifiable individual, social and structural factors, most of which, it should be emphasised are outwith the control of those directly affected' (Bramley and Fitzpatrick, 2017: 17).

Figure 14.2: Health inequalities: theory of causation

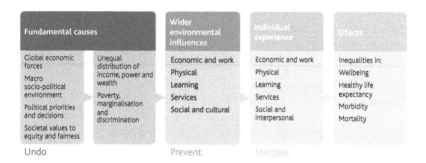

Source: © NHS Health Scotland (reproduced with permission)

The Scottish Government engaged in a national conversation during 2015/16 on what makes a 'fairer' Scotland and what steps need to be taken to achieve the vision of a fairer Scotland by 2030 (Scottish Government, 2015b). There is undoubted political commitment to social justice and tackling inequality, as reflected in the current Programme for Government (Scottish Government, 2016). The challenge has always been translating that into actions that deliver change for individuals, families and communities.

In summary, homelessness, and particularly repeat homelessness, is often an extreme form of social exclusion and inequality; the visible iceberg of a much larger issue of complex disadvantage lying below the waterline. Therefore, all policies that seek to address poverty (lack of resources for life) and health inequalities across the life course make an important contribution to the prevention of homelessness. Raising awareness and understanding about homelessness as a late manifestation of social and health inequity will help to make the life–course approach to its prevention more explicit.

Restoration

The fourth 'R' is 'Restoration' and reflects both the time, space and personal recovery that needs to take place in order for a homeless individual to recover sufficient personal agency to hold down a tenancy and regain a purposeful life. Life can be hard on all of us, and recovery, recuperation and regeneration are a necessary part of the human condition. Like sleep, it cannot be short-cut or made more efficient. Healing from life's daily knocks takes time, and the journey from homelessness back to well-being takes much more. Substance misuse and mental health services have led the research into the importance of the recovery journey. However, the principles and importance of fostering time, space and essential service continuity in the restorative journey of clients is equally valid for the homeless community, who often have multiple social and behavioural issues to address. 'Restoration' requires the underpinning provision of 'Rafters', 'Relationships' and 'Resources'; a safe secure place plus the trusting sustained therapeutic relationships of holistic support services and facilitated access to resources such as personal skills training, education, employability and sufficient finances are all necessary components of the restorative process. Inherent in this is the need for 'sticky services' that do not easily give up on clients, but 'stick' with them for as long as the healing process dictates for that person. This requires highly motivated and supported staff and re-emphasises the core value of taking a holistic psychologically informed approach to homelessness recovery.

The background to this approach stems from the 'Hard edges' report, which mapped severe and multiple disadvantage in England (Bramley et al, 2015). The term 'severe and multiple disadvantage' was used to signify the problems faced by adults involved in homelessness, substance misuse and the criminal justice system in England. It found considerable overlap between these three populations and highlighted the need for greater collaboration between these sectors as professionals are often working with the same people 'viewed through different lenses' (Bramley et al, 2015: 44). Poor educational achievement, experience of difficult family relationships and childhood trauma puts people at greater risk of severe and multiple disadvantage than others in similar circumstances of deprivation and poverty. This data-linking work highlighted the need for professionals to recognise that they are very often working with the same people, 'viewed through different lenses' but facing complex and highly disempowered and disconnected lives.

Service responses to this insight include the development of Housing First as the 'housing option' that has been found to deliver more effective outcomes for those with the most complex needs who have experienced difficulties in sustaining tenancies (Pleace, 2011, 2013). The main elements of the model are that a secure tenancy is provided as well as multi-agency 'sticky' support. It is important that sites identified for Housing First are scattered, and that support and the tenancy is maintained for the person regardless of behaviour such as substance misuse. Evaluations of the approach in Glasgow and Renfrewshire support international evidence that it provides the best model to resolve homelessness in around 80% of those with complex needs (Johnsen and Fitzpatrick, 2012). By providing a stable home for people to build their lives from, along with support that 'sticks' with the person, those with the most complex needs are being supported to overcome cycles of homelessness. As mentioned previously, peer support workers are recognised as a significant component of the Housing First model of recovery for the most multiply excluded homeless people to navigate support: 'People with complex needs are at serious risk of falling through the cracks in service provision. There needs to be an integrated response across health, housing and social care' (McDonagh, 2011: 1).

An important finding from the research by Fitzpatrick et al (2012), which has important implications both for service responses and for homelessness prevention, is that visible homelessness often happens very late, and following contact with non-housing services such as mental health, substance misuse and criminal justice. This finding highlights critical points in a person's journey into multiple exclusion homelessness and the opportunities for services such as mental health and substance misuse to identify those at risk of future homelessness and make provision for early preventive support.

All services need to respond to this new evidence with earlier detection of 'at-risk' individuals and families, and identify appropriate prevention pathways. In a report commissioned by Public Health England into the prevention of homelessness, engaging with schools, educational establishments and early years services by housing and health professionals was identified (Homeless Link, 2015). Such engagement can raise awareness and help to share effective cross-professional practice in identifying those at risk of homelessness and providing person–centred and sometimes assertive anticipatory support.

In Scotland, the revision of the role of school nurses provides a timely opportunity to embed homelessness prevention into school nursing, as well as protecting the health and well-being of children, young people and families experiencing homelessness. Similarly as council housing and homelessness services transition to a more preventive 'housing options' approach, there is an opportunity to embed new service styles into training modules for client-facing housing staff.

Resilience

The last 'R' is 'Resilience' and this develops when the other four 'Rs' are to be found in a person's life. Resilience captures the human capacity to take life's knocks, bounce back and carry on. It is the very lack of this capacity that leads individuals to spiral downwards through negative experiences and personal behaviours that can ultimately result in the state of homelessness. Thus, the building or rebuilding of personal resilience is the sum outcome of the recovery journey out of homelessness and its underlying social and behavioural drivers.

A focus on resilience also highlights the importance of taking an assets-based approach to the homeless client. The homeless individual is traditionally labelled by his or her problems or support needs. This can strip the client of dignity, self-worth and, most importantly, self-agency. An assets-based approach, however, chooses to emphasise the capabilities and potential of the person and seeks to build on their inherent personal strengths and abilities. This approach is evidenced in the success of the street soccer movement and Homeless World Cup initiatives (Homeless World Cup, no date).

Resilience and dignity are closely aligned to the rebuilding of a personal sense of self-worth. Thus, in the discourse of homelessness, there is a need to identify opportunities where an early intervention can avert a loss of dignity or foster a greater sense of personal value and capacity. We describe these as 'safety nets' and 'springboards', which communities and public services can provide to those at high-risk transition or trigger points in their lives.

The appropriate springboard or safety net will vary according to the circumstance but the timely provision of benefits for someone leaving prison is clearly a classic example of an appropriate safety net. The introduction by the Scottish Prison Service of 'Throughcare Support Workers' (TSOs) – prison officers who are assigned to work individually with short-stay prisoners from six weeks prior to their release and out into the community for up to three months post-release – is a good example of a 'springboard'-style service. The TSO will meet the released prisoner at the gate and accompany them through the complexity of the release day when applications for GP registration, temporary accommodation, welfare benefit claims and more are required to be set up.

There are a growing number of services that are taking an assets-based approach to rebuild resilience in those who have faced the indignity of homelessness. In turn, a number of those individuals have found new dignity, purpose and self-worth in acting as peer support workers and service navigators in homelessness services.

Summary

We are fortunate in Scotland to have such a strong rights-based legislative framework for the homeless. The current political commitment to increase affordable social housing, act on the recommendations of the Commission on Housing and Wellbeing and consult widely on a 'socially just Scotland' bode well for the policy environment that underpins the root social and economic determinants of homelessness. Inequity drives disadvantage and consequently health inequality, which is seen in its most extreme in the appalling health outcomes experienced by the multiply excluded homeless in our society. There are promising signs that with increased understanding about routes into homelessness and action to prevent adversity in childhood, we can prevent the negative causes and consequences of homelessness. New ways of working between health, social care and housing, alongside such partners as the Scottish Prison Service, Alcohol and Drug Partnerships, Employability Services and the Department for Work and Pensions (DWP), to name but a few, can empower us to prevent, intervene earlier and mitigate against homelessness.

References

Anna Evans Housing Consultancy (2014) 'Homelessness and complex needs in Glasgow'. Available at: www.aehousing.co.uk/uploads/ FINAL%20DETAILED%20ON%20AEHC%20WEB%2030.1.15. pdf

Bellis, M.A,.Hughes, K., Leckenby, N.,Hardcastle, K.A., Perkins, C. and Lowey, H. (2014) 'Measuring mortality and the burden of adult disease associated with adverse childhood experiences in England: a national survey', *Journal of Public Health*, 37(3): 445–54. Available at: http://jpubhealth.oxfordjournals.org/content/early/2014/08/30/ pubmed.fdu065.full

Bramley, G., Fitzpatrick, S., Edwards, J., Ford, D., Johnsen, S., Sosenko, F. and Watkins, D. (2015) 'Hard edges: mapping severe and multiple disadvantage', The LankellyChase Foundation. Available at: http:// lankellychase.org.uk/multiple-disadvantage/publications/hard-edges/

Bramley, G. and Fitzpatrick, S. (2017) 'Homelessness in the UK: Who is most at risk?', *Housing Studies*, DOI: 10.1080/02673037.2017.1344957

Breedvelt, J.F. (2016) *Psychologically informed environments: A literature review*, London: Mental Health Foundation.

Centers for Disease Control and Prevention (no date) *About the CDC-Kaiser ACE study*, Atlanta, GA: CDC. Available at: www.cdc.gov/violenceprevention/acestudy/about.html

Commission on Housing and Wellbeing (2015) 'A blueprint for Scotland's future'. Available at: http://housingandwellbeing.org/assets/documents/Commission-Final-Report.pdf

Council on Community Pediatrics (2013) 'Providing care for children and adolescents facing homelessness and housing insecurity', *Pediatrics*, 131(6): 1206–10.

Crisis (2011) *Homelessness: A silent killer. A research briefing on mortality amongst homeless people*, London: Crisis.

Dahlgren, G. and Whitehead, M. (1991) *Policies and strategies to promote social equity in health. Background document to WHO strategy paper for Europe*, Stockholm: Institute for Futures Studies. Available at: www.iffs.se/en/publications/working-papers/policies-and-strategies-to-promote-social-equity-in-health/

Dahlgren, G. and Whitehead, M. (2008) *Policies and strategies to promote social equity in health*, Copenhagen: World Health Organization.

Department for Communities and Local Government (2012a) 'Making every contact count: a joint approach to preventing homelessness'. Available at: https://www.gov.uk/government/uploads/system/uploads/attachment_data/file/7597/2200459.pdf

Department for Communities and Local Government (2012b) 'Psychologically informed services for homeless people: good practice guide'. Available at: http://www.rjaconsultancy.org.uk/6454%20CLG%20PIE%20operational%20document%20AW-1.pdf

Dore, E. (2005) *Insights: Prison leavers and homelessness*, Glasgow: IRISS. Available at: www.iriss.org.uk/sites/default/files/insight29_prisonleavers.pdf

Edidin, J.P., Ganim, Z., Hunter, S.J. and Karnik, N.S. (2012) 'The mental and physical health of homeless youth: a literature review', *Child Psychiatry and Human Development*, 43(3): 354–75.

Fazel, S, Geddes, J.R. and Kushel, M. (2014) 'The health of homeless people in high-income countries: descriptive epidemiology, health consequences, and clinical and policy recommendations', *Lancet*, 384(9953): 1529–40.

Felitti, V.J., Anda, R.F., Nordenberg, D., Williamson. D.F., Spitz, A.M., Edwards, V., Koss, M.P. and Marks, J.S. (1998) 'Relationship of childhood abuse and household dysfunction to many of the leading causes of death in adults. The Adverse Childhood Experiences (ACE) Study', *American Journal of Preventive Medicine*, 14(4): 245–58. Available at: http://www.ajpmonline.org/article/S0749-3797(98)00017-8/abstract

Fitzpatrick, S., Johnsen, S. and White, M. (2011) 'Multiple exclusion homelessness in the UK: key patterns and intersections', *Social Policy*, 10(4): 501–12.

Fitzpatrick, S., Bramley, G. and Johnsen, S. (2012) *Multiple exclusion homelessness in the UK: an overview of findings*, Briefing paper no 1, Edinburgh: Heriot-Watt University.

Hart, J.T. (1971) 'The inverse care law', *Lancet*, 1(7696): 405–12.

Homeless Link (2014) *The unhealthy state of homelessness: Health audit results*, London: Homeless Link. Available at: www.homeless.org.uk/sites/default/files/site-attachments/The%20unhealthy%20state%20of%20homelessness%20FINAL.pdf

Homeless Link (2015) *Preventing homelessness to improve health and wellbeing: Evidence review into interventions that are effective in responding to health and wellbeing needs amongst households at risk of homelessness*, London: Homeless Link. Available at: www.homeless.org.uk/sites/default/files/site-attachments/20150708.Public%20Health%20England%20-%20Rapid%20Review.pdf

Homeless World Cup (no date) 'Homepage'. Available at: https://www.homelessworldcup.org/

Hwang, S.W. (2001) 'Homelessness and health', *CMAJ Canadian Medical Association Journal*, 164(2): 229–33.

Hwang, S.W. and Burns, T. (2014) 'Health interventions for people who are homeless', *Lancet*, 384(9953): 1541–7.

Johnsen, S. (2014) 'Turning Point Scotland's Housing First project evaluation', Turning Point Scotland. Available at: www.turningpointscotland.com/wp-content/uploads/2014/05/TPS-Housing-First-Executive-Summary-2.pdf

Johnsen, S. and Fitzpatrick, S. (2012) *Turning Point: Scotland's Housing First project evaluation – interim report*, Edinburgh: Heriot-Watt University.

Johnson, R. and Haigh, R. (2010) 'Social psychiatry and social policy for the 21st century – new concepts for new needs: the "psychologically-informed environment"', *Mental Health and Social Inclusion*, 14(4): 30–5.

Kirkman, M., Keys, D., Bodzak, D. and Turner, A. (2010) '"Are we moving again this week?" Children's experiences of homelessness in Victoria, Australia', *Social Science and Medicine*, 70(7): 994–1001.

McDonagh, T. (2011) *Tackling homelessness and exclusion: Understanding complex lives*, York: Joseph Rowntree Foundation.

Morrison, D. (2009) 'Homelessness as an independent risk factor for mortality: results from a retrospective cohort study', *International Journal of Epidemiology*, 38(3): 877–83.

New Economics Foundation (2008) *Work it out: Barriers to employment for homeless people*, London: New Economics Foundation. Available at: www.yooyahcloud.com/MOSSCOMMUNICATIONS/p57s4/WORK_IT_OUT_-_Barriers_to_employment_for_homeless_people.pdf

Office of the High Commissioner for Human Rights (2008) 'The right to health', Fact sheet no. 31. Available at: www.who.int/hhr/activities/Right_to_Health_factsheet31.pdf

Pleace, N. (2011) 'Ambiguities, limits and risks of Housing First from a European perspective', *European Journal of Homelessness*, 5(2): 113–27.

Pleace, N. (2013) 'Consumer choice in Housing First', *European Journal of Homelessness*, 7(2): 329–39.

Rafferty, J. (2013) 'Homeless children and families in Edinburgh. Business case proposal', unpublished.

Scottish Executive (2005) 'Health and homelessness standards', Edinburgh. Available at: www.gov.scot/Publications/2005/03/20774/53761

Scottish Executive (2007) *A literature review on multiple and complex needs*, Edinburgh: Scottish Executive. Available at: www.gov.scot/Resource/Doc/163153/0044343.pdf

Scottish Government (2009) *Prevention of homelessness guidance*, Edinburgh: Scottish Government. Available at: www.gov.scot/Publications/2009/06/08140713/0

Scottish Government (2015a) 'The Scottish Government response to the recommendations of the Commission on Housing and Wellbeing'. Available at: http://housingandwellbeing.org/assets/documents/Scottish-Government-Response-to-Commission.pdf

Scottish Government (2015b) 'Fairer Scotland blog'. Available at: https://blogs.gov.scot/fairer-scotland/about-us/

Scottish Government (2016) *A plan for Scotland*, Edinburgh: Scottish Government. Available at: www.gov.scot/Resource/0050/00505210.pdf

Shelter (2010) *Value for money in housing options and homelessness services*, London: Shelter.

St Mungo's (2013) *Health and homelessness: Understanding the costs and role of primary care services for homeless people*, London: St Mungo's. Available at: www.mungos.org/documents/4153/4153.pdf

Wright, N.M. and Tompkins, C.N. (2006) 'How can health services effectively meet the health needs of homeless people?', *British Journal of General Practice*, 56(525): 286–93.

FIFTEEN

Local authority perspectives on community planning and localism: a case study

Joyce Melican

Introduction

"*One life-changing event away from homelessness*", said the facilitator as I was sitting in a training session while working at the London Borough of Croydon. That is my story in a nutshell; relationship breakdown and loss of home and job had sent me to my local authority in need of help with housing. As I had a three-year-old son, I was entitled to a home under the Housing Act 1985. While my case was investigated, I was put into temporary accommodation and, subsequently, given a secure tenancy.

My emotions on being rehoused are hard to describe. I was delighted and relieved, and could see a settled future for my son and I. In that instant, I realised that secure housing is the very foundation stone of society, and that without it, people are doomed to an insecure and unhealthy life. The brutal fact is that street homeless people die at a much younger age than the national average, and while the headline cause of these deaths is often drug and alcohol abuse, it is hard to oversee the chicken-and-egg nature of substance abuse and a lack of stable housing. Without a stable abode, many lack the self-respect and security to seek the treatment needed to overcome these lifestyle issues.[1]

Besides the obvious negative effects of rough or insecure sleeping, in a broader sense, family stability, mental and physical welfare, employment and educational opportunities, and a true sense of worth and belonging are essential prerequisites for a healthy and happy society. The cost implications of marginalising any section of society are great, and homelessness, as well as being hugely distressing and stressful to those suffering from it, has a ripple effect as it occasions expensive and time-consuming interventions. In short, it is less expensive to house people adequately and securely than it is to deal with them once they are on the streets.

When I returned to work in 1990, I went into a local authority housing office as a receptionist, quickly becoming fascinated by the subject, and began a career progression that took me through positions as a housing officer, a homeless persons officer, a residents participation coordinator and a housing project leader. Moving my way from the day-to-day groundwork into shaping policy at a council level, I gained a comprehensive view of the sector from the operational and the strategic perspective, deepening my knowledge by acquiring an advanced qualification in housing in the process.

Social housing policy: a brief history

In the immediate post-war years, 'council housing' was intended to be available to everyone who needed or wanted it. Yet, in the 1970s, there was a political sea-change in which it became considered the responsibility of the individual to provide for their own housing needs unless they are incapable of so doing. Thus, since 1977, entitlement to social housing in the UK has been needs-based, with 'priority need' originally defined in the Housing (Homeless Persons) Act 1977, while criteria have since been refined and expanded in England and Wales, as well as Scotland (where it was abolished altogether at the end of 2012) (see Chapter Fourteen). As a general rule, an applicant must belong to one of the following categories in order to be considered for a social-sector property:

- a pregnant woman;
- dependent children;
- someone vulnerable as a result of old age, mental illness or physical disability, or other special reason;
- someone homeless or threatened with homelessness as a result of an emergency, such as flood, fire or other disaster;
- aged 16 and 17 years old;
- aged under 21 years old who were in local authority care between the ages of 16 and 18;
- aged 21 and over who are vulnerable as a result of leaving local authority care;
- vulnerable as a result of leaving the armed forces;
- vulnerable as a result of leaving prison; and
- vulnerable as a result of fleeing domestic violence or the threat of domestic violence.

People in these groups frequently require intervention by social services, tenancy managers and estate managers to sustain their tenancies successfully; this makes providing social housing, by definition, an expensive and time-consuming service. There is no way around the issue, if social housing is not provided for these groups, they will be forced into precarious circumstances and will be afflicted by above-average rates of homelessness. Local authorities are acutely aware of this, both because of their statutory responsibilities to house those in need and because the knock-on effects of homelessness are visible in the communities they serve and the services they provide.

Nevertheless, the local authority perspective on housing is both complex and political. The shift in policy emphasis as a council changes from one party to another is palpable. On a broader level, until recent years, social housing has not been a priority for politicians and the electorate. It is expensive and has not yet been a vote-winner; indeed, it is only recently that the lack of affordable housing, in particular, in London and the South, has become the hot topic it is now.

The results of many years of neglect and underfunding have become abundantly clear as local authorities and housing associations struggle to reconcile an increase in demand and the statutory obligations placed on them by central government with an ever-decreasing housing stock. Yet, becoming a political priority does not make housing any less of a political football. The recent 'Housing White Paper' (DCLG, 2017) is symptomatic of the state that we are in: openly acknowledging that the entire housing market is 'broken' – an almost unprecedentedly candid admission – the White Paper closes by berating councils for not building more social housing. Given the unprecedented cuts to local authority funding since 2010 and the fact that Westminster policy is still forcing councils to shed stock, this is a staggeringly baseless exhortation.

This crisis has a wide variety of causes, which are – in my view as a housing professional – best summed up as follows:

- The loss of social housing stock through the Right to Buy (the original legislation made no provision to replace dwellings lost).
- The lack of political will, desire or motivation to ensure that remaining stock is maintained and increased, resulting in dwindling and poorly maintained dwellings.
- Light-touch regulation in the private rented sector. The Housing Act 1988 introduced – and later extended – the Assured Shorthold Tenancy, making it easier for landlords to repossess properties. While there will always be a tension between the rights of owners and tenants, there is now broad consensus that the pendulum has swung

too far in favour of landlords, creating a high degree of insecurity in the market. Rents have also risen to a very high level.

- The rise in house prices, putting home-ownership out of reach for many average earners.
- The incursion of free-market forces into social housing provision. Politically, it has long been considered opportune to transfer existing council stock to housing associations and to use development consortiums to regenerate housing estates. As government funding does not cover the full costs of regeneration, some properties need to be sold to finance projects, leading to a loss of local authority stock while sub-par compulsory purchase orders force many owner-occupiers to leave their areas (a particular issue in London redevelopments).

This last point is illustrative of the political consensus vis-à-vis social housing that has prevailed since the 1980s: every government from those of Margaret Thatcher through the New Labour years and into the recent Coalition and Conservative administrations has sought to channel social housing out of the public and into the private sector. At some times, this aim has been preserved by overt force as funding is cut severely; at others, there has been more carrot than stick as headline grants to local authorities were actually going up. Yet, the direction has never changed.

In 2000, for instance, the Blair/Brown governments set a target that they would:

> ensure that all social housing meets set standards of decency by 2010, by reducing the number of households living in social housing that does not meet these standards by a third between 2001 and 2004, with most of the improvement taking place in the most deprived local authority areas ... (Anon, 2000, ch 24, p 61, para 13)

It was, *prima facie*, a well-intentioned attempt to upgrade many ignored and dilapidated council estates; government money was to be spent on improving the living conditions of their residents. However, the language of what became known as the 'Decent Homes' target (NAO, 2010) was deceptively simple. The delivery models suggested to councils by the government were:

- using their own resources and those made available through the newly introduced major repairs allowance and the single capital pot;

- transferring their housing stock to one or more housing associations;
- setting up an arm's-length management organisation (ALMO); and
- pursuing a private finance initiative (PFI) scheme.

It was made clear to councils that there would be no extra funding available for authorities who selected the first option, effectively ruling out publically funded regeneration. The PFI option was considered and rejected by most councils (it had failed in the London Tube regeneration), so the options were narrowed to stock transfer or creating an ALMO so that they could apply for funding to implement the Decent Homes standards (Haringey Council, 2004).

Neither of these two options was particularly palatable to either local authorities or their residents, and yet there was no other way to secure funding. Despite the fact that these were the fiscally expansive New Labour years, funding to councils was, in real terms, stagnant; as such, the non-public options presented as choices – for which residents would be required to vote following extensive participation exercises – were, in reality, ineluctable.

At that time, I worked for the London Borough of Merton, which opted for the stock transfer option. This entailed consulting with residents, finding or creating a suitable housing association partner, and holding a referendum. Merton residents voted in line with council's suggestion for stock transfer, and so the stock was transferred, and funding obtained – at the price of the local authority losing control of its housing stock to another landlord.

Yet, complicated situations often arose. The London Borough of Sutton – the local authority for the Roundshaw Estate, on which I live – also consulted with and balloted its residents, with the result that the residents voted for stock transfer; the remaining Sutton residents, however, voted for the creation of an ALMO. It was felt that the remaining council-owned stock on Roundshaw should also be transferred in order to regularise the situation. The majority of the 1,900 homes belonged to Roundshaw Homes, partners in the regeneration under way at the time, and the remaining 681 were transferred.

The management of the remaining stock was passed to the management of the ALMO, Sutton Housing Partnership (SHP). The Decent Homes work was undertaken but not without difficulties. SHP was awarded its two-star rating (a prerequisite for Decent Homes funding) in 2010; however, by this stage, the political winds had changed and the Coalition government then deferred the funding until 2011. The Sutton Tenants and Residents Association, together with the local Liberal Democrat MPs, the leader of the council and Lord Graham Tope, lobbied long and hard for the funding.

They also announced that:

> Sutton Council has joined forces with four other councils and the Local Government Association to seek a Judicial Review of a Government decision to defer funding for their Decent Homes programmes for 2009/10 and 2010/11 together with not guaranteeing money in the following years.[2]

The funding was reinstated and the work was carried out.

The complexity of the process, however, lasting a full 12 years from the Decent Homes announcement to work being carried out, was bewildering to outsiders; in the process, the London Borough of Sutton was forced to divest itself of its housing stock. This is a story repeated in hundreds of local authorities across the country.

From Right to Buy to Pay to Stay

This was not however the first attempt to change the face and ownership of social housing, and it built on far-reaching changes to the legal framework under which councils provided social housing. The Thatcher government, for example, introduced compulsory competitive tendering (CCT), one of the key privatisation measures of the Conservative governments of 1979–97. This cost-saving measure changed how local authorities maintained their stock and introduced a high degree of uncertainty for providers in what had previously been a sector marked by long-term planning and consistency.

Pursuant to the shift to CCT, every housing department was obliged to tender to the private sector to supply services of all kinds (caretaking, repairs, etc). The process was closely overseen by Michael Heseltine, as Environment Secretary, and was not confined to housing. There were three rounds of tendering, and the council that I worked for at the time, the London Borough of Croydon, was in round three, with Sutton in round two. Sutton's service was won by Serco, but Croydon received no tenders, so had to retain its services in-house. However, Sutton Serco, the company set up specifically to win the tendering process, went on to fail, along with many other companies of its ilk, and the service was brought back in-house, only to be outsourced once again – along with the housing stock itself – a decade later (see earlier).

Aside from large-scale outsourcing initiatives and stock transfers, however, local authorities have been steadily losing stock due to the effects of another long-lived element of central government policy: the Right to Buy, enshrined in the Housing Act 1980 (Anon, 1980). The basic tenet of the Right to Buy – which survives more or less unchanged to this day – is that a secure social housing tenant may make an application to buy the property; the Act, however, makes no reference to the funding of the purchase – a crucial omission. It also, notably, did not ensure that the receipts from Right-to-Buy sales would be used to build more homes. While this failure to ring-fence the proceeds for replacement council housing is frequently – and not incorrectly – cited as the key flaw of the idea, it is worth noting that even in the Right-to-Buy boom conditions of the 1980s and 1990s, it is very unlikely that there would ever have been like-for-like replacement: the discounts applied by law to the sale prices would have meant that yields, even fully ring-fenced, would have been insufficient.

The first of these omissions has led to widespread abuse of the system. Intended to give tenants the right to buy their home, it has often turned tenants into willing or unwitting frontmen and women as others have put up the money to buy their heavily discounted home. There have even been situations in which family members have bought a tenant's home and gone on to evict their own kith and kin; there is also a flourishing market in companies offering tenants considerable sums of money to buy the house, which then passes into the company's ownership. The rent is raised, and when the tenant runs out of money, they are evicted for rent arrears; the home is then re-let at a very high rent. Frequently, the ex-tenants will apply to the council as homeless and in need of rehousing. The second omission has meant that the sector has lost approximately 1.5 million homes since 1980 without replacement; unsurprisingly, these lost dwellings tend to be the most desirable homes in the best locations, frequently family homes.

It is notable that, following a consultation in 2012, the Scottish Government has now abolished the Right to Buy; since its introduction in 1980, Scotland has seen approximately 500,000 social homes sold. The Welsh Assembly intends to bring a Bill in its next legislative session to do the same. This is a clear difference in policy from the current government, whose Housing and Planning Bill 2015 (DCLG, 2015) has extended the Right to Buy to all social homes – that is, including those transferred to or built by housing associations. In view of the widely acknowledged lack of social housing – and the evidence-based decisions taken in Edinburgh and Cardiff – it is hard to see those decisions as anything other than a political assault on social housing; it is even harder to see in the recent White Paper's berating of councils for not building enough homes anything more than naked cynicism.

Besides the flagship extension of the Right to Buy, the Housing and Planning Bill 2015 was passed with the stated intention of increasing the rate of house building and reversing the downward trend in home-ownership. Its other provisions include:

- starter homes for first-time buyers;
- lifetime secure tenancies to be phased out;
- councils to be obliged to sell off their high-value stock;
- 'Pay to Stay' to encourage higher-earning tenants to leave social housing; and
- councils to be required to have a local plan for increasing housing supply.

It should also be noted that the recent move by the government to force councils and housing associations to cut their rents by 1% a year from 2016/17 to 2019/20 has severely damaged their business plans; in a lot of cases, this will mean that the Housing Revenue Account will fall into deficit in coming years as tenants pay less while costs remain constant or increase. Examining each of these provisions in detail, it becomes clear that current government housing policy represents a clear and present danger to what remains of social housing provision:

- *Right to Buy extended to housing associations.* As has happened in the council sector, this can and will lead to a reduction in homes available for social housing. Housing associations are anxious about their future; there is also a probity issue in as much as the government is forcing charities and not-for-profit organisations to sell their assets, an unprecedented breach of ownership rights in a democratic society. The scheme is being piloted in five Housing Associations at present: L&Q, Riverside, Saffron, Sovereign and Thames Valley. It will run until January 2017, with an evaluation report expected in September 2016. No date for the extension has been announced.
- *Starter homes for first-time buyers.* First-time buyers aged 23–40 can apply for this scheme and are offered a 20% discount off one of the 100,000 starter homes to be specifically built. With the price in London likely to be about £400,000, the discount would be about £80,000. The money will come from reducing the section 106 monies due to councils from developers for improvements to an area affected by building work. This policy therefore further weakens local authorities' finances. Furthermore, by only imposing a

minimum of five years' ownership before the 20% funding is written off, the policy potentially creates an incentive for the first-time buyers to sell their discounted properties at a particularly handsome profit precisely five years and one month after signing.

- *Phasing out of lifetime secure tenancies.* In 2012, the government offered housing associations the discretion to offer fixed-term tenancies to new tenants. The take-up was very low and many councils decided against it as it was felt to be very detrimental to tenants who are, by definition, vulnerable. On a more practical note, it was felt that the administration of such a scheme would be extremely burdensome on departments that were cash-strapped and shedding staff. The Housing and Planning Bill makes it a duty for councils and housing associations to offer new tenants fixed-term tenancies only.

- *Councils obliged to sell off their high-value housing.* Councils are expected to sell off high-value homes and pass the proceeds to the government to fund the Right to Buy for housing associations. After opposition from the House of Lords, this was changed to impose a levy on councils to pay for their high-value stock. After this policy was announced, the National Housing Federation offered a voluntary scheme to the government, which was accepted as it solved some of the issues of compensation for the loss of properties, as well as the ability to refuse to sell some.

- *'Pay to Stay' for higher-earning tenants.* The original plan was to make it compulsory for tenants earning £40,000 per household in the London area, and £31,000 elsewhere, to pay a higher rent; the aim was to get them to vacate social housing in order to free it up for others in need and it may be seen as the flanking manoeuvre to the phasing out of lifetime tenancies. However, given the potential administrative chaos of trying to define household earnings in specific time frames and fix higher rents – not to mention the insecurity generated for higher-earning tenants and the economic disincentive to earn more – this policy has been quietly made discretionary and is unlikely to be enforced by many councils.

In a sector in which operational staff have learned to become grateful for small mercies, the shelving of this latter policy has been greeted by a mild form of rapture. Yet, as tempting as it might be to look for one, this is no sea-change, no genuine realisation dawning in Westminster that social housing has become perhaps the defining social issue of our day.

In 2012, many saw just such a sea-change in the government pledge to replace council homes sold under the Right to Buy. This meant, however, that local authorities would need to build 21,000 homes every year to achieve this goal, with no extra funding and only the low sales proceeds from homes sold (see earlier). From April 2015 to March 2015, the number of replacement homes built was 2,055.

In an attempt to increase the supply of social housing, local authorities are being forced to become creative. Sutton Council, for example, has set up a Local Authority Trading Company, called Sutton Living (Anon, 2015), which is in the process of acquiring land and planning permission for new homes. These companies, which have been set up by many councils, can trade as a commercial company but are wholly owned by the council, thus sidestepping the effective decades-long ban on local authorities owning stock imposed by the Right to Buy, CTT and the ineluctable ALMO/stock transfer route. Importantly, they can trade with other organisations beside the council, and as not-for-profit organisations, reinvest any surpluses that they do make. They are increasingly being seen as the model for delivery.

What is needed in housing policy

The need for social housing has not gone away. In fact, as property prices rise out of the reach of all but the highest earners and the private rental sector continues to benefit from light-touch regulation, it is increasing. Yet, the shrinking of the sector will result in those who require its services being pushed over the edge into homelessness and need, and the nigh-on inevitable downward spiral that this entails.

Recently, councils' supply of temporary accommodation for the homeless has become so scarce that families are being placed in 'out of borough' placements, often many miles from the home borough, with all the upheaval that brings to what is already a chaotic family situation. The situation has been exacerbated by the reduction of Local Housing Allowances, meaning that councils can only look at the lowest third of available accommodation to house the homeless (formerly, it was the lower half).

Increasingly, younger people in the volatile private rented sector either have to be helped out by their parents in order to buy or, if that is not possible, return home to try and save for a deposit. Patterns of residency that used to be the norm for young persons – that is, either buying a home in the early years of a career or moving into council housing if this option proved impossible – have become ever rarer.

Concurrently, besides the high costs of renting generally, landlords have become wary of tenants on housing benefit as payments are no longer made directly from authorities to the landlord, but to the tenant; as this group is, by definition, worse off and more vulnerable than those able to pay rent without state support, this effectively means that landlords are entering into a far greater deal of risk. They prefer to let to tenants with a proven ability to pay – who nevertheless have to pay some of the highest rents in the Western world relative to their salaries in an unregulated sector in which annual 'rent reviews' see the landlord's takings rise and push ever more tenants to the edge (and, potentially, into difficult circumstances that may, perversely, see them ending up as claimants of housing benefit).

So, what about the future? It is, to put it mildly, highly unlikely that we will see a return to the social housing heyday of the 1960s, with the construction and provision of council properties in an upward cycle of expansion. Both in my view and that of most experts and practitioners, the recent Housing White Paper does not help the situation in the least as it does little to address any of the most pressing needs, namely:

- a significant increase in the provision of financial resources for social housing;
- acknowledgement of public sector housing staff (both culturally and financially) in order to stop the negative recruitment spiral;
- a reduced focus on home-ownership at the expense of affordable rented accommodation;
- real sanctions to prevent the practice of 'land banking' – that is, speculatively withholding building plots in expectation of increasing prices (and thereby helping to push prices up);
- increased protection for tenants in the private sector from ever-rising rents and unscrupulous landlords; and
- reform of a housing benefit system that actively encourages private landlords to overcharge.

Beyond idle talk, the 2017 Housing White Paper (DCLG, 2017) offers no concrete measures on any of these issues. The sharp decline in the supply of social housing that I have experienced since the beginning of my career looks set to continue; combined with constant cuts to subsidies, this decline has created a situation in which local authorities are now struggling to fulfil their legal obligations and being forced ever deeper into the private sector in an attempt to satisfy the needs of their residents.

Housing our population is a matter of huge concern, and I fear that the effects of the drive to home-ownership and the relentless political pressure towards the private sector have resulted in huge personal gain and healthy profits for some while ignoring the needs of the most vulnerable and helpless in our society. A glance at social housing websites will show that my view is all too prevalent at the present time. It saddens me that, as a society, we feel able to allow this to happen. It seems hard to avoid the conclusion that if all the money and energy that had been sunk into these privatisation initiatives had been put into the provision and maintenance of housing stock, we may well have more available housing than we do now. The thrust towards privatisation has been constant, and continues unrelenting.

The mark of a civilised society is how it treats its poor and vulnerable, and the current landscape does not bode well for this group. If we choose to ignore their housing needs, we not only push them ever further towards the edge, but, in the long-term, increase the cost to society as interventions from various agencies to try and contain and control their difficulties become very expensive.

It is hard to see how I would have been able to have a successful second career and send my son to one of the world's top universities without the stable home that I was given when I most needed it. In other words, if I were 30 years younger, I fear that my life – and that of my son – may have taken a very different path.

Notes

1. See: http://www.crisis.org.uk/data/files/publications/Homelessness%20kills%20 -%20Executive%20Summary.pdf
2. See: http://researchbriefings.files.parliament.uk/documents/RP94-40/RP94-40. pdf

References

Anon (2000) 'Spending Review: Public Service Agreements'. Available at: http://webarchive.nationalarchives.gov.uk/20121013052506/ http://archive.treasury.gov.uk/sr2000/psa/psa.pdf

Anon (2015) 'Sutton Living Ltd'. Available at: https://beta. companieshouse.gov.uk/company/09897512/officers

DCLG (Department for Communities and Local Government) (2015) 'A decent home: definitions and guidance. 200DCLG: Housing and Planning Bill'. Available at: http://services.parliament.uk/ bills/2015-16/housingandplanning.html

DCLG (2017) 'Housing White Paper'. Available at: https://www.gov. uk/government/collections/housing-white-paper

Haringey Council (2004) Report to Haringey Council, November, https://www.minutes.haringey.gov.uk/Data/Cabinet/20041221/ Agenda/$Item%2014%20Decent%20Homes%20and%20Stock%20 Options%20Appraisal%20Appendix%20D.doc.pdf)

NAO (National Audit Office) (2010) 'The Decent Homes programme'. Available at: https://www.nao.org.uk/report/the-decent-homes-programme/

Housing (Homeless Persons) Act 1977, c 48. Available at: www.legislation.gov.uk/ukpga/1977/48/pdfs/ukpga_19770048_en.pdf

Housing Act 1980. Available at: www.legislation.gov.uk/ukpga/1980/51

Housing Act 1988. Available at: www.legislation.gov.uk/ukpga/1988/50/contents

Part Five
Supporting people at the edge of the community

Education, employment and housing services, as noted in previous sections of this book, promote the development of healthy individuals and communities. People with complex needs require support from statutory and third sector health and social service agencies. This section will provide an insight into the needs of people with mental health and cognitive disabilities. These needs are often associated with housing needs and limited access to appropriate health and social care. The multiple complex needs of homeless people include mental health, substance misuse, relational problems and skill deficits. Providing support for these often disengaged people has many challenges due to the problems of lack of collaborative working between the tiers of local government, the National Health Service (NHS) and the third sector. The development of 'Inclusion Health' pathways into primary care is an innovative approach, underpinned by an understanding of the psychological dimensions of both those who are homeless and those providing support for the homeless.

SIXTEEN

Towards an integrative theory of homelessness and rough sleeping

Nick Maguire

Introduction

The reasons why people become and remain homeless are complex; this is perhaps why, in the 21st century in a highly developed industrial society, we still have people living and dying on the streets. A single solution has not yet been found; nor is it likely to be, given the wide range of factors implicated in rough sleeping specifically and homelessness generally, as well as the multiple populations who are considered to make up the 'homeless'.

Referring to 'homelessness' itself is an issue. There is a danger of oversimplifying the understanding of the issue in terms of a single population of people and therefore a single set of causes and effects. There are, of course, many issues that lead people to become homeless, the differences being idiosyncratic depending on the people and circumstances involved. For many, deprivation, poverty and financial issues may conspire to make sustaining housing all but impossible. For others, it may be that the housing situation was untenable because of domestic violence. For others, it may be that an inability to sustain rent payments due to funding drug addiction results in eviction. The term 'homeless' is therefore applied to a highly diverse group of people who are defined only by where they are, or are not, found.

This chapter will briefly cover a number of the main psychological factors theorised to be implicated in the causation and maintenance of homelessness. It is not possible to cover all factors in depth, but the point is to highlight them in enough detail that a model may be developed, which is presented near the end of this chapter. First, however, we need to consider what a good theory or model may do.

A useful theory

Any useful theory or model in this area needs to be useful enough to have predictive as well as explanatory power, but also needs to be loose enough to encompass the diversity of experience leading to homelessness, including different levels of factors, from genetic to societal influences. This chapter develops such a theory, which may then be useful in unpacking the psychological factors and concomitant interventions that may be useful in enabling people to break out of behavioural patterns that maintain a cycle of rough sleeping and homelessness.

Factors at different levels

A starting point is to consider factors that impact on the likelihood of people becoming and staying homeless on a number of levels by making use of a framework increasing in 'reductionism'. Reductionism involves describing phenomena in terms of increasingly small 'building blocks', or fundamental aspects of that phenomenon. In terms of homelessness, the most reductionistic level at which we could start at may be a genetic one, which influences individual differences in terms of, for example, emotional reactivity. Behaviour could be described in terms of neurological connections and innervated muscles, and emotions in terms of cortisol, adrenaline or endocrinal factors. This may be useful for some questions (eg around cognitive dysfunction, brain injury, etc) but can never fully or even partially account for why people become and stay homeless. Further down a reductionistic continuum, we can make use of psychological models, which more broadly consider cognitive and emotional content and processes rather than using a neurological perspective. This will be the focus of Chapter Seventeen and so will not be covered in detail here. Still less reductionistic may be more macro-factors, for example, environmental, policy and societal factors, such as housing quality, housing quantity, economic policy and structural factors like those that affect geographically specific poverty (see Bramley et al, 2015).

A psychological approach to homelessness

Psychology is the scientific study of mind and behaviour; it stresses the interaction between the individual and their environment. Applied psychology, among other things, seeks to understand human problems within psychological frameworks, which may lead to empirically testable theories and interventions that may be evaluated in terms of how effective they may be.

Interaction between the environment and the individual

This is a particularly useful way of thinking when attempting to account for why people become and remain homeless. For many years, the dominant model accounting for homelessness has been a housing one, and homelessness numbers certainly do seem to correlate with housing availability to some extent (Park, 2000). However, this masks a number of issues, such as the different subgroups of people who become homeless, linked to the reasons that they become homeless in the first place. For example, families who become homeless may be suffering problems linked to economic or other structural and societal issues, such as employment, redundancy and poverty. Their immediate need is for secure and affordable housing. However, many single homeless people may have been provided with a tenancy, private or otherwise, and may not have been able to maintain it due to adverse situations relating to isolation or exploitation and other issues associated with mental health problems. The issue here is much more complex, with only one aspect being the appropriateness of the housing solution. It may be that the mental health issues suffered involve the use of illegal substances, of which the landlord may or may not become aware. Awareness of such illegal activity would invariably lead to loss or threat of loss of that tenancy.

Therefore, the provision of housing is just one factor in the increasing likelihood of a person becoming and staying homeless. For many single people, the things that they do and whether these behaviours contravene tenancy rules may also contribute to homelessness. Of course, it is not just single people who may be evicted due to rule-breaking; families may also experience tenancy loss through this route. Families are inherently complex systems that add another dimension to the set of factors that result in homelessness. We will now move on to consider, first, single homeless people and the way in which they interact with their environments, making use of psychological theories, frameworks and research to propose an overall model of this interaction.

The psychology of environment–individual interaction

A psychological approach is ideally suited to describing an interactional way of thinking. People 'construct and construe' their environments (Safran and Segal, 1996), meaning that they not only perceive, or form beliefs about, what is going on around them, but also behave in ways to shape their environment. As an example, in interpersonal relationships, this is simply described as perceiving (having thoughts about) what others are saying (or doing) and why they are saying (or doing) it. An attempt is made to elicit reactions that make sense to the individual, thereby making the world more predictable and less anxiety-provoking. Mental health problems, particularly those associated with childhood adversity, will shape the way in which people experience and perceive the world. This will be dealt with in more detail later. A useful metaphor to describe this interaction is the idea that we are dealt a hand of cards, in terms of being born into a particular environment, that shape one's early life (see Chapter One). It is then up to us how we play that hand, limited or full as it may be. Psychological (or other) interventions may augment the skills that people have in playing that hand.

Environmental factors

The effect of environmental and contextual factors will briefly be covered before moving on to psychological factors. There is a significant evidence base around the effect of the design of the built environment on mood and behaviour, particularly in health settings (for a detailed consideration, see: http://ebdjournal.com). Physical environments and the geography in hostels and private rented accommodation may have a significant effect on, for example, isolation, the maintenance of negative beliefs about self and others, and so on.

It is therefore useful to think about how different environments may interact with particular behaviours, particularly those associated with severe and enduring mental health problems (eg complex trauma experiences and adult diagnoses of personality disorder). There may be some environments in which some behaviours are tolerated, whereas in others, they are not. For example, one way of guiding organisational responses to drug-use behaviours is with a risk policy. Conservative risk policies may mean that such behaviours, even if covert, result in punitive consequences. Factors that may generally govern the conservatism in risk policies and residence rules may be the physical environment, staffing levels and expertise, the inclusiveness of the organisation mission statement, and so on.

Psychological factors

Assuming that homelessness is an interaction of individual and environmental factors, as argued earlier, it is possible to theorise about those individual factors and the behavioural components that are implicated in tenancy loss. If we assume that there are basically two reasons why tenancies are lost – that is, (1) people 'abandon' (leave) their residence or (2) they are evicted – we may be able to formulate (describe) the reasons why this happens, making use of psychological frameworks. Theories of attachment are covered in detail elsewhere; what follows is a very brief description of some of the main points (for detailed coverage, the reader is particularly directed to Mikulincer, Shaver and Pereg [2003]; see also Chapter One of this book).

We have reasonable evidence from a number of sources which indicates that a high proportion of people who are homeless have suffered significant childhood trauma, including physical, emotional and sexual abuse and neglect (eg Simons and Whitbeck, 1991). This is associated with adult presentations that may be diagnosed within a medical model as personality disorder, or described in a more useful way as complex trauma (eg Herman, 1992).

A significant issue for people who have experienced trauma as children is that attachment systems may be disrupted. Horowitz, Rosenberg and Bartholemew (1993) usefully reconceptualise Bowlby et al's (1989) original taxonomy of avoidant, anxious, disorganised and secure attachments along two dimensions, formulating the experiences that may lead to higher or lower avoidant and/or anxious attachment. The theory is that high on both aspects may be understood as 'disorganised' in that aspects of both sets of coping behaviours are evident, but not in any strategic way. Low on both aspects is conceptualised as a more secure attachment style.

Other evidence-based theories then link attachment to the capacity to regulate emotions (Mikulincer et al, 2003), expressing attachment as an evolved emotion-regulation strategy. Modern humans give birth to peculiarly immature young when compared to our primate cousins in that they cannot crawl or cling, or even see properly in the first few months of life. In our evolutionary past, they were therefore vulnerable to predation and needed constant attention in order to survive. The theory is that attachment is the process that drives proximity or closeness between mother[1] and baby; if they are separated, they both experience high anxiety that is only abated on reunification. Thus, attachment is an evolved survival process in that emotion regulation (calming) through mother–young proximity drives that proximity and increased rate of survival. A failure to attend to the expressed emotion of a distressed baby, or an unpredictable response, may therefore result in later experiences of 'others' not being sources of safety and calm (avoidant attachment), or a constant uncertainty of whether others will be available (anxious attachment) and difficulties developing the skills to regulate emotions internally. What follows in adult life are attempts to cope with difficult emotions via extrinsic means, typically ingesting substances or self-harming to change the internal emotional state (for coverage of these processes and their links with a number of mental health problems, see Aldao et al, 2010).

Psychological therapies that have a focus on enabling the development of emotion-regulation skills are particularly useful in this area. There is a sizeable research base for the effectiveness of dialectical behaviour in this area, as well as a National Institute for Health and Clinical Excellence guideline (NICE, 2009) specifying dialectical behaviour therapy (DBT) where self-harming associated with emotion regulation is a target for therapy. It may also be that therapies that directly target the attachment experience may be useful, though there is no evidence yet supporting this mechanism of change.

Attachment and interpersonal issues

Attachment difficulties do, of course, also have a highly detrimental effect on interpersonal relationships. This has been well documented and is the focus of many psychological therapies. The difficulties may be mediated by three main processes: (1) attachment itself and the sense of safety and closeness felt when in the presence of people who we trust or otherwise feel close to; (2) the content of thoughts in terms of beliefs about what others think about us, what they may do and whether they are a threat or not (this is covered in more detail later); and (3) cognitive processes that govern the way in which we 'process' information about ourselves and the world.

A great deal of literature details the sense of safety associated with the attachment process as important (eg Bowlby et al, 1989). This will not be detailed here, but, briefly, it is theorised that securely attached children are able to take risks when they have a predictably safe 'base' in the form of an attentive parent. This generalises to other situations, including interpersonal behaviours later in life, when trusting that another will not behave contrary to one's needs becomes important in establishing functional relationships. Avoidant attachments may result in lack of affection or difficulty in attending to the needs of others;

anxious attachment may result in difficulties in trusting others, over-controlling and checking behaviours, and so on.

In any case, establishing and maintaining long-term relationships may be difficult for people who have suffered trauma in childhood, resulting in difficult emotions and coping behaviours that result in negative feedback and vicious cycles, which maintain the original difficulties. This theoretical approach is exemplified in Chapter Twelve, which contains self-reports from two homeless people (see also the case study in Chapter Fifteen).

Cognitive functioning

Evidence indicates that people who are homeless suffer a range of cognitive difficulties, associated with a range of factors that affect brain function. Heavy drinking, particularly when associated with a poor diet, may result in Korsakov's Syndrome, seriously affecting memory and other cognitive functions (eg Darnton-Hill and Truswell, 1990). Traumatic brain injuries (TBIs) are common (Oddy et al, 2012), having occurred before people became homeless but also as a result of being vulnerable to attack or injury on the street. Impulsivity is an issue, particularly engaging in risky behaviours that may lead to harm or illegal behaviours. This may be associated with frontal lobe syndrome (again associated with TBIs and/or alcohol or substance abuse) or impoverished early environments as skills in the consideration and articulation of consequences are not learned. This set of issues is reviewed in Chapter Eighteen.

Negative beliefs

We have clinical evidence that fundamental ways of thinking about oneself and the world (cognitive content) are implicated in the maintenance of behaviours that may be implicated in homelessness. At a fundamental level, clinical and theoretical evidence indicates a prevalence of negative core beliefs about self, such as being worthless, unlovable, inferior, vulnerable, a failure and bad (eg Safran et al, 1986). The cognitive model accounts for these as being related to early experience and governing the way in which people perceive the actions of others and resultant coping behaviours. This simple framework is useful in understanding the internal world of those who may have suffered traumatic childhoods. If someone has a fundamental belief that they are a failure and inferior, reinforced by repeated messages to this effect from parents and teachers, they may not engage in activities that risk 'activating' this core belief and the concomitant negative emotions. Thus, they may avoid work or training opportunities as these are the kinds of situations that may be interpreted in black-and-white terms as success or failure and are unlikely to be seen as successful. These kinds of avoidance behaviours may, in turn, be incomprehensible to staff, who may, of course, not see the individual's belief leading to them, but just the loss of a recovery opportunity.

Ellis's (1977) Antecedents, Beliefs, Consequences (ABC) model (see Table 16.1, with the previous example used) is a simple way of understanding the cognitive model, formulating the relationship between perceptions about the world and resulting behaviours and emotions. This is invaluable to both service users and staff to understand their internal world.

Table 16.1: ABC cognitive model

Activating event	Belief	Consequences
Work placement organised for Monday morning	'I'll fail' 'People will think I'm stupid, incompetent' 'I'm a complete failure, will never succeed at anything'	*Emotions:* Anxiety, fear, embarrassment
	'They shouldn't do this, they know I'll fail'	Anger, frustration *Behaviours:* Drink heavily on Sunday night, don't turn up to appointment

Source: Ellis (1977)

Summary

To summarise, theory and early research evidence indicate that early childhood trauma is prevalent in populations of people who are homeless, and that this is related to attachment difficulties. Early trauma is also associated with difficulties in regulating emotions and impulses, compounded by fundamental negative views of self, which are, in turn, linked with asocial behaviours that may lead to loss of tenancy through eviction or abandonment. Impairments in cognitive functioning may be an additional problem for some. Interpersonal relationships are negatively affected by early experience, which may also contribute to behaviours that lead to tenancy breakdown. These issues are just some of the factors that may contribute to a possible pathway to homelessness; there are many other factors that have not yet been targets of research.

Proposed model of repeat homelessness

Taking all of the factors discussed earlier, it is possible to propose a model that explicitly links macro, societal factors through psychological, mediating factors to those around the individual. It can be seen that the way in which people have been taught to experience the world in terms of early traumatic experience leads to an increased likelihood of behaviours that may lead to tenancy breakdown of one form or another. Once the behaviours have been identified, a number of interventions become possible.

As has been iterated, psychological factors in themselves are not deemed wholly responsible for homelessness, but rather identify one possible pathway into homelessness, taking into account macro- and micro-factors.

Figure 16.1: A proposed model of repeat homelessness

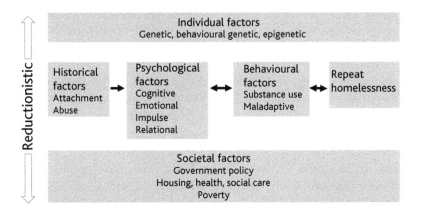

Figure 16.1 represents the macro–micro continuum between societal and individual factors that may be implicated in homelessness. Psychological factors associated with early traumatic abuse are theorised to be linked to a range of behaviours that have been found to be linked to repeated tenancy breakdown and homelessness. Psychological factors

resulting from trauma experience are therefore positioned as providing a link between the person and their context.

As discussed earlier, the model is deliberately simplified for ease of use, but is intended to be complex enough to enable some form of predictive value. It perhaps does not yet have the status of a formal theory as there may be many factors to consider, but as a model, it does make use of evidence, allows an understanding of a possible pathway into homelessness and enables some prediction of the kinds of behaviours that may be manifest. It is the identification of these behaviours and the factors that may underpin them that may be useful in developing interventions.

Psychological interventions

By focusing on the behaviours that lead to homelessness, we may adapt existing psychological interventions to suit the needs of homeless people. However, we also need to build in, where appropriate, treatments for predisposing factors (such as ongoing reactions to complex trauma) and the related antecedents to particular maladaptive behaviours (eg negative beliefs about others' intentions, difficulties in coping with rejection, significant people leaving, etc).

DBT has an excellent theory and language that, in part, focuses on the acquisition of skills such as emotion regulation and the management of relationships, as well as cognitive skills by making use of mindfulness techniques (Linehan, 2014). The problem of homelessness being ameliorated by the acquisition of new skills seems a very hopeful narrative, which moves away from one which blames either the individual or society. The basic formulation leading to an understanding of maladaptive behaviours is that people will choose external ways of regulating emotions if they were not able to develop them in childhood. So, the function of such behaviours is primarily an emotion-regulation one, although, for example, social, care-eliciting and identity functions may also serve to maintain the behaviours (for a comprehensive coverage of these ideas, see Gross and Thompson, 2007). The intervention that follows is the teaching of such skills, meaning that at least some functions are served with more adaptive behaviours. The issues are complex, of course, and other interventions may be needed, such as community or inpatient care.

Cognitive behaviour therapy (CBT) (eg Westbrook et al, 2011) has an excellent language around thought content and processes, which may be particularly useful if people react quickly to what they think are others' negative intentions. 'Urge-surfing' (ie recognising an urge to behave in an unhelpful way and staying with it until it passes) is a phrase common to both DBT and CBT. Many forms of CBT also enable the individual to develop metacognitive awareness skills (the ability to think about what one is thinking), question the validity of thoughts and/or notice helpful and unhelpful ways of thinking. Testing out beliefs with behavioural experiments is a change process that is concrete and easily learned. The cognitive practice of mindfulness has become popular in itself and as part of cognitive-behavioural interventions, which although perhaps more abstract than cognitive content challenge, many people understand and like.

Both of these models focus on clear behavioural and emotional change, which is obviously significantly stressed in the model. A key intervention that is sometimes neglected, however, is one that will support engagement in the process of change. Both do have languages and techniques designed to engage, but arguably they are not as well developed as that of motivational interviewing (MI) (Miller and Rollnick, 2012).

MI is a non-directive counselling technique based on the sound, empirically validated self-determination theory (Deci and Ryan, 2008). It has a particularly well-developed language for working with people at the 'pre-contemplative' stage of change (Prochaska and DiClemente, 1992), that is, when change seems unimportant or perhaps hopeless, and motivation to engage in behavioural change is low.

By making use of interventions that have strengths at different stages of change and/or that have a good, empirically sound theoretical reason for being effective, we may increase the effectiveness of psychological therapies. The model described earlier may help with the focus of therapies given the complexity of many of the issues faced by homeless people. Keeping in mind behaviour change as the ultimate goal of interventions may be part of this process.

Measuring outcomes and economic evaluation

When considering behaviour change, it is important to focus on a specific component in the evaluation of the impact of any intervention. The sector as a whole does not have a well-developed literature on research and evaluation. A contributory factor here may be the complexity of the issues and identifying outcomes that are meaningful, for both the organisation and also the individual. The use of a realist approach, reviewed in Chapter Twelve, provides an opportunity to understand what works for whom, where and when.

Measures of behavioural incidence rates, that is, how often a behaviour with a prosocial or asocial consequence occurs, may provide a partial solution. If an individual is enabled to discuss what they are doing that is getting in the way of where they want to be (assuming that they are actively 'contemplating' change), they may identify target behaviours that can be counted over time (eg behaviours that result in arrest, hospitalisation, eviction, etc). If an individual tends to be involved in violent behaviour and work is done to enable the person to reduce these behaviours, both the individual and the organisation may be able to describe success. The individual is able to see progress on something that they have highlighted as problematic, and the service is able to gather data on reduction in, for example, antisocial behaviours. The organisation may then aggregate these reductions across the population of people they work with to count average reductions for a given time period.

Furthermore, the costs of many consequences of asocial behaviours are known. For example, the costs of arrest, hospital days, psychiatric hospital stays, ambulance calls and emergency department visits are all known. Any reductions in the cost associated with these behaviours may be calculated across a population, thereby demonstrating financial return on investment.

Most people work in this area as they want to contribute, and such economic evaluation may or may not be meaningful. However, at an organisational level, demonstrating success is becoming more essential. The provision of such data may help commissioners make evidence-based decisions on how to commit increasingly scarce resource. Arguably, robust evaluation and data-driven commissioning are two of the most significant factors in driving up the quality of homelessness services on a national level.

Conclusions

It is argued here that a psychological approach, generating an understanding of the relationship between the individual and their environment, may be useful in understanding the behaviours that lead to homelessness and rough sleeping. It acknowledges that answers are not to be found in either a sociological view or individual one, but in understanding the interaction. Engagement in this complexity and making use of empirically based theory and practice are essential if we are to make significant progress in reducing homelessness. This chapter has proposed a model that may make these complexities clear, and has utility in that sense. It may also propose research questions around the links between traumatic experiences and later behaviours that lead to and maintain homelessness.

Note

1. In our evolutionary past, it would have mainly, but perhaps not exclusively, been the female giving care. Arguably, the pressures in our language-mediated, post-industrial society are different and men may equally be primary attachment figures.

References

Aldao, A., Nolen-Hoeksema, S. and Schweizer, S. (2010) 'Emotion-regulation strategies across psychopathology: a meta-analytic review', *Clinical Psychology Review*, 30(2): 217–37.

Bowlby, J., May, D.S. and Solomon, M. (1989) *Attachment theory*, Lifespan Learning Institute.

Bramley, G., Fitzpatrick, S., Edwards, J., Ford, D., Johnsen, S., Sosenko, F. and Watkins, D. (2015) 'Hard edges: mapping severe and multiple disadvantage', The LankellyChase Foundation. Available at: http://lankellychase.org.uk/multiple-disadvantage/publications/hard-edges/

Darnton-Hill, I. and Truswell, A.S. (1990) 'Thiamin status of a sample of homeless clinic attenders in Sydney', *The Medical Journal of Australia*, 152(1): 5–9.

Deci, E.L. and Ryan, R.M. (2008) 'Self-determination theory: a macrotheory of human motivation, development, and health', *Canadian Psychology/Psychologie Canadienne*, 49(3): 182.

Ellis, A. (1977) 'The basic clinical theory of rational-emotive therapy', *Handbook of Rational-Emotive Therapy*, 1: 3–34.

Gross, J.J. and Thompson, R.A. (2007) 'Emotional regulation: conceptual foundation', in J.J. Gross (ed) *Handbook of emotional regulation*, New York: Guilford Press, pp 3–24.

Herman, J.L. (1992) 'Complex PTSD: a syndrome in survivors of prolonged and repeated trauma', *Journal of Traumatic Stress*, 5(3): 377–91.

Linehan, M.M. (2014) *DBT® skills training manual*, New York: Guilford Publications.

Mikulincer, M., Shaver, P.R. and Pereg, D. (2003) 'Attachment theory and affect regulation: the dynamics, development, and cognitive consequences of attachment-related strategies', *Motivation and Emotion*, 27(2): 77–102.

Miller, W.R. and Rollnick, S. (2012) *Motivational interviewing: Helping people change*, New York: Guilford Press.

NICE (National Institute for Health and Clinical Excellence) (2009) *Borderline personality disorder: Treatment and management*, CG78, London: National Institute for Health and Clinical Excellence.

Oddy, M., Moir, J.F., Fortescue, D. and Chadwick, S. (2012) 'The prevalence of traumatic brain injury in the homeless community in a UK city', *Brain Injury*, 26(9): 1058–64.

Park, J.Y.S.H. (2000) 'Increased homelessness and low rent housing vacancy rates', *Journal of Housing Economics*, 9(1/2): 76–103.

Prochaska, J.O. and DiClemente, C.C. (1992) 'Stages of change in the modification of problem behaviors', *Progress in Behavior Modification*, 28: 183.

Horowitz, L.M., Rosenberg, S.E. and Bartholomew, K. (1993) 'Interpersonal problems, attachment styles, and outcome in brief dynamic psychotherapy', *Journal of Consulting and Clinical Psychology*, 61(4): 549.

Safran, J. and Segal, Z.V. (1996) *Interpersonal process in cognitive therapy*, Oxford: Jason Aronson, Incorporated.

Safran, J.D., Vallis, T.M., Segal, Z.V. and Shaw, B.F. (1986) 'Assessment of core cognitive processes in cognitive therapy', *Cognitive Therapy and Research*, 10(5): 509–26.

Simons, R.L. and Whitbeck, L.B. (1991) 'Sexual abuse as a precursor to prostitution and victimization among adolescent and adult homeless women', *Journal of Family Issues*, 12(3): 361–79.

Westbrook, D., Kennerley, H. and Kirk, J. (2011) *An introduction to cognitive behaviour therapy: Skills and applications*, Oxford: Sage Publications.

SEVENTEEN

Mental health and multiple exclusions

Claire Luscombe

Introduction

Throughout history, health (or, more specifically, poor health) and exclusion have been intrinsically linked. From the leper, to those inflicted with venereal disease, to the mad confined to 'Ships of fools', to the poor and the homeless, 'the game of exclusion', as Foucault (1972: 6) called it, has linked these two concepts, with the result that over the centuries, people have been confined in buildings or places where they all have been treated in 'oddly similar fashion[s]'. These social inequalities in health arise because of inequalities in the conditions of daily life and because of the fundamental drivers that give rise to them, that is, inequalities in power, money and resources (Wilkinson and Marmot, 2003). Mental health is a key component to this process of exclusion.

The World Health Organization defines mental health as 'a state of well-being in which every individual realizes his or her own potential, can cope with the normal stresses of life, can work productively and fruitfully, and is able to make a contribution to her or his community' (WHO, 2011). Mental health (or, more specifically, mental ill health) is a significant societal problem in the UK, accounting for 23% of the total burden of ill health; it is also the largest cause of disability. Annually, £2 billion is spent on social care for people with mental health problems and the cost of mental health to the economy in England alone has been estimated at £105 billion, with treatment costs expected to double over the next 20 years (HMG and DH, 2011).

Poor mental health is both a contributor to and a consequence of exclusion. It is well established as a significant risk factor for poorer health and economic and social outcomes (the level of adversity of these outcomes varying with the disorder and socio-economic status of the individual in question), as well as a direct cause of mortality and morbidity (Friedli, 2009; IHME, 2013).

Good mental health is a vital component of an individual's capabilities, resilience and capability to adapt; it enables them to manage adversity and reach their full potential. Good mental health and resilience are fundamental to our physical health, relationships, education and work. In fact, it is essential to all aspects of an individual's self and potential, and, as such, has wider social and economic effects. It is therefore a key aspect of facilitating inclusion (see Chapter Nineteen). Individuals with mental health problems are less likely to be able to sustain themselves in employment, particularly when there is high unemployment (McNaught and Bhugra, 1996).

Defining multiple exclusions

Multiple exclusion is a concept that progressed from the idea of deep exclusion, which itself evolved from New Labour and their championing of social exclusion. The term 'deep exclusion' was first introduced by David Miliband in a speech given in 2005 (Miliband, 2006: 6). Individuals are in deep exclusion if they experience exclusions over multiple dimensions. The first significant government initiative to tackle this issue was the Adults Facing Chronic Exclusion (ACE) programme initiated by New Labour and run between 2007 and 2010. Following this, there has been no direct successor commissioned by central government, in no small part due to the localism agenda; however, there have been key strategies such as *Social justice: Transforming lives* (DWP, 2012a) and the follow-up *Social justice outcomes framework* (HMG and DWP, 2012), in which a key element is providing 'support for the most disadvantaged adults' (HMG and DWP, 2012: 7). These strategies relate to homeless people, offenders, those with mental health problems and drug and alcohol dependency, and those in debt (MEAM and RDA, 2011). This term, along with 'multiple disadvantage adults' (referring to individuals or families who experience low income, poor health or no qualifications) (HMG/DWP, 2012), has been used increasingly to describe disadvantaged groups.

More recently, individuals have been identified as having multiple needs and exclusions. In its vision paper, the Making Every Adult Matter Coalition (2009) identified those with multiple needs and exclusions as being any individual facing multiple problems who has ineffective contact with services, and who, as a result, has a chaotic lifestyle. Factors such as mental ill health, homelessness, drug and alcohol misuse, offending and family breakdown have been identified as key issues. What is known is that most individuals who are experiencing multiple needs and exclusions are to be found in either the prison or the homeless population (MEAM, 2009), although there is no universal definition of what and who makes up this group of individuals, despite there being requests for statutory bodies to agree one (MEAM and RDA, 2011, 2012). Critically, the 'multiple needs and exclusion' group is growing. Across England alone, 60,000 people are thought to be facing multiple needs and exclusion (MEAM, 2009: 8).

Homelessness has been theorised to be an extreme form of exclusion (Pleace, 1998) and has been given a central role within the multiple excluded group (McDonagh, 2011). Since most individuals who find themselves with multiple needs and exclusions are known to be within this population (MEAM, 2009), understanding their needs and exclusions seems critical to any improvement in their well-being and situation. However, the issue of homelessness is not just one of having no home. The complex needs of those individuals affected mean that it is not just a case of giving homeless people somewhere to live. Homeless people are among the most marginalised in our society and experience varied and challenging issues. Factors such as the associated lack of social networks and inferior cognitive functioning largely associated with mental health problems, substance misuse and psychotic disorders influence both the experience of homelessness and the likelihood of a successful resettlement.

For a majority of the 'homeless', their homelessness should not be the dominant issue of need. Homeless individuals with mental health disorders need all their issues to be given equal attention, not just the visible presenting need of having no house. This is a mindset that needs to be re-evaluated across the sector.

Understanding which factors of exclusion could indicate mental health disorders is useful when looking at the development of needs assessments, not only at a local level for services to identify client need, but also at the commissioning level to identify service needs. There needs to be awareness about the interactive nature of exclusion factors and the mental health of homeless people, and the resulting requirement for needs assessments that embrace not only the health and social care needs of the individual, but also the wide domains of relationships, criminal and antisocial activity, and individual factors, as well as negative childhood and lifetime experiences.

Research about people experiencing homelessness

Despite the extensive developments in both exclusion and mental health policy, there is a scarcity of research on their impact on and interaction with each other. Nor is there much robust evidence of mental health need within the homeless population and the impact of multiple exclusions on successful recovery. Wright and Stickley (2013) found only 36 studies eligible for review, and while they acknowledge the limitations of their study design (using only English-language papers and requiring mental health and social exclusion to be explicit terms used within the papers' keywords), this dearth of robust studies is unexpected. They further found there to be little research to support the conceptual development of what is meant by the terms 'social exclusion/inclusion' within the field of mental health and very little work on practice-based interventions (Wright and Stickley, 2013). Curran et al (2007) carried out a systematic review of the literature on mental health and social exclusion. The authors reported that any conclusions made in their review about the links between social exclusion and mental health were limited by the diversity of approaches used in defining social exclusion in the selected studies and by the complexity of the concepts being defined (of the 1,000 studies randomly taken from their initial screening, only 72 were found by them to be of sufficient rigour). They felt that the review was further compounded by the cross-disciplinary nature of the topic (Curran et al, 2007). Their review summarises the issues and problems arising from the use of social exclusion well and perhaps outlines why it has encountered such difficulties in establishing itself as fundamental concept. It touches so many disciplines of research, not only within the social sciences, but also across clinical and treatment settings, that it is hardly surprising that consensus is difficult.

It should be noted that there is a substantial amount of research on mental health and the specific dimension of exclusion, investigating its causal and treatment effect, but its authors have simply not classified it as being research into the broader concept. Examples include research on mental health and employment (Bartley, 1994; Kiely and Butterworth, 2013), social networks (Corrigan and Phelan, 2004; Kogstad et al, 2013) and family relationships.

When considering the health needs of homeless individuals, researchers often acknowledge in their writings the poor physical and mental health that characterises this population (Wright and Tompkins, 2006; Morrison, 2009; Fitzpatrick-Lewis et al, 2011). The most common health needs reported among its members are drug and alcohol dependence and mental illness, with co-occurring disorders being frequent (Griffiths, 2002; Wright and Tompkins, 2006).

Common physical health conditions among the homeless include chronic obstructive pulmonary disease, musculoskeletal disorders and arthritis. Diabetes, anaemia and hypertension are often managed ineffectively, and respiratory tract infections are very common. Intravenous drug-using homeless individuals will also have disorders commonly associated with injecting, for example, deep vein thrombosis and blood-borne viruses such as hepatitis (Hwang, 2001; Wright et al, 2004). Poverty, delays in seeking treatment, noncompliance with treatment, cognitive impairment and the unfavourable conditions of the homeless lifestyle are all factors that are known to contribute to these disorders and to the severity of illness experienced by homeless people (Wood, 1992).

Prevalence of mental health disorders within the population

Despite being acknowledged as a common health disorder, the prevalence of reported mental health issues within the homeless population varies significantly (Fazel et al, 2008). This is a reflection both of Fitzpatrick and Christian's (2006) observation regarding weak quantitative research and also of the different understandings expressed in studies on mental health regarding what being homeless actually is. This was certainly a finding of the research by Fazel et al (2008), who carried out a systematic review of the literature, investigating the prevalence of mental disorders among homeless people in Western countries. It is important to note that of the 29 studies identified, only eight had been carried out in the UK, the most recent of which had been conducted in 2000 on homeless individuals in Glasgow (Kershaw et al, 2000). When investigating further, the most recent study carried out across the widest geographical spread within the UK was that by Gill et al (1996), which was carried out across Great Britain (Northern Ireland was excluded). Coincidentally, this is the last major study recognised on homeless individuals within the UK (Fitzpatrick et al, 2013). This demonstrates how infrequently robust studies are commissioned within the UK into this population.

In part, this is likely because the needs of homeless people are thought to be well known; however, the true complexity of these individuals is very much underplayed. In her recent PhD, Luscombe (2015) investigated factors of social exclusion and their association with mental health disorders within people experiencing homelessness as part of the Collaborative Study into Homeless People (CoSHoPe). As part of this study, the prevalence of mental health disorders found within the homeless population under investigation was compared with the psychiatric mobility survey's findings within the general population (McManus et al, 2009). It was further compared to the study by Gill et al (1996) (see Table 17.1). These results clearly demonstrate this increased prevalence of mental health disorders within the homeless population (CoSHoPe data collection was completed within 2008/09) and the significantly higher prevalence compared to the general population although carried out during the same period (Luscombe, 2015).

Table 17.1: Prevalence of mental health disorders within the general population compared to homeless individuals within Gill et al (1996) and CoSHoPe's populations (2008/09)

Disorder	General population (McManus et al, 2009)	Homeless (Gill et al, 1996)	CoSHoPe (2008/09) (Luscombe, 2015)
Psychiatric illness	0.4	4	5.8
Depressive episode	2.3	12	20.9
Alcohol dependence	5.9	16	33.5
Drug dependence	3.9	11	25.4
Common mental disorders (CMDs)	16.2	–	38.4

Why is understanding multiple exclusions important?

How to work effectively with these individuals is a key concern. Not only do those with mental health issues experience discrimination and hence exclusion because of their mental ill health, but they also experience exclusions if seeking services for other health conditions. It is acknowledged that when dealing with the most disadvantaged:

- services focus on single presenting needs to the exclusion of multiple needs;
- contract culture induces providers to 'cream off' those easier to help, even within high-need groups;
- some easier-to-manage needs are prioritised over others, regardless of the impact on the individual; and
- by their very nature, these individuals are chaotic and so their engagement with services is episodic and often driven by their immediate needs (McNeil, 2012).

This pattern has a substantial impact on their life expectancies (Rethink, 2013), with the annual cost of unscheduled care for the homeless estimated to be eight times that of the housed population (Hewett et al, 2012). Whether at an individual or at the service level, unmet need is central to this, and identifying this need is critical to reducing unnecessary economic and social burden.

Multiple excluded individuals need services that are tailored to their needs, of which having nowhere to live is just one. Exploring how exclusion indicators are associated within this group would seem to be very beneficial, particularly in relation to developing an appropriate needs assessment for this group. As with many concepts within social policy, definitions adopted very much depend on the motivation and priorities of the governments or bodies attempting to address the issue. As stated previously, multiple exclusion is one such concept, as was social exclusion (a forerunner to this concept), where there is no definitive definition and hence no agreed indicators or markers explaining it (Levitas, 2006). Therefore, to explore this, Luscombe (2015) drew from the work of Percy-Smith (2000), who carried out an extensive review of social exclusion in 2000, as well as work done by the Multiple Exclusion Homelessness Research Project (Fitzpatrick et al, 2011, 2013), and identified 21 markers of exclusion from these. In Table 17.2, the factors identified are listed, as are the percentages of people experiencing homelessness that reported having experienced them.

In reviewing Table 17.2, the depth of the issues and nature of the difficulties for people experiencing homelessness can be clearly seen. This is a very complex population of people.

Implications for service delivery

In considering services, understanding the effect of these interactions seems very important, particularly when considering the effects that this may have on the severity and range of needs that a person presents to services with, and the subsequent 'treatment' pathway provided. Quality assessment is central to this. Services are needed that not only place the emphasis on the individual and their health needs, but are also tailored to the homeless client group. Individuals with these multiple needs, however, are too often being defined by their 'societal' need or issue (eg being an ex-prisoner, homeless, a substance misuser, unemployed). Within the key policy issue areas of substance misuse and criminal justice, there is wide acceptance of the need for holistic health services and comprehensive assessments of need, with alcohol

Table 17.2: Percentage of homeless individuals who reported having experienced each of the social exclusion markers

Factor	% of individuals	Factor	% of individuals
Never worked	6.9	Loss of self-esteem/ confidence	49.4
Never been employed for more than six months	18.4	Any institutional care (combined)	61.7
No reported positive relationship with parents in childhood	18.5	Positive for substance misuse (diagnostic)	23.8
No current contact with own children	40.4	Ever arrested and charged with anti-social behaviour or any anti-social activity	40.0
No positive relationship with close family now	13.3	Any distressing event within your life	71.5
First-time homeless	51.5	Exposure to violent injury	36.9
Ever arrested and charged with any violent crime	55.2	Homeless before the age of 18	24.8
Ever arrested and charged with any non-violent crime	63.0	Survivor of abuse or neglect during childhood	53.2
Left school with no qualifications	37.5	Suspended from school ever	44.0
Ever been to prison	54.2	Any experience of the care system	9.8
Ever treated in a psychiatric hospital	23.8		

treatment (NICE, 2011), drug treatment (NICE, 2001) and criminal justice (Day, 2010) being key areas of public health concern. However, homeless individuals are not afforded the same health and social care provision or assessment as the general population. Multidisciplinary services and assessments are needed for these complex individuals that cover both health and social care issues in their widest context. It could be argued that the fact that an individual has nowhere to live is one of the easier exclusionary factors to resolve (admittedly, keeping them in their home might be more complicated). Perhaps this is why so much focus is placed on this aspect of homelessness to the detriment of other issues; as noted by Widdowfield (1999), homelessness is visible, and providing temporary hostel accommodation is quite a simple, quick-win solution.

When working with homeless individuals, health services have been dominated by policies and legislation in relation to the management of risk, resulting in services being focused on criminal justice and crime prevention (Joly et al, 2011). Drug services offer the best example of this. Policies have been enacted in which the police and law enforcement agencies are taking the lead within services, with the result that both the individual's health and public health are being neglected (RSA, 2007). The problem is that despite the belief that there is common understanding between professionals and services, the concept of integrated care has not been clearly defined or completely understood (Eyrich et al, 2008), and one could argue that this lack of understanding could be partly due to insufficient awareness of the needs of homeless individuals. Assessment is key to this understanding and the assessment must encompass the multidimensional needs of the individuals.

The way out of exclusion is to promote inclusion. For those with mental health issues, inclusion begins when there is engagement and benefit from statutory and non-statutory support structures and services. Inclusion involves more than support, however; belonging and participating in the community are key aspects (Bonner, 2006). The importance of an individual participating in society cannot be underestimated, nor can the healing potential of this action; indeed, non-participation is recognised as a risk factor in poor mental health (RCP, 2009).

A key component of this participation for successive UK governments is the emphasis on work as a means to participation. For some, however, the emphasis that the government is placing on 'work' as the route out of exclusion is perpetuating the very issues that they are trying to escape. So, too, are the 'conditionality and sanctions' being enforced on this group as a result of welfare reform, not only because of their economic impact, but also because of the political discourse (which labels the homeless as part of a 'moral underclass') attached to them. A disproportionate number of homeless people are subject to sanctions (31% of homeless people compared to 3% of other claimants) (Homelesswatch, 2013). However, there is evidence to suggest that the majority of homeless people want to work but face a number of barriers that prevent them from doing so, and those most excluded are least likely to be able to gain access to sustained employment (Singh, 2005). Consideration must certainly be given to the impact that an individual's mental ill health will have on their ability to meet the requirements placed on them. While there has been an increasing awareness of the role that mental health has on job exclusion (DWP, 2012b), for many homeless individuals, their welfare status is not appropriate for their 'health' status.

Within the homeless sector, it is housing support workers within the voluntary sector who provide a large proportion of support to these individuals. Cornes et al (2011) reviewed the interagency working practices of services working with multiple excluded homeless people. Their study mirrored Cameron's (2010) findings regarding the breadth of work carried out by housing support workers because they said other professionals have retreated from this client group. This has to stop; without appropriate support, this complex group will only get bigger and more complex. The prevalence of mental health disorders has previously been demonstrated to have increased (Luscombe, 2015). The uncomplicated homeless have been rehoused due in no small part to programmes such as Supporting People, which has been credited with radically changing the delivery and assistance offered to some of the most vulnerable within society (Homelesslink, 2013). Those that are left should have the support of a multidisciplinary team of professionals able to meet their complex needs, rather than that of a single housing worker filling a gap. With the reforms to the Health and Social Care Act 2012 (see Chapter Twenty-two), Health and Wellbeing Boards (HWBs) are central to this, not only because of their role in commissioning services, but also because of the multidisciplinary make-up of the board itself. However, the decisions made by HWBs are informed by joint needs assessments, and without good-quality information on this client group, relevant services will not be commissioned.

Concluding remarks

As a sector, there is a need to accept the need for quality data. Education about the importance of quality data and the consequences of not having this, particularly with the reforms to health and social care provision, need to be understood. Homelessness should be (properly) recognised as a public health concern, with the resulting funding and robust reporting requirements placed upon it. Services need to be routinely linked to primary health-care provision and not, as all too often happens for this client group, only when a crisis occurs. It needs to be noted that there are already very good examples of specialist treatment services for the homeless that work effectively with complex individuals; indeed, this was noted in a recent review commissioned by the Department of Health investigating the use of primary health services by the homeless (St Mungo's, 2013). An example of good practice in this sector includes double-length appointments to enable the assessment and treatment of the broad range of needs that are presented (St Mungo's, 2013). Interestingly, however, the most pertinent finding from this review indicated that while successful models exist, data to demonstrate effective outcomes and financial benefit were not routinely collected, and as a consequence, there is no evidence to inform commissioning (St Mungo's, 2013). A more robust means of data collection is needed and this needs to be addressed not only within these services, but also across the homeless support sector as a whole, and as a sector, services need to recognise the need for quality assessments. The breadth of the exclusionary issues that homeless people face and the complexity that this brings to their potential well-being requires services adequate and appropriate to needs. The sector needs to embrace and take responsibility for this, which historically there seems to have been a reluctance so to do; it seriously needs to develop appropriate evidence-gathering processes for service development and the assessment of individuals' needs.

References

Bartley, M. (1994) 'Unemployment and ill health: understanding the relationship', *Journal of Epidemiology and Community Health*, 48: 333–7.

Bonner, A. (2006) *Social exclusion and the way out: An individual and community response to human social dysfunction*, Chichester: John Wiley and Sons.

Cameron, A. (2010) 'The contribution of housing support workers to joined-up services', *Journal of Interprofessional Care*, 24: 100–10.

Cornes, M., Joly, L., Manthorpe, J., O'Halloran, S. and Smyth, R. (2011) 'Working together to address multiple exclusion homelessness', *Social Policy and Society*, 10: 513–22.

Corrigan, P. and Phelan, S. (2004) 'Social support and recovery in people with serious mental illnesses', *Community Mental Health Journal*, 40: 513–23.

Curran, C., Burchardt, T., Knapp, M., Mcdaid, D. and Li, B. (2007) 'Challenges in multidisciplinary systematic reviewing: a study on social exclusion and mental health policy', *Social Policy & Administration*, 41: 289–312.

Day, E. (2010) *Routes to recovery via criminal justice: Mapping user manual*, London: The National Treatment Agency for Substance Misuse.

DWP (Department for Work and Pensions) (2012a) *Social justice: Transforming lives*, London: Department for Work and Pensions.

DWP (2012b) 'Working for wellbeing in employment: a toolkit for advisers'. Available at: https://www.gov.uk/government/uploads/system/uploads/attachment_data/file/49878/mh-toolkit.pdf (accessed 17 September 2013).

Eyrich, K.M., Cacciola, J., Carise, D., Lynch, K. and Mclellan, A. (2008) 'Individual characteristics of the literally homeless, marginally housed and impoverished in a US substance abuse treatment seeking sample', *Society of Psychiatry and Psychiatric Epidemiology*, 43: 831–42.

Fazel, S., Khosla, V., Doll, H. and Geddes, J. (2008) 'The prevalence of mental disorders among the homeless in Western countries: systematic review and meta-regression analysis', *PLoS Med*, 5: e225.

Fitzpatrick, S. and Christian, J. (2006) 'Comparing homelessness research in the US and Britain', *European Journal of Housing Policy*, 6: 313–33.

Fitzpatrick, S., Johnsen, S. and White, M. (2011) 'Multiple exclusion homelessness in the UK: key patterns and intersections', *Social Policy and Society*, 10: 501–12.

Fitzpatrick, S., Bramley, G. and Johnsen, S. (2013) 'Pathways into multiple exclusion homelessness in seven UK cities', *Urban Studies*, 50: 148–68.

Fitzpatrick-Lewis, D., Ganann, R., Krishnaratne, S., Ciliska, D., Kouyoumdjian, F. and Hwang, S. (2011) 'Effectiveness of interventions to improve the health and housing status of homeless people: a rapid systematic review', *BMC Public Health*, 11: 638.

Foucault, M. (1972) *History of madness*, London: Routledge.

Friedli, L. (2009) *Mental health, resilience and inequalities*, Copenhagen: World Health Organization.

Gill, B., Meltzer, H., Hinds, K. and Petticrew, M. (1996) *OPCS surveys of psychiatric morbidity in Great Britain report 7 – Psychiatric morbidity among homeless people*, London: HMSO.

Griffiths, S. (2002) *Addressing the health needs of rough sleepers: A paper to the Homelessness Directorate*, London: HMSO.

Hewett, N., Halligan, A. and Boyce, T. (2012) 'A general practitioner and nurse led approach to improving hospital care for homeless people', *BMJ*, 345, doi: https://doi.org/10.1136/bmj.e5999

HMG (Her Majesty's Government) and DH (Department of Health) (2011) *No health without mental health: A cross-government mental health outcome strategy for people of all ages*, London: Department of Health.

HMG and DWP (Department for Work and Pensions) (2012) *Social justice outcomes framework*, London: Department for Work and Pensions.

Homelesslink (2013) 'Supporting people'. Available at: http://homeless.org.uk/supporting-people#.UiNEiCBwZdg

Homelesswatch (2013) 'A high cost to pay: the impact of benefit sanctions on homeless people', London.

Hwang, S. (2001) 'Homelessness and health', *Canadian Medical Association Journal*, 164: 229–33.

IHME (Institute for Health Metrics and Evaluation) (2013) *The global burden of disease: Generating evidence, guiding policy*, Seattle: Institute for Health Metrics and Evaluation.

Joly, L., Goodman, C., Froggatt, K. and Drennan, V. (2011) 'Interagency working to support the health of people who are homeless', *Social Policy and Society*, 10: 523–36.

Kershaw, A., Singleton, N. and Meltzer, H. (2000) *Survey of the health and well-being of homeless people in Greater Glasgow. Summary report*, London: National Statistics.

Kiely, K.M. and Butterworth, P. (2013) 'Social disadvantage and individual vulnerability: a longitudinal investigation of welfare receipt and mental health in Australia', *Australian and New Zealand Journal of Psychiatry*, 47: 654–66.

Kogstad, R., Mönness, E. and Sörensen, T. (2013) 'Social networks for mental health clients: resources and solution', *Community Mental Health Journal*, 49: 95–100.

Levitas, R. (2006) 'The concept and measurement of social exclusion', in C. Pantazis, D. Gordon and R. Levitas (eds) *Poverty and social exclusion in Britain*, Bristol: The Policy Press.

Luscombe, C. (2015) 'Mental health and social exclusion in people experiencing homelessness: the case for improved assessment', PhD dissertation, The University of Kent.

McDonagh, T. (2011) *Tackling homelessness and exclusion: Understanding complex lives*, York: Joseph Rowntree Foundation.

McManus, S., Meltzer, H., Brugha, T., Bebbington, P. and Jenkins, R. (2009) *Adult psychiatric morbidity in England, 2007: Results of a household survey*, London: The NHS Information Centre for Health and Social Care.

McNaught, A. and Bhugra, D. (1996) 'Models of homelessness', in D. Bhugra (ed) *Homelessness and mental health*, Cambridge: Cambridge University Press.

McNeil, C. (2012) *The politics of disadvantage: New Labour, social exclusion and post-crash Britain*, London: Institute For Public Policy Research.

MEAM (Making Every Adult Matter Coalition) (2009) 'A four-point manifesto for tackling multiple needs and exclusions', London.

MEAM (Making Every Adult Matter) and RDA (Revolving Doors Agency) (2011) 'Turning the tide: a vision paper for multiple needs and exclusions', London.

MEAM and RDA (2012) 'Progress on multiple needs and exclusions', London.

Miliband, D. (2006) *Social exclusion: The next steps forward*, London: Office of the Deputy Prime Minister.

Morrison, D.S. (2009) 'Homelessness as an independent risk factor for mortality: results from a retrospective cohort study', *International Journal of Epidemiology*, 38: 877–83.

NICE (National Institute for Clinical Excellence) (2001) 'Quality standard for drug use disorders', NICE quality standard.

NICE (2011) 'Alcohol use disorders: diagnosis, assessment and management of harmful drinking and alcohol dependence', NICE clinical guideline.

Percy-Smith, J. (ed) (2000) *Policy responses to social exclusion. Towards inclusion?*, Maidenhead: Open University Press.

Pleace, N. (1998) 'Single homelessness as social exclusion: the unique and the extreme', *Social Policy & Administration*, 32: 46–59.

RCP (Royal College of Psychiatrists) (2009) *Mental health and social inclusion: Making psychiatry and mental health services fit for the 21st century*, position statement by the RCP Social Inclusion Scoping Group, London: Royal College of Psychiatrists.

Rethink (2013) *Lethal discrimination*, London: Rethink Mental Illness.

RSA (Royal Society for the Arts) (2007) *Drugs – Facing the facts: The report on the RSA Commission on Illegal Drugs, Communities and Public Policy*, London: RSA.

Singh, P. (2005) *No home, no job: Moving on from transitional spaces*, London: Off the Streets and into Work (OSW).

St Mungo's (2013) *Health and homelessness: Understanding the costs and role of primary care services for homeless people*, London: St Mungo's.

WHO (World Health Organization) (2011) 'WHO mental health factfile; mental health: a state of wellbeing', World Health Organization.

Widdowfield, R. (ed) (1999) *The limitations of official homelessness statistics*, London: Arnold.

Wilkinson, R. and Marmot, M. (2003) *Social determinants of health: The solid facts* (2nd edn), Geneva: World Health Organization.

Wood, D. (ed) (1992) *Delivering health care to homeless persons: The diagnosis and management of medical and mental health conditions*, New York, NY: Springer Pub.

Wright, N. and Stickley, T. (2013) 'Concepts of social inclusion, exclusion and mental health: a review of the international literature'. *Journal of Psychiatric and Mental Health Nursing*, 20: 71–81.

Wright, N. and Tompkins, C. (2006) 'How can health services effectively meet the health needs of homeless people?', *British Journal of General Practice*, 56: 286–93.

Wright, N.M.J., Tompkins, C., Oldham, N.S. and Kay, D.J. (2004) 'Homelessness and health: what can be done in general practice?', *Journal of the Royal Society of Medicine*, 97: 170–3.

EIGHTEEN

Brain injury and social exclusion

Michael Oddy, Sara da Silva Ramos
and Deborah Fortescue

Social disadvantage and brain injury

There is growing evidence that those in socially peripheral and disadvantaged groups are more likely to have suffered an acquired brain injury (ABI), particularly a traumatic brain injury (TBI). What is less clear is whether this association is due to common risk factors for social exclusion and for brain injury, or whether each increases the risk of the other. Of course, the likely answer is that these factors are not mutually exclusive and that each factor or combination of factors plays some part in increasing this association. It is the aim of this chapter to examine the current evidence in order to understand this association better and to look at the implications of this analysis in terms of intervention for both the prevention and treatment of brain injury and for addressing social exclusion.

The most common form of ABI (brain injury that occurs after birth) is TBI. TBI is caused by physical impact to the head, either by sudden acceleration or sudden deceleration. TBI often leads to a characteristic pattern of deficits that makes the demands of life more difficult to meet. Common problems include cognitive deficits, such as memory, concentration and executive problems. Executive problems affect a person's ability to problem-solve, plan and organise goal-directed behaviour. In addition, certain non-cognitive neurobehavioural changes are common, such as reduced ability to regulate emotion, disinhibition, impulsivity and problems with social cognition. The latter affect a person's ability to read social cues and to moderate their behaviour so that it is appropriate to the situation.

It is easy to speculate about how these deficits could lead the individual to become marginalised by society as they affect many of the core skills required to conform to accepted patterns of behaviour. Cognitive problems make it difficult to maintain work in the open market. Other neurobehavioural deficits make it difficult to maintain social relationships, both at work and outside work. Such difficulties can therefore clearly have an impact on the likelihood of becoming homeless, falling foul of the law and failing to cope adequately with the demands of civilian life after time spent in the structured and regulated world of the military. TBI appears likely to be one possible risk factor for social exclusion, which, in combination with other known risk factors, such as social milieu, poor education and drug misuse, can lead an individual to be marginalised.

If brain injury is a significant factor in taking people to the edge of society, what are the implications of this? The impact of brain injury on cognitive abilities such as memory and learning suggests that different approaches, informed by an understanding of the effects of brain injury, need to be taken in order to support such individuals. This support could be offered at different stages in the cycle. The ideal is to prevent brain injury in the first place. This can be achieved through the better protection of pedestrians and the use of helmets for cycling, skateboarding and other activities where head trauma is clearly a risk. However, it could also be addressed through interventions to prevent falls and non-accidental injuries. Addressing alcohol and drug misuse can also reduce the incidence of brain injury.

The next stage at which there is an opportunity to prevent the potential impact of brain injury is in the provision of better support and rehabilitation in the acute and post-acute phases of recovery. Interventions at this stage, though expensive, have the potential to help the individual cope with the demands of life, maintain employment and avoid falling into criminality or homelessness. The final phase is to address the problems arising from brain injury after the person has fallen into the criminal justice system or has become unemployed or homeless.

Screening for brain injury

The evidence for an increase in the prevalence of TBI comes mainly from self-report studies rather than studies involving the medical documentation of brain injury. This, of course, raises the question as to whether such a methodology allows us to have confidence in the findings.

There has been an explosion of studies using self-report of brain injury in recent years. However, there has been little attention to the psychometric properties of the screening tools used. Many studies simply design their own questions and use this without any check on validity, reliability, sensitivity or specificity. There are a small number of exceptions to this, such as the Ohio State University Traumatic Brain Injury – Identification (Corrigan and Bogner, 2007), Help Emergency Lose Problems Sicknesses (Picard et al, 1991; Hux et al, 2009) and the Traumatic Brain Injury-4 (Olson-Madden et al, 2014), where some attempt has been made to gather psychometric data to support the use of such instruments.

Our research group, sponsored by The Disabilities Trust Foundation (TDTF), has been developing a tool, the Brain Injury Screening Index (BISI), over the last few years. This 11-item self-report tool focuses on the occurrence of a TBI rather than the consequences of a TBI, as in mild TBI these are non-specific and overlap with the symptoms of a number of other conditions. The BISI asks whether the person has experienced a 'serious blow to their head' and the frequency of having suffered such blows. It asks about immediate effects such as feeling dizzy, unsteady or dazed. It asks about the presence of post-traumatic amnesia (i.e. a gap in the memory for events immediately after the blow to the head), the presence and duration of loss of consciousness, and any treatment sought or received. While it is TBI that is particularly over-represented in these groups, the BISI also asks about other ABIs as the consequences are similar and it makes little sense to exclude those with other forms of ABI from any services that are provided. Associated problems (prior diagnosis of epilepsy, Attention Deficit Hyperactivity Disorder [ADHD], learning disabilities [LDs], mental health problems) are asked about as these will influence the interpretation of the symptoms reported by the individual.

Initial findings of a statistical association between screening positive on the BISI and scoring lower on formal tests of cognition are initial evidence for its validity (Pitman et al, 2015). A study of the homeless population in Glasgow has confirmed the results of studies using the BISI and other self-report methods of a higher prevalence of TBI in this population, even when hospital records are used to identify those with a TBI (McMillan et al, 2015). Further studies investigating the reliability and validity of the BISI are ongoing in both a male prison and a female prison. Initial findings suggest that the BISI has good psychometric properties (O'Sullivan, 2015).

Homelessness and brain injury

It has long been acknowledged that LDs and mental health problems are more prevalent among those without homes (Silver et al, 2001; Solliday-McRoy et al, 2004; Spence et al, 2004). ABI has been mentioned in studies whose focus has been on LDs or mental health, but it is only within the last 10 years that brain injury has become a focus in its own right. The first such study was that of Hwang et al (2008), who investigated the homeless population of Toronto. Using a self-report methodology, they found a lifetime prevalence of 53% among 904 homeless individuals. The authors noted that this is five times the prevalence in the general population of the US. While the direction of causality is unclear, for 70% of homeless individuals with TBI, the injury preceded the onset of homelessness, suggesting that TBI could perhaps be a risk factor for homelessness. Oddy, Moir, Fortescue and Chadwick (2012) replicated this study in Leeds in the UK, this time with a comparison group matched for age, gender and education. Those who were homeless had a prevalence rate of TBI of 48%, very similar to that found by Hwang et al (2008). This compared to a rate of 21% in the matched comparison group, so the prevalence was more than double. Once again, a large proportion (90%) had sustained their brain injury before becoming homeless.

Clearly, both these studies can be criticised for their reliance on a self-report methodology. However, the study in Glasgow which matched hospital admission records for head injury with those of homelessness compiled by general practitioners found that the frequency of admission to hospital for head injury was found to be five times higher in the homeless group than in the general Glasgow population. There was a prevalence rate of 13.5% among the homeless, compared to 2.7% in the general Glasgow population (McMillan et al, 2015). In absolute terms, the prevalence rate in the Glasgow study using medical records was lower than the Leeds and Toronto studies using self-reports. However, relative to the general population, the Glasgow study found an even greater increase in the prevalence of brain injury among those who were homeless than that found in self-report studies. The Glasgow study also found that those who were homeless and had been hospitalised for head injury had increased mortality rates of 33.6% during the seven-year period of the study, compared to 13.9% for those who were homeless but had not had a head injury. The reasons for this are unclear and the subject of further research.

It is also unclear as to whether homelessness is a risk factor for brain injury or brain injury raises the risk of being homeless. Indeed, the risks may be raised in both directions. Certainly, those who currently have no home are more at risk of assault. However, it is true that a brain injury can make it more difficult to cope with the demands of daily life and may make it more likely that a person loses their home. Clearly, there are other factors that raise the risk of both brain injury and homelessness. Alcohol and drug misuse are the most obvious factors.

Substance misuse can raise the incidence of brain injury through falls or by putting the individual at risk of assault. It can also increase the risk of becoming homeless through the loss of work or financial priorities switching from paying rent to funding the drug or alcohol habit. Despite the complexities, addressing one or more of the predisposing factors may reduce the cycle of deprivation and enable the person to hold down work and escape from homelessness.

Offending and brain injury

A similar situation prevails in relation to offenders and those committed to custodial care. There is rapidly increasing evidence from around the world that there is a higher prevalence of TBI among those who engage in criminal behaviour than in the rest of the population (Williams, 2012). TBI is also related to earlier onset of criminal behaviour, repeat offending and greater violence. Similarly, there is an increased prevalence of TBI in people in custody across the world, especially in the case of those with more severe injuries

However, the picture is at least as complex as in the case of homelessness. Alcohol and drug taking are also related to violent crime. There is a high prevalence of other conditions, such as post-traumatic stress disorder (PTSD), self-harm, depression and anxiety, among prisoners. ADHD is a risk factor for both TBI and offending. However, once again, there may be an opportunity to intervene and prevent the cycle from continuing.

The Linkworker system

It is clear that with competing demands for government finance, an expensive solution is unlikely to be implemented. Ideally, a solution needs to be cost-effective in the sense that the cost of an intervention must be no more than that which can be saved through the individual's avoidance of the criminal justice system. With this in mind, TDTF has been developing a low-cost, low-intensity intervention known as the Linkworker system. The concept of a Linkworker is that a recent graduate, with aspirations to become a social care or health professional, is recruited. They are provided with basic training that enables them to understand the impact of ABI, to be aware of the key principles of brain injury rehabilitation, and to know what interventions can be used to mitigate the problems that a prisoner may experience. In addition to induction training, they are provided with a manual that provides guidance and resources to help them in their task and receive supervision from a clinical psychologist experienced in brain injury rehabilitation. Thus equipped, they are able to provide a time-limited, low-intensity intervention supplementing, not replacing, existing prison services. Due to the cognitive problems (including memory, learning and problem-solving), the Linkworker intervention is designed to take these difficulties into account and provide a form of offender rehabilitation that can benefit those with a brain injury.

On reception, new prisoners are screened with the BISI, and where found to be positive for brain injury, are referred to the Linkworker. The Linkworker may provide direct help to such prisoners, developing goals that the prisoner wants addressed. This direct help may involve enabling the prisoner to understand his or her injury and develop strategies to compensate for any difficulties that they experience as a result. In addition to direct support, the Linkworker may identify services both inside the prison and following release that can help the prisoner cope with the effects of their brain injury. The Linkworker may work with staff to help them manage difficulties that the prisoner may experience or exhibit and often participates in meetings (Multi-Agency Public Protection Arrangements [MAPPAs]) to assist in case planning.

Following release from prison, the Linkworker provides 'through-the-gate' support for prisoners returning to the local community. There may be face-to-face and telephone support sessions for a limited period, with the aim of helping former prisoners to apply in the community the skills learned through their brain injury support plans in prison. The Linkworker can make necessary referrals to agencies in the community able to offer support and assistance to those who have had a brain injury. Finally, the Linkworkers develop 'portable profiles' with prisoners. These are documents that identify their brain injury-related difficulties and suggested solutions. They can provide advice to individuals and organisations who are involved with the individual following their release.

A recent independent review of the Linkworker system has concluded that screening was able to identify those who had had a brain injury, that the service was meeting its key aims and that it was acceptable and valued by both prisoners and staff (Williams and Chitsabesan, 2016).

Further trials of the Linkworker system are under way and these are designed to tease out the separate effects on prisoners of training prison staff to have an awareness of brain injury and the introduction of a Linkworker. The Linkworker model can equally be applied with minor modifications to other groups with a high prevalence of TBI, such as those who are homeless and ex-military personnel. Studies are under way with both these groups. So far, the focus has been on male prisoners but, once again, the system is being adapted and applied to female prisoners in several locations.

Discussion

There is growing and convincing evidence that TBI is over-represented in socially marginalised groups such as offenders, those who are homeless and ex-military personnel. Much of this evidence has been based on self-reports of brain injury. Until recently, little attention has been given to ensuring that this methodology provides valid and reliable findings. This situation is changing and there is now evidence that self-reports can provide valid and useful findings. Pitman et al (2015) have demonstrated that self-reports of TBI correlate with cognitive deficits on formal neuropsychological assessment. McMillan et al (2015) have demonstrated that in a homeless population, medical records of TBI confirm the finding of a higher prevalence compared to the general population. Considerable development has gone into one particular self-report tool, the BISI, and initial findings suggest this to have psychometric properties of reliability and validity (O'Sullivan, 2015).

Once accurate screening methods have been developed, it becomes possible to ensure that appropriate supports and services are targeted towards those who have experienced a brain injury. There are opportunities to break cycles of deprivation at several points. Clearly, the best interventions would be those that prevent the TBI from occurring in the first place. However, beyond this, there are opportunities to target interventions at this group. The emphasis in this chapter has been on low-intensity, low-cost interventions as these are much more likely to be feasible and adopted. Staff training and 'Linkworker' systems have been described and discussed. The Linkworker system, although brief and conducted by staff with limited training, does still involve one-to-one contact. Although this can have important non-specific value in psychological therapy, it is possible that group interventions could be even lower in cost and more effective. Well-structured and well-led groups can take advantage of the effects of social approval and support, of peer understanding, and of sharing common experiences. At their best, such interventions can be very powerful, but they require expert leadership.

With minor adaptations, these can be applied to any socially deprived group. Research is ongoing to determine whether such interventions can be effective. Can they influence rates of recidivism and reduce homelessness and stress? Initial informal evidence suggests that, at least in some cases, they can. If low-intensity services can make a difference to such outcomes, it is a huge opportunity not to be missed. The prizes of success are well worth pursuing. The ramifications of diverting one individual from homelessness or a criminal path are considerable, embracing the offender, the victims and their respective families.

References

Corrigan, J.D. and Bogner, J. (2007) 'Initial reliability and validity of the Ohio State University TBI identification method', *Journal of Head Trauma Rehabilitation*, 22(6): 318–29.

Hux, K., Schneider, T. and Bennett, K. (2009) 'Screening for traumatic brain injury', *Brain Injury*, 23(1): 8–14. Available at: www.informaworld.com/10.1080/02699050802590353

Hwang, S.W., Colantonio, A., Chiu, S., Tolomiczenko, G., Kiss, A., Cowan, L., Redelmeier, D. and Levinson, W. (2008) 'The effect of traumatic brain injury on the health of homeless people', *Canadian Medical Association Journal*, 179(8): 779–84. Available at: http://doi.org/10.1503/cmaj.080341

McMillan, T.M., Laurie, M., Oddy, M., Menzies, M., Stewart, E. and Wainman-Lefley, J. (2015) 'Head injury and mortality in the homeless', *Journal of Neurotrauma*, 32(2): 116–19. Available at: http://doi.org/10.1089/neu.2014.3387

Oddy, M., Moir, J.F., Fortescue, D. and Chadwick, S. (2012) 'The prevalence of traumatic brain injury in the homeless community in a UK city', *Brain Injury*, 26(9): 1058–64. Available at: http://doi.org/10.3109/02699052.2012.667595

Olson-Madden, J.H., Homaifar, B.Y., Hostetter, T.A., Matarazzo, B.B., Huggins, J., Forster, J.E. Schneider, A.L., Herbert, B.A., Nagamoto, T., Corrigan, J.D. and Brenner, L.A. (2014) 'Validating the traumatic brain injury-4 screening measure for veterans seeking mental health treatment with psychiatric inpatient and outpatient service utilization data', *Archives of Physical Medicine and Rehabilitation*, 95(5): 925–9. Available at: http://doi.org/10.1016/j.apmr.2014.01.008

O'Sullivan, M. (2015) 'Utility of the Brain Injury Screening Index in identifying female prisoners with a traumatic brain injury and associated cognitive impairment', Doctoral thesis, University of Surrey, UK.

Picard, M., Scarisbrick, D. and Paluck, R. (1991) *International Center for the Disabled, 9/91*, TBI-NET Grant #H128A00022, US Department of Education, Rehabilitation Services Administration.

Pitman, I., Haddlesey, C., Ramos, S.D.S., Oddy, M. and Fortescue, D. (2015) 'The association between neuropsychological performance and self-reported traumatic brain injury in a sample of adult male prisoners in the UK', *Neuropsychological Rehabilitation*, 25(5): 763–79. Available at: http://doi.org/10.1080/09602011.2014.973887

Silver, J.M., Kramer, R., Greenwald, S. and Weissman, M. (2001) 'The association between head injuries and psychiatric disorders: findings from the New Haven NIMH Epidemiologic Catchment Area Study', *Brain Injury*, 15(11): 935–45. Available at: http://doi.org/10.1080/02699050110065295

Solliday-McRoy, C., Campbell, T.C., Melchert, T.P., Young, T.J. and Cisler, R.A. (2004) 'Neuropsychological functioning of homeless men', *The Journal of Nervous and Mental Disease*, 192(7): 471–8. Available at: http://www.ncbi.nlm.nih.gov/pubmed/15232317

Spence, S., Stevens, R. and Parks, R. (2004) 'Cognitive dysfunction in homeless adults: a systematic review', *Journal of the Royal Society of Medicine*, 97(8): 375–9. Available at: http://doi.org/10.1258/jrsm.97.8.375

Williams, W.H. and Chitsabesan, P. (2016) 'Young people with traumatic brain injury in custody: an evaluation of a Linkworker service', London: Barrow Cadbury Trust. Available at: https://www.barrowcadbury.org.uk/wp-content/uploads/2016/07/Disability_Trust_linkworker_2016Lores.pdf

NINETEEN

What works to improve the health of the multiply excluded?

Nigel Hewett

Introduction

Inclusion Health (IH) is a research, service and policy agenda that aims to prevent and redress health and social inequities among the most vulnerable and marginalised in a community (Luchenski et al, forthcoming). This includes people with experiences of homelessness, drug use, imprisonment and sex work, as well as Gypsies, Travellers and vulnerable migrants. IH target populations face common adverse life experiences and risk factors that lead to deep social exclusion, poverty and multiple co-morbidities, with extreme levels of morbidity and mortality across all categories of disease (Hayward et al, 2017) and poor access to mainstream services. From an intervention perspective, IH may be thought about in terms of access to, integration with and trust in essential systems, services and institutions to promote, protect and improve health (Luchenski et al, forthcoming). This chapter focuses particularly on homeless people as exemplars for IH.

A significant challenge is that poor physical and mental health is compounded by the failure of mainstream health and social care services to respond effectively. We often dismiss groups as 'hard to reach'; this chapter considers the extent to which the services, and not the patients, are 'hard to reach', and how we might change this situation.

After prolonged exclusion, people on the margins of society frequently experience severe and complex ill health, often characterised by tri-morbidity: the combination of physical and mental ill health with drug or alcohol misuse (O'Connell et al, 2010). There is often a history of institutional care, including childcare and prison. The emerging concept of syndemic interactions may offer an approach to understanding the resulting complexity (Singer Merrill, 2009). The traditional biomedical approach is to consider each disease in isolation, so co-morbidity is two conditions in the same person, treated separately.

A syndemic is two or more diseases that interact, synergistically, to increase the negative health effects. Syndemics tend to occur in conditions of poverty, stress and health inequalities.

A core flaw in society's response is fragmented and inadequately funded health and social care systems, resulting in perverse incentives to protect budgets by refusing to provide services for people who never quite meet the criteria for inclusion. The consequence is that care is too often characterised by crisis management at multiple disconnected points of episodic care, so that excluded people end up in the most expensive parts of the system – hospitals and prisons. Exclusion from access to health and social care is commonly associated with negative stereotyping by health and social care professionals. Fragmented and uncoordinated crisis management continues in the acute and social care system, further compounding the distress and unproductive expense.

Why special effort is needed

Homelessness is more hazardous than poverty alone (Hwang et al, 2009) and has been shown to be an independent risk factor for death from specific conditions. For example, a homeless person admitted to hospital with complications of drug misuse is seven times more likely to die over the next five years than a housed person with the same drug-related health problem (Morrison, 2009). Widening inequalities in society (Wilkinson and Pickett, 2010) should encourage us to re-examine the inverse care law – 'availability of good medical care tends to vary inversely with the need for it in the population served' (Tudor Hart, 1971) – and rebalance the provision of health care to benefit those who need it most.

A study of pathways into homelessness in seven UK cities (Bramley, 2015) revealed that the most complex forms of multiple exclusion homelessness (MEH) are associated with childhood deprivation and psychological trauma; this is followed by mental health problems and substance misuse well before homelessness and associated adverse life events. However, other groups have significantly fewer MEH experiences; this is particularly true for people who migrated to the UK as adults. This group is much less likely to have experienced mental illness or substance misuse. This finding mirrors the observation from a large mortality study in Boston, USA (Baggett et al, 2013), which showed higher mortality in white homeless people, associated with more complexity and trauma going back to childhood, compared to African-Americans, whose problems were more directly related to poverty and discrimination.

An additional consideration is the effect of an ageing homeless population. New York demographic research (Culhane et al, 2010) has suggested that adults born in the second half of the 'baby boom' (mid-1950s to 1964) have experienced a sustained elevation in their risk of experiencing homelessness. This may represent a generational effect of reduced employment and housing opportunities due to the crowding in of the early baby-boomer group combined with repeated recessions in the late 1970s and early 1980s. The compounding effect of drug abuse and involvement in the criminal justice system may have reduced opportunities to form new families, resulting in an underlying susceptibility to homelessness. Increased demand then further stretched limited welfare services, exacerbating the downward spiral. Syndemic outcomes are confirmed by US evidence that geriatric syndromes are more commonly observed in older homeless adults than in the general population (Brown et al, 2012), and by descriptions of previously undiagnosed depression and cognitive impairment among Canadian elderly homeless men revealed by simple testing in primary care (Joyce and Limbos, 2009). This cohort effect raises the very real concern that the 2008 recession and subsequent welfare cuts and austerity measures scheduled to continue until 2020 may have a similar effect, and produce another lost generation at high risk of homelessness.

It might be assumed that health-care systems that are provided free at the point of delivery improve outcomes for those on the margins of society. Regrettably, the evidence does not support this assumption. In Canada, with free access to health services for all citizens, a study of users of homeless services (Bonin et al, 2007) who met DSM-IV (*Diagnostic and Statistical Manual of Mental Disorders*, 4th edition) criteria for affective or psychotic disorders found that health service uptake was still predicted by socio-demographic characteristics, illness characteristics and social networks. Health service uptake was less likely if male, older, with little social support and homeless rather than simply impoverished. Further evidence is provided by a study of homeless women (Cheung and Hwang, 2004) in seven cities across England, Canada, Denmark and the US. The study found that the risk of death among younger homeless women was five to 30 times higher than among their housed counterparts, with no observable effect on mortality of health insurance and therefore access to free health care in the different countries. It is not enough to simply assume that universal access to health care will result in universal uptake.

Health-care systems will never respond effectively to the needs of excluded groups if our understanding is limited to enumerating the ways in which complex patients fail to adapt to our service delivery systems. As health inequalities grow, we must find ways to respond to the health consequences of the social determinants of health or our health-care systems will collapse under the resulting pressure. This duty to provide a systematic response to improving health equity has been accepted by all the clinical professional groups in England, coordinated by the Institute for Health Equity (Allen et al, 2013).

A common personal and institutional response to overwhelming demand is to retreat into professional silos, with an increasing proportion of limited resources being expended on a bureaucratic effort to justify the denial of care to individuals who do not quite fit defined criteria. This seems particularly problematic when health and social care systems are not joined up, and weighs disproportionately on those on the margins of society who may lack documentary proof of rights to treatment or care. A review funded by the Scottish Government's Multiple and Complex Needs Initiative (Gallimore et al, 2008) examined qualitative research papers looking at service users' views. The review concluded that people with complex needs want what anyone wants, and what differentiates those with multiple and complex needs is not the nature of demand for services but the barriers to accessing those services. This issue is further explored by a review of key texts published by the Lankelly Chase Foundation (Duncan and Corner, 2012), and their 'Hard edges' report (Bramley, 2015). They confirm a huge overlap between the offender, substance misusing and homeless populations. For example, two thirds of people using homeless services are also either in the criminal justice system or in drug treatment in the same year. An important consideration for future generations is the finding that the majority are in contact with or are living with children. These papers propose 'severe and multiple disadvantage' as a preferable term because it recognises the social nature of disadvantage, described as the experience of disadvantages that most others do not experience. This avoids the focus on the individual, which results from the discussion of 'needs'. This may offer a useful perspective for health-care providers and help to overcome negative assumptions. The problem is not inherent in the person, but in the particular circumstances in which they find themselves.

Not simply a housing problem

Both a right of access to health care and a right of access to housing are necessary to address health inequalities, but neither is sufficient in isolation. A growing body of evidence supports 'Housing First'

(Woodhall-Melnik and Dunn, 2016; see also Chapters Fourteen and Sixteen).

What works

Prevention

Most of the evidence for interventions to reduce health harms involves substance use disorder (SUD). Multi-component harm reduction programmes, including needle and syringe programmes, behavioural interventions, treatment for SUD, and syringe disinfection have been shown to reduce the risk of hepatitis C virus infection by as much as 75%, although single-component interventions are minimally effective. Using mobile outreach to deliver needle and syringe programmes has been shown to reach younger clients and those with a higher risk profile than static programmes. Opioid overdose prevention programmes involve training people with SUD and their contacts to recognise overdose and administer naloxone to reverse the effects of opioids. Studies have reported 85–100% survival after naloxone administration, and areas with high uptake of opioid overdose prevention programmes have lower levels of heroin overdose-related deaths. Supervised injecting sites (where trained medical personnel provide harm reduction equipment and supervise drug consumption) have also been shown to reduce overdose deaths and ambulance call-outs for overdose, as well as decrease unsafely discarded needles, public injecting and needle sharing. Supervised injecting sites are not associated with increases in crime, or numbers of people injecting drugs. Targeted screening in primary care, the training of primary care practitioners, the use of dried blood spot testing and outreach all improve uptake of hepatitis C virus testing (Luchenski et al, forthcoming).

Pharmacological interventions

Opioid replacement therapy, particularly methadone maintenance, is highly effective for people with opiate dependency, and can improve outcomes for other conditions when provided concurrently. For example, Inclusion Health target populations (IHTPs) have an increased risk of contracting tuberculosis, hepatitis C virus and human immunodeficiency virus (HIV) infections. Integrating opioid replacement therapy with HIV treatment or hepatitis C treatment for drug users with these infections improves outcomes. Contingency management (vouchers for adherence) is also effective; improving outcomes for people with SUD needing HIV treatment, improving tuberculosis treatment compliance for homeless people as well as those leaving prison or using drugs, and promoting behaviour change for people who use cocaine and other psychostimulants. However, in every situation, the benefit only lasts until the support ceases.

Service organisation

If an effective response to health inequalities is to be mounted, we need to consider the evidence about innovative approaches to the delivery of care. A recent King's Fund study of five UK-based services included a non-systematic review of the literature (Goodwin et al, 2013). Core features included a named care coordinator supported by a multidisciplinary team, care that went beyond narrow clinical targets and focused on what the patient needed, and a lot of effort to support communication across networks in the community and hospital; overall, an approach nicely summarised by the phrase 'low tech, high touch'. Interestingly, all of the services studied felt 'outside the system'. Perhaps the greatest challenge is to find ways of bringing these approaches inside the system.

A key component of all of these health interventions is case management, and there is a broad supporting evidence base (Luchenski et al, forthcoming). Case management aims to improve the coordination and delivery of health and social care services and can be most simply understood by its functions: assessment, planning, linking, monitoring and advocacy. In homeless populations, case management is associated with improvements in mental health symptoms and SUD compared with usual care. Case management with assertive community treatment (eg delivered by a multidisciplinary team with low caseloads, community-based services and 24-hour coverage) reduces homelessness with a greater improvement in psychiatric symptoms when compared to standard case management for the treatment of homeless populations with severe mental illness.

Models of service delivery

Hwang et al have synthesised the evidence supporting interventions intended to improve the health of homeless people (Hwang et al, 2005; Fitzpatrick-Lewis et al, 2011; Hwang and Burns, 2014). Specialist primary care services are popular with patients and 'may' produce better outcomes. Specialist mental health services generally produce better outcomes as well as improved access and engagement.

Interventions that provide case management and supportive housing have the greatest effect when they target individuals who are the most intensive users of services. Critical time interventions provide effective support from a case manager who has formed a therapeutic relationship with the patient for the transition from inpatient to outpatient care. Assertive community treatment (ACT) provides multidisciplinary support through a case manager with a small caseload (10–15 clients) and improves symptoms and reduces homelessness, but not hospital admissions. Housing First, with the immediate provision of housing in independent units with support, improves outcomes for individuals with serious mental illnesses. For homeless individuals with chronic alcoholism and frequent emergency department use, case management with supportive housing that permits drinking is effective in ending homelessness and reducing service costs. For chronically mentally ill homeless adults being discharged from hospital, the provision of case management and supportive housing is effective in the reduction of hospital use. Medical respite programmes that provide homeless patients with a suitable environment for recuperation and follow-up care on leaving the hospital reduce the risk of readmission to hospital and the number of days spent in hospital. Many interventions are effective in the reduction of substance misuse compared with no intervention, but there is little evidence to indicate the superiority of any particular programme over another.

Health-care providers need to be familiar with the full range of local community programmes and resources for homeless people, or work closely with staff who have this expertise. Adapted clinical guidelines are available to help health-care providers make necessary adjustments to their practice (Bonin et al, 2010). Clinicians in accident and emergency departments need to develop systems that ensure appropriate follow-up in the community. When homeless individuals are admitted to hospital, proactive two-way communication between hospital-based and community-based providers is essential to facilitate smooth transitions of care. Provision of health care should include active outreach to homeless people, and collaboration should result in health-care teams that can provide general medical care, mental health care and addiction treatment, as well as housing services. When care is provided for an individual with a mental illness, the individual should be connected with whatever services are available locally rather than trying to precisely match the individual to a specific programme. Health-care providers can be advocates for the establishment and maintenance of evidence-based interventions to improve the health of people who are homeless. Although health-care providers understandably focus on interventions that address illness and risk factors for homelessness at the individual level, they should also seek to address social policies and structural factors that result in homelessness.

Looking beyond the existing evidence base, experience suggests some additional emerging themes. For example, many services are built around multi-agency working, which often requires new and unconventional partnerships (O'Connell et al, 2005). Where professionals from different 'tribes' do find a way to put their professional concern for the individual back at the centre of their efforts, everyone benefits through the provision of integrated care (Hewett et al, 2012). Most importantly, the patient has a better experience, but, in addition, the professionals reconnect with the core values that brought them into the caring professions and outcomes and efficiency are improved (Ham and Walsh, 2013). Advocacy within the health-care system might best be supported by Marmot's concept of proportionate universalism (Marmot et al, 2010). To reduce the steepness of the social gradient in health, actions must be universal but with a scale and intensity that is proportionate to the level of disadvantage. IH embraces creative efforts to make services more accessible to those most in need, based on an understanding of their situation. A growing response is 'home visits' on the streets and into hostels and hospitals, aiming to improve access to care and to nurture the physician–patient relationship (O'Connell, 2004). This includes Street Medicine (Howe et al, 2009), pathway hospital care coordination (Dorney-Smith et al, 2016) and other forms of hospital in-reach, health-care services (including primary care, psychiatric and psychological treatment, and secondary care outpatient treatment) provided in hostels, in day centres and on the streets, and special medical respite facilities that provide medical and nursing care for homeless people who are too sick to be on the streets or in traditional shelters but do not need inpatient hospitalisation.

Young people also value tailored services. A recent Cochrane review examined a range of interventions compared to standard care for street-connected children and young people (children who work or sleep, or both, on the streets and may or may not necessarily be adequately supervised or directed by responsible adults) (Coren et al, 2013). Inclusion and reintegration (the primary outcomes of the review) were not measured in any of the reviewed studies, and no consistent results were found within the domains of psychosocial health, SUD and risky sexual behaviour. The authors conducted a subsequent systematic review and found that neither length nor quality of service engagement could account for the lack of significant difference between interventions developed specifically for street-connected youth and standard services. The authors noted that, in contrast, qualitative research findings consistently emphasise youth's appreciation of engagement-related aspects of interventions, such as safe environments and caring relationships, indicating their value irrespective of other outcomes (Hossain and Coren, 2015).

Although conclusive evidence is lacking, there are potentially promising results for family-based therapy, cognitive behavioural therapy and brief interventions for a range of outcomes for youth. For children in care, foster care may help to reduce criminal activity and improve mental health outcomes (Luchenski et al, forthcoming).

A key component of effective health interventions for excluded groups is peer involvement. Trained and supported peers bring a unique perspective to any interaction and can be a key part of ensuring engagement with services (Boisvert et al, 2008). Support by trained peers improves access to health care for service users, reduces unplanned care and improves outcomes for the peers themselves (Finlayson et al, 2016).

What works – values

> T'Ain't What You Do (It's the Way That You Do It), that's what gets results. (Song written by jazz musicians Melvin 'Sy' Oliver and James 'Trummy' Young, 1939)

What we do to improve health inequalities is important, but perhaps more important is how we set about it. Improving outcomes requires an understanding of the point of view of the service user, and how that may be affected by past experience, and a mindful reassessment and repeated challenge of the role of care providers. Is it simply that the patient is non-compliant or that the system is insufficiently responsive to their needs? The association between childhood psychological trauma and MEH is clear. Those who have suffered neglect or abuse, particularly in childhood, are more likely to perceive threat and less likely to be able to regulate the resultant emotions (Gilbert, 2009). Difficulty in regulating emotions may result in behaviours that are perceived as 'antisocial', which may then drive exclusion behaviours. Front-line health-care practitioners working with excluded groups frequently observe that a compassionate approach is fundamental to establishing a therapeutic relationship. The key to engagement lies in the values that inform services. Ultimately, it is only by responding compassionately to the needs of excluded groups that we can change health and social care systems for the benefit of us all.

Social determinants of health

There is growing evidence of the widening gap in life expectancy between the richest and poorest in society (Mayhew and Smith, 2016). Over the 60 years to the Second World War, the gap narrowed as improved plumbing and mass vaccination helped everyone, but particularly benefited the poor. Over the last 60 years, although average life expectancy has risen, the inequality gap has not improved, and has recently widened again, particularly for men. This is due to the burden of chronic disease associated with smoking, exercise and diet. The challenge seems to be improving the choices available to poor people – or, better still, eradicating poverty. Growing numbers of destitute people in the UK must be part of this picture. A recent report (Fitzpatrick et al, 2016) suggests that 1,252,000 people, including 312,000 children, were destitute at some point during 2015. Contrary to popular expectations, 79% were born in the UK. Key triggers include debt repayment (usually to public authorities), benefit delays and sanctions. Evidence-based responses include deinstitutionalised housing support (such as Housing First), support into employment, whole-family approaches and policies to reduce structural disadvantages faced by people, households and communities living in persistent or recurrent poverty (Luchenski et al, forthcoming).

Conclusions

Health inequalities are a direct result of social inequality and can only ultimately be prevented by eradicating poverty. The most effective long-term prevention policy is likely to be to reduce poverty among families with children (Luchenski et al, forthcoming). However, given the recent decades of widening inequalities, an enduring duty will persist for health and social care systems to ameliorate the health consequences of this injustice.

Health-care systems in the developed world must evolve to address the challenges of multi-morbidity, long-term conditions, widening inequality and financial constraints. The solutions that are emerging in the field of IH exemplify approaches that are likely to benefit health-care systems at every level. Above all, responding to health inequalities will require a rediscovery of compassionate patient-focused care, which can only improve health-care systems for us all.

References

Allen, M., Allen, J., Hogarth, S. and Marmot, M. (2013) 'Working for health equity: the role of health professionals', UCL IHE, March.

Baggett, T.P., Hwang, S.W. and O'Connell, J.J. (2013) 'Mortality among homeless adults in Boston shifts in causes of death over a 15-year period', *JAMA Intern Med*, 173(3): 189–95. Available at: doi:10.1001/jamainternmed.2013.1604

Boisvert, R.A., Martin, L.M., Grosek, M. and Claire A.J. (2008) 'Effectiveness of a peer-support community in addiction recovery: participation as intervention', *Occupational Therapy International*, 15(4): 205–20.

Bonin, J.P., Fournier, F. and Blais, R. (2007) 'Predictors of mental health service utilization by people using resources for homeless people in Canada', *Psychiatric Services*, 58(7): 936–41.

Bonin, E., Brehove, T. and Carlson, C. (2010) *Adapting your practice: General recommendations for the care of homeless patients*, Nashville: Health Care for the Homeless Clinicians' Network, National Health Care for the Homeless Council. Available at: www.nhchc.org/resources/clinical/adapted-clinical-guidelines/ (accessed 17 September 2014).

Bramley, G., Fitzpatrick, S., Edwards, J., Ford, D., Johnsen, S., Sosenko, F. and Watkins, D. (2015) 'Hard edges: mapping severe and multiple disadvantage', The LankellyChase Foundation. Available at: http://lankellychase.org.uk/multiple-disadvantage/publications/hard-edges/ (accessed May 2016).

Brown, R.T., Kiely, D.K., Bharel, M. and Mitchell, S.L. (2012) 'Geriatric syndromes in older homeless adults', *Journal of General Internal Medicine*, 27(1): 16–22. Available at: doi:10.1007/s11606-011-1848-9

Cheung, A.M. and Hwang, S.W. (2004) 'Risk of death among homeless women: a cohort study and review of the literature', *CMAJ*, 170(8): 1243–7.

Coren, E., Hossain, R., Pardo, J.P., Veras, M.M., Chakraborty, K., Harris, H., Coren, M.A.J. and Hossain, R. (2013) 'Interventions for promoting reintegration and reducing harmful behaviour and lifestyles in street-connected children and young people', *Evidence-Based Child Health*, 8: 1140–272.

Culhane, D.P., Metraux, S. and Bainbridge, J. (2010) 'The age structure of contemporary homelessness: risk period or cohort effect?', Penn School of Social Policy and Practice Working Paper.

Dorney-Smith, S., Hewett, N., Khan, Z. and Smith, R. (2016) 'Integrating health care for homeless people: experiences of the KHP Pathway Homeless Team', *British Journal of Healthcare Management*, 22(4): 215–24.

Duncan, M. and Corner, J. (2012) 'Severe and multiple disadvantage: a review of key texts', Lankelly Chase Foundation, July. Available at: www.lankellychase.org.multiple-disadvantage/publications/severeand-multiple-disadvantage-literature-review/

Finlayson, S., Boelman, V., Young, R. and Kwan, A. (2016) 'Saving lives, saving money. How homeless health peer advocacy reduces health inequalities', Groundswell. Available at: http://groundswell.org.uk/wp-content/uploads/2016/03/Saving-Lives-Saving-Money-Full-Report-Web.pdf (accessed May 2016).

Fitzpatrick, S. et al (2016) 'Destitution in the UK', Joseph Rowntree Foundation, April. Available at: https://www.jrf.org.uk/report/destitution-uk (accessed June 2016).

Fitzpatrick-Lewis, D., Ganann, R., Krishnaratne, S., Ciliska, D., Kouyoumdjian, F. and Hwang, S.W. (2011) 'Effectiveness of interventions to improve the health and housing status of homeless people: a rapid systematic review', *BMC Public Health*, 11: 638. Available at: www.biomedcentral.com/1471-2458/11/638

Gallimore, A., Hay, L. and Mackie, P. (2008) *What do those with multiple and complex needs want from health, social care and voluntary sector services?*, Musselburgh: East Lothian CHP.

Gilbert, P. (2009) 'Introducing compassion-focused therapy', *Advances in Psychiatric Treatment*, 15: 199–208.

Goodwin, N., Sonola, L., Thiel, V. and Kodner, D.L. (2013) 'Co-ordinated care for people with complex chronic conditions. Key lessons and markers for success', The King's Fund. Available at: www.kingsfund.org.uk/publications/co-ordinated-carepeople-complex-chronic-conditions (accessed January 2014).

Ham, C. and Walsh, N. (2013) 'Making integrated care happen at scale and pace', King's Fund, March. Available at: www.kingsfund.org.uk/publications/making-integrated-care-happen-scale-and-pace (accessed January 2014).

Hayward, A. et al (2017, forthcoming) 'The health impact of social exclusion: a review and meta-analysis morbidity and mortality from homeless, prison, work and substance populations in high-countries', *Lancet* series 1, submitted February.

Hewett, N., Halligan, A. and Boyce, T. (2012) 'A general practitioner and nurse led approach to improving hospital care for homeless people', *BMJ*, 345: e5999.

Hossain, R. and Coren, E. (2015) 'Service engagement in interventions for street-connected children and young people: a summary of evidence supplementing a recent Cochrane–Campbell review', *Child Youth Care Forum*, 44(3): 451–70.

Howe, E., Buck, D. and Withers, J. (2009) 'Delivering health care on the streets: challenges and opportunities for quality management', *Quality Management in Health Care*, 18(4): 239–46.

Hwang, S.W. and Burns, T. (2014) 'Health interventions for people who are homeless', *Lancet*, 384: 1541–7.

Hwang, S.W., Tolomiczenko, G., Kouyoumdjian, F.G. and Garner, R.E. (2005) 'Interventions to improve the health of the homeless: a systematic review', *Am J Prev Med*, 29: 311–19.

Hwang, S.W., Wilkins, R., Tjepkema, M., O'Campo, P.J. and Dunn, J.R. (2009) 'Mortality among residents of shelters, rooming houses and hotels in Canada: 11 year follow-up study', *BMJ*, 339: b4036.

Joyce, D.P. and Limbos, M. (2009) 'Identification of cognitive impairment and mental illness in elderly homeless men, before and after access to primary health care', *Can Fam Physician*, 55: 1110–1. e1–6.

Luchenski, S. et al (forthcoming) 'What works in Inclusion Health: overview of effective interventions for marginalised and excluded populations', *Lancet*.

Marmot, M., Allen, J. and Goldblatt, P. (2010) *Fair society, healthy lives: The Marmot Review. Strategic review of health inequalities in England post-2010*, London, February. Available at: www.instituteofhealthequity. org/resources-reports/fair-society-healthy-lives-the-marmot-review (accessed January 2014).

Mayhew, L. and Smith, D. (2016) 'An investigation into inequalities in adult lifespan', Cass Business School, Faculty of Actuarial Science and Insurance, City University London, May. Available at: www. cass.city.ac.uk/__data/assets/pdf_file/0019/317314/ILC-UK-An-investigation-into-inequalities-in-adult-lifespan__9_5_16.pdf (accessed June 2016).

Morrison, D.S. (2009) 'Homelessness as an independent risk factor for mortality: results from a retrospective cohort study', *International Journal of Epidemiology*, 38: 877–83.

O'Connell, J.J. (2004) 'Dying in the shadows: the challenge of providing health care for homeless people', *CMAJ*, 170(8): 1251–52.

O'Connell, J.J., Mattison, S., Judge, C.M., Allen, J.S., Howard, K. and Koh, A. (2005) 'Public health approach to reducing morbidity and mortality among homeless people in Boston', *Journal of Public Health Management Practice*, 11(4): 311–16.

O'Connell, J.J., Oppenheimer, S.C., Judge, C.M. et al (2010) 'The Boston Healthcare for the Homeless program: a public health framework', *American Journal of Public Health*, 100(8): 1400–8.

Singer Merrill, S. (2009) *Introduction to syndemics: A systems approach to public and community health*, San Francisco, CA: Jossey-Bass.

Tudor Hart, J. (1971) 'The inverse care law', *Lancet*, 297(7696): 405–12.

Wilkinson, R. and Pickett, K. (2010) *The spirit level: Why equality is better for everyone*, London: Penguin Books.

Woodhall-Melnik, J.R. and Dunn, J.R. (2016) 'A systematic review of outcomes associated with participation in Housing First programs', *Housing Studies*, 21(3): 287–304.

Part Six
The socio-political environment

This section focuses on the geopolitical aspects of health and health inequalities, and the health-related issues of migrants entering the UK and the demand on health services as a result of poor migration policies. The Care Act 2014 offered the potential to address health and social inequalities by refocusing care from a deficits to an assets approach. 'Well-being' was seen as a new organising principle. Despite the best intentions of the Care Act, the UK austerity economic planning is undermining the activities in the care and health sectors. The main agency for delivering health care, the National Health Service (NHS), has significant problems in addressing its aims due to increasing demands by the community, funding deficits and the need for organisational reform.

TWENTY

Geopolitical aspects of health: austerity and health inequalities

Clare Bambra, Kayleigh Garthwaite and Amy Greer Murphy

Introduction

This chapter examines the effects of austerity on geographical inequalities in health using case studies of the North–South health divide in England and inequalities in health between local neighbourhoods. The chapter is divided into three sections. First, it introduces how geography matters for health, outlining the two case studies – the North–South divide and local inequalities. It then outlines the austerity and welfare reforms that have been enacted in England since 2010 and the effects that these policies are having upon these spatial health divides. The latter section draws on previous international research into welfare retrenchment, as well as qualitative data about the lived experiences of people at the sharp end of austerity. The chapter concludes by arguing that austerity measures are having uneven implications for health across localities, as well as across different socio-demographic groups, further increasing existing health inequalities.

Health and place

Health varies spatially – between countries, regions, cities and even neighbourhoods. This section examines two key examples of such spatial variations: the North–South health divide in England and inequalities in health between local neighbourhoods. It then examines explanations for the relationship between health and place with a focus on political and economic approaches.

North–South divide

Northern England (commonly defined as the North-East, North West and Yorkshire and Humber regions) has persistently had higher all-cause mortality rates than the South of England, with people in the

North consistently found to be less healthy than those in the South, across all social classes and among men and women (Dorling, 2010). This is demonstrated through life expectancy at birth (see Figure 20.1). Since 1965, this has amounted to 1.5 million excess premature deaths (Whitehead et al, 2014). A baby born today in the North-East will live, on average, six years less in good health than one born in the South-East (ONS, 2014). Likewise, the life expectancy gap (how long someone is expected to live, on average, based on contemporary mortality rates) between the two regions is over two years for both men and women.

These spatial inequalities in health between North and South have been documented since the mid-18th century and have fluctuated over time (Hacking et al, 2011; Bambra et al, 2014). In the 1950s, the health gaps between areas of England were smaller, and continued to decrease through to the 1970s before rising from the 1980s onwards (Dorling and

Figure 20.1: Map of life expectancy by region for men in England, 2011

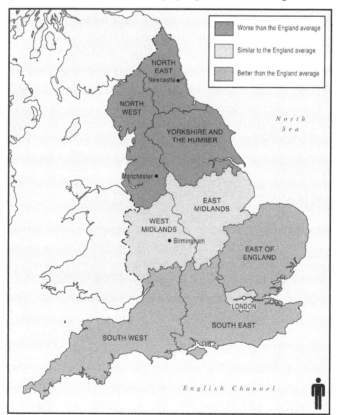

Thomas, 2009). Indeed, health inequalities between the North and the South, and also between local neighbourhoods, are now at levels only previously seen in the 19th century (Dorling, 2013). Since 1965, the 'health penalty' paid by the North has amounted to 1.5 million excess premature deaths (Whitehead and Doran, 2011). These inequalities between North and South are also part of a more extensive regional gradient in health – which encompasses all of England – whereby, generally speaking, average levels of health and life expectancy decline the further north you travel (Dorling, 2010). Although England is not alone in experiencing such spatial health inequalities, they are some of the largest in Europe – greater, for example, than those between the former East and West Germany (Bambra et al, 2014).

Local neighbourhood inequalities

The North–South health divide is supplemented by a second, more widespread, divide in health within regions and within towns and cities – a divide between affluent and deprived local neighbourhoods. By way of example, Table 20.1 shows the relationship between life expectancy and healthy life expectancy (how long someone can be expected to live, on average, in good or very good health) for men and women by neighbourhood deprivation decile (bands of 10%) in England.

Deprivation is measured in terms of area-level income, employment, health, education, crime, access to services and the living environment (DCLG, 2011). Neighbourhoods that are the most deprived have worse health than those that are less deprived, and this follows a spatial gradient, with each increase in deprivation resulting in a decrease in average health. In England, the gap between the most and least deprived areas is nine years average life expectancy and 18 years average healthy life expectancy for men, and around seven and 19 years, respectively, for women. Deprived and affluent areas with such differences in health outcomes can be located very closely together, even a few miles apart.

These smaller-scale local health inequalities related to deprivation are particularly large within Northern towns and cities. The town of Stockton-on-Tees in the North-East region, for example, has a 17-year gap in life expectancy for men and 11 years for women between its most and least deprived areas (Public Health England, 2015). This is the largest gap in life expectancy within a single local authority in England. Local health inequalities in Stockton-on-Tees are returned to later in this chapter.

Table 20.1: Life expectancy and healthy life expectancy for men and women by neighbourhood, England, 2011–13

Deprivation Decile*	Life Expectancy (LE), at birth, years		Deprivation Decile*	Health Life Expectancy (HLE), at birth, years	
	Male	Female		Male	Female
1 Most deprived	74.1	79.1	1 Most deprived	52.2	52.4
2	76.2	80.7	2	56.2	56.3
3	77.3	81.5	3	58.4	59.6
4	78.5	82.3	4	61.6	61.6
5	79.5	83.2	5	62.8	64.2
6	80.1	83.6	6	65.5	65.7
7	81.0	84.2	7	66.5	67.0
8	81.5	84.5	8	67.5	68.0
9	82.0	85.1	9	68.5	69.4
10 Least deprived	83.1	86.0	10 Least deprived	70.5	71.3
Gap	9.0	6.9	Gap	18.3	18.9

Place matters

These spatial inequalities in health are a result of a complex mix of economic, social, environmental and political processes, coming together in particular places. Places can be health-promoting (salutogenic) or health-damaging (pathogenic) (Bambra, 2016). The academic sub-discipline of health geography has conventionally presented two main explanations as to why these health inequalities exist: compositional and contextual (Macintyre et al, 2002). The compositional explanation argues that the health of a given area, such as a town, region or country, is a result of the individual characteristics of the people who live there.

It is argued that it is the demographic (age, sex and ethnicity), risky health behaviours (smoking, alcohol, physical activity, diet, drugs) and socio-economic (income, education, occupation) profiles of the people living within a place that determine its health outcomes. The contextual explanation argues that area-level health is determined by the nature of the place itself in terms of its economic, social and physical environment. The relationship between health and place has therefore been thought of in terms of 'Who lives here?' (compositional) and 'What is this place like?' (contextual).

Drawing on political science and political geography, it is increasingly being acknowledged that compositional and contextual determinants of health are themselves shaped by political factors and that health inequalities between people and places are thus politically determined (Bambra, 2016). The political approach to explaining health divides focuses on the 'social, political and economic structures and relations' that may be, and often are, outside the control of the individuals or the local areas they affect. Compositional and collective factors, such as income levels, public services and employment rates – many of the issues that dominate political life – are key determinants of health and well-being (Bambra et al, 2005). Why some places and people are consistently privileged while others are consistently marginalised is a political choice. Political choices can therefore be seen as the fundamental causes of health inequalities. Austerity is examined in this chapter as a case study of such political causes of health inequalities.

Austerity, health and place

In economics, 'austerity' refers to reducing budget deficits in economic downturns by decreasing public expenditure, particularly on welfare, and/or increasing taxes. It is, in part, a set of economic and social policies purported to reduce the budget deficit (Konzelmann, 2014). In the UK, since 2010, this has been characterised by large-scale cuts to central and local government budgets, continued National Health Service (NHS) privatisation, and cuts in welfare services and benefits.

Shrinking the safety net

The economic recession has been used as an excuse for implementing a massive restructuring of the state. The UK government (a Conservative–Liberal Democrat coalition from 2010 to 2015) introduced several benefit reductions and restrictions through the Welfare Reform Act 2012. This included caps on levels of entitlement, the 'under-occupancy charge' (or 'bedroom tax' as it is more commonly known) for Housing Benefit recipients, longer waiting periods between unemployment and benefit eligibility, and the establishment of local welfare assistance to replace the discretionary social fund. This is set against a backdrop of 'ubiquitous conditionality' (Dwyer and Wright, 2014) – sanctions, delays and changes to benefits, which have led to increasing numbers of people using food banks (Loopstra et al, 2015). These changes to welfare benefits in the UK from 2010 to 2015 are listed in Table 20.2. Further welfare reforms have been announced since the 2015 general election (which returned a majority Conservative government), and include: Universal Credit tapers and thresholds; a further reduction in the benefit cap to £23,000 a year in London and £20,000 elsewhere; the end of automatic entitlement to Housing Benefit for out-of-work 18–21 year olds; and a four-year freeze in the value of most working-age benefits.

The effects of these welfare changes and reductions in local government budgets (which impact on services such as libraries and social care) have been unequally spatially distributed, hitting the poorest parts of the country hardest (Taylor-Robinson et al, 2013). This is demonstrated in Figures 20.2 and 20.3, where the disproportionate impact on the older industrial areas in the North of England is evident (Beatty and Fothergill, 2016). Beatty and Fothergill (2016) report that older industrial areas, less prosperous seaside towns, some London boroughs and a number of other Northern cities have been the hardest hit by austerity.

By contrast, much of Southern England outside London escapes relatively lightly. For example, Blackpool (North-West) will experience an estimated loss as a result of welfare reforms of more than £900 a year per working-age adult. Local government spending has also fallen by around a third since 2008 and the worst-hit local authority areas – mainly located in the North (eg Middlesbrough, North-East – £470 less per working-age adult) – have lost far more than the authorities least affected by the cuts – located exclusively in the South (eg Hart, Hampshire – £50 per working-age adult).

The effect of tax and benefit reforms has also largely been socio-economically regressive, with low-income households of working age losing the most, particularly low-income women (Fawcett Society, 2014). Beatty and Fothergill (2016) estimate that couples with two or more dependent children will lose an average of £1,450 a year; lone parents with two or more dependent children lose an average of £1,750 a year. A total of 83% of the overall financial loss falls on families with children. A number of the new reforms affect tenants in council and housing association properties, who are set to lose more than £6 billion a year, or nearly half the entire loss from the new reforms. On average, working-age social sector tenants lose more than five times as much as working-age owner-occupiers. Low-income households of working age are losing the most and are disproportionately located in deprived neighbourhoods (De Agostini et al, 2014). Austerity measures have therefore not affected all places or people equally.

Table 20.2: Austerity-driven welfare reform in the UK, 2010–15

Date	Measure
January 2011	Child Trust Fund abolished.
April 2011	Child Benefit frozen until 2015.
April 2012	A one year time limit to the receipt of contributory ESA for people in the Work Related Activity Group. Tax credits withdrawn from 'middle income' families.
May 2012	Lone Parent Obligations introduced.
October 2012	Conditionality, sanctions and hardship payments introduced.
January 2013	Child Benefit withdrawn from individuals earning more than £50,000.
March 2013	Housing Benefit/Local Housing Allowance restricted to the Consumer Price Index – as are other benefits.
April 2013	Childcare costs covered by Working Tax Credit cut from 80% to 70%. Councill Tax Benefits – 10% reduction for welfare recipients in total payments to local authorities. Up-rating of working-age benefits not related to disability restricted to 1% (inflation 3.5%). Household Benefit Cap (set at £26,000 maximum). Social Fund replaced by locally determined schemes for crisis loans and community care grants. Under occupancy change or 'Bedroom Tax' if claimant has one spare bedroom (14% reduction) or more (25% reduction). Restrictions in access to legal aid.
April 2013-October 2017	Migration of all existing working-age Disability Living Allowance (DLA) claimants onto Personal Independence Payments (PIP).
June 2013	Replacement of DLA by PIP for all new claimants
October 2013	Universal Credit - new claims and changes
December 2013	PIP reassessment of DLA claims
April 2014	Universal Credit – transfer existing clients
February 2015	Roll out of Universal Credit
July 2015	Tax credits and family benefits under Universal Credit limited to the first two children. Working age benefits frozen for four years from 2016. Working element of Employment and Support Allowance (ESA) payments reduced to Job Seeker's Allowance (JSA) levels. The benefit cap reduced to £20,000. Housing Benefit entitlement restricted for those aged between 16 and 21. Those earning more than £30,000 pay more if they rent social housing.

Figure 20.2: Map of per head welfare reductions for English local authorities, 2010–15

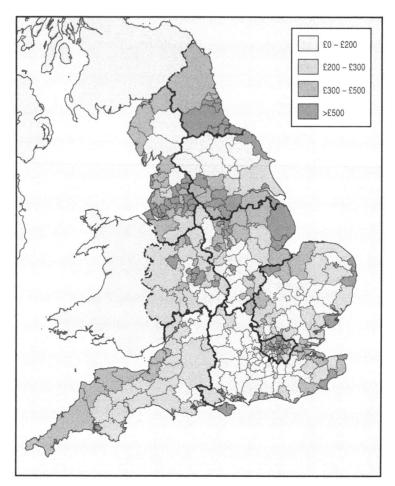

Increasing the health gap

In terms of health inequalities, emerging evidence suggests that the socially and spatially concentrated effects of austerity are beginning to negatively impact on the health of the most vulnerable. Taylor-Robinson et al (2013) observed that austerity measures hit the sickest hardest, and across England, there has been an increase in indicators of poor mental health since 2010, and evidence nationally of widening inequalities in mental health. While population mental health usually declines during an economic recession and then recovers, this has not been the case in the current period. Mental health continues to be affected, including an increase in rates of suicides, with 2013

Figure 20.3: Map of per head reductions in local authority budgets, England, 2010–15

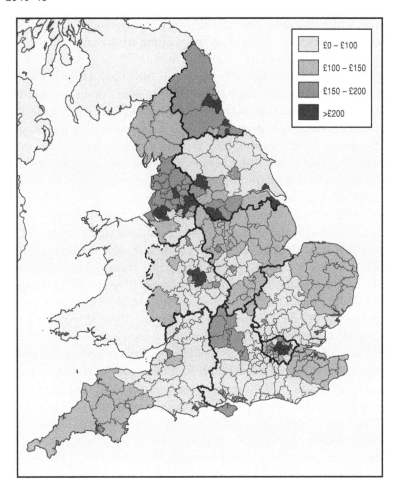

witnessing the highest male suicide rate since 2001 (ONS, 2015). Across England, inequalities in mental health have been exacerbated by ongoing austerity and welfare reform in the UK, with evidence suggesting that the effect of tax and benefit reforms has largely been regressive (Barr et al, 2015). Similarly, in their study on self-harm, Barnes et al (2016: 132) reported that economic hardships resulting from the recession and austerity measures accumulated or acted as a 'final straw' to trigger 'self-harm', emphasising that 'changes in welfare benefits may have contributed' to this rise.

Niedzwiedz et al (2016) found that reductions in spending levels and increased conditionality may adversely affect the mental health of disadvantaged social groups. Austerity measures in England have also affected vulnerable old-age adults (Loopstra et al, 2016). They found that rising mortality rates among pensioners aged 85 years and over were linked to reductions in spending on income support for poor pensioners and social care. Moffatt et al (2015: 1) found that the bedroom tax 'has increased poverty and had broad-ranging adverse effects on health, wellbeing and social relationships' in the community. Loopstra et al (2015) found that the rise in food bank use is associated with cuts to local authority spending and central welfare spending.

Evidence from previous international research on reductions in welfare has also shown that where welfare services are cut, inequalities in mortality and morbidity increase, while overall population health is generally unaffected – cuts in welfare have a detrimental impact on the health of the poorest. A US study found that while premature mortality (deaths under age 75) and infant mortality rates (deaths before age one) declined overall in all income quintiles from 1960 to 2002, inequalities by income and ethnicity decreased only between 1966 and 1980, and then increased between 1980 and 2002 (Krieger et al, 2008). The reductions in inequalities (1966–80) occurred during a period of welfare expansion in the US (the 'War on Poverty') and the enactment of civil rights legislation that increased access to welfare state services. The increases in health inequalities occurred during the Reagan–Bush period of neoliberalism, when public welfare services (including health-care insurance coverage) were cut, the funding of social assistance was reduced, the minimum wage was frozen and the tax base was shifted from the rich to the poor, leading to increased income polarisation.

Research into the health effects of Thatcherism (1979–90) has also concluded that the large-scale dismantling of the UK's social-democratic institutions and the early pursuit of 'austerity-style' policies increased socio-economic health inequalities. Thatcherism deregulated the labour and financial markets, privatised utilities and state enterprises, restricted social housing, curtailed trade union rights, marketised the public sector, significantly cut the social wage via welfare state retrenchment, accepted mass unemployment, and implemented large tax cuts for the business sector and most affluent. In this period, while life expectancy increased and mortality rates decreased for all social groups, the increases were greater and more rapid among the highest social groups, so that inequalities increased. Area inequalities also increased in this period, with the North and Scotland falling behind the rest of the UK (Scott-Samuel et al, 2014).

International research into the effects of welfare reform also suggests that existing spatial inequalities in health within towns and cities will increase. This is evident, for example, in studies of New Zealand in the 1980s and 1990s, when major welfare reform (including a less redistributive tax system, targeted social benefits, the introduction of a regressive tax on consumption, the privatisation of major utilities and public housing, user charges for welfare services, and a more deregulated labour market) resulted in a rapid increase in spatial inequalities in health (Pearce et al, 2006). Since the mid-1990s, when the New Zealand economy improved and there were some improvements in services (eg better access to social housing, more generous social assistance and a decrease in health-care costs), regional inequalities stabilised (Pearce and Dorling, 2006).

These historical increases in social and spatial health divides were not inevitable; in the UK – like the US and New Zealand – inequalities in mortality declined from the 1920s to the 1970s as income inequalities were reduced and the welfare state was expanded. Taken together, these early signs and previous international experience suggest that austerity will have differential spatial effects on health. Areas such as the North of England, with its higher rates of poverty, unemployment and welfare receipt, are suffering disproportionately, as are poorer neighbourhoods and vulnerable socio-demographic groups. This is explored further in the following section.

Lived experiences of austerity

Emerging qualitative research that explores the lived experiences of austerity offers immediate and intimate insights into how it is being experienced on the ground and how it is influencing health and well-being (Elliot et al, 2015). Some indicative data from our 'Local health inequalities in an age of austerity: the Stockton-on-Tees study' is presented in the following with regards to the rise of food banks – the poster child of austerity Britain – and also in respect of mothers living in deprived neighbourhoods – the group arguably most negatively affected financially by austerity and the associated welfare cuts.

Stockton-on-Tees is in the North-East of England and has the highest neighbourhood-level local health inequalities in England for both men (at a 17.3-year difference in life expectancy at birth) and for women (11.4-year gap in life expectancy) (Public Health England, 2015). The borough has a population of 191,600 residents and demonstrates high levels of social inequality, with some areas of the local authority having low levels of deprivation (eg Ingleby Barwick and Yarm) and others nearby characterised by very high levels of deprivation (eg Hardwick and Port Clarence). This proximity is illustrated in Figure 20.4.

Food bank use and health inequalities

Almost half of food bank users cite austerity-led welfare changes as their reason for service use. Benefit delays, sanctions and the 'bedroom tax' are central factors in the significant increase in the numbers of people accessing food banks. Often, people who used the food bank experienced a range of mental health problems, from anxiety and depression to paranoid schizophrenia and personality disorders (Perry et al, 2014; Garthwaite et al, 2015; Garthwaite, 2016), which can place people at a greater risk of having their benefits sanctioned. People using the food bank regularly spoke of the associated health problems of living on a low income at a time of austerity.

Naomi, aged 36, had been receiving Employment and Support Allowance (ESA) and Disability Living Allowance (DLA) for five years due to her physical and mental health problems. Naomi was also recovering from a heroin addiction that she has been dealing with since she was 18. Speaking about having to choose between food and heating her home, Naomi said:

> "I've been there many a times, it's like do I starve or go without electric, or do I freeze but have something to eat? I do get that but a lot of people use meters in my situation so you know what you're using. I remember in ma last flat, summat happened with the company I was with, I told them I wanted a key meter and they never put one in. Next thing I know I was £700 in debt, so I actually had no gas for about three, four year and I ended up nearly dying in hospital with pneumonia."

Research has regularly shown that those on benefits or the statutory minimum wage have insufficient money to buy the food that they need for health, however carefully they budget and shop (Davis et al, 2014). This has long-term health consequences in terms of obesity, diabetes and other dietary-related diseases, such as high cholesterol, as food bank volunteer and user Simon pointed out after a recent visit to his general practitioner:

> "Dr, I'm unemployed – I'm not eating meat, I'm eating chips, ready meals – my cholesterol is going to go up. If I make mashed

potatoes I put margarine in, blue top milk, plenty of salt and pepper to give it some taste."

Figure 20.4: Map of Stockton-on-Tees study neighbourhoods

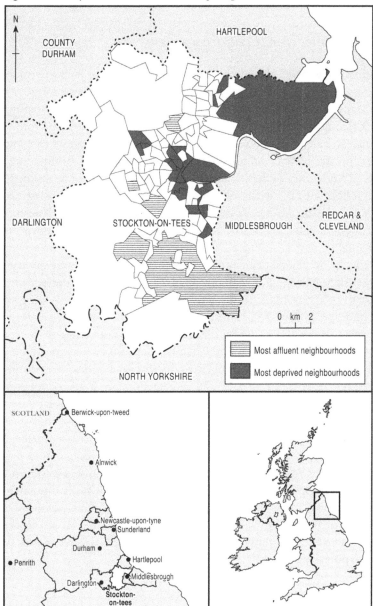

The negotiation of living on a low income could often result in mental health problems for people accessing a food bank (Perry et al, 2014; Garthwaite et al, 2015), with pre-existing health problems interweaving with complex factors such as relationship breakdown, job loss and welfare reform.

Mothers, austerity and health inequalities

Emphasis has been placed on the distinct challenges facing women due to austerity policies (Fawcett Society, 2014; Greer Murphy, 2016). Austerity is creating a 'triple jeopardy' through welfare cuts, rising work insecurity and public sector service cuts and job losses. Women are placed in a difficult position: societal expectations around care and work, greater reliance on public sector employment and services, high rates of underemployment and part-time work, and a more sustained interaction with the benefits system means that austerity threatens to widen the inequalities they face. The provision of affordable housing, fairly compensated work, labour bargaining power, universal education and quality public services have been gradually eroded for several decades by neoliberal principles applied to policymaking, and austerity is intensifying this (Schrecker and Bambra, 2015). For gender equality, some of the gains made in the past decades are at risk.

There is a lack of insight into the intersecting nature of gendered and spatial inequalities stemming from these processes (Greer Murphy, 2016). Patterns of inequality between women and men are not linear, and have changed in complex ways in recent decades, not simply for better or worse (Walby, 1997). Intersectionality, a key concept in feminist discourse, provides an important prism through which to view this. In the borough of Stockton-on-Tees, empirical research with mothers is exploring the complex pathways of women's inequalities across the life cycle. These are found to be spatiality concentrated in deprived areas of the borough and exacerbated by socio-economic position, education status, debt, disability and poor health, tenancy, and household type. This research is finding that the intersections of these inequalities both create the conditions for and exacerbate the lived experiences of poor health, debt and multiple disadvantages. As Chloe discussed:

> "Our house is rented, so we don't have much of a say in what goes on with it. But it's fine for us and it's better than what we were living in before. We were living in a two-bedroom bungalow that was cold, it had damp, I had a bad chest the whole time we

lived there. We're lucky we've managed to move on. But we got the boys' diagnosis, and I managed to get Carer's Allowance. Before, when your children still have something different about them, you still have to look after them but you don't get Carer's Allowance. I couldn't get Job Seeker's, I couldn't get any Income Support, I could get nothing. I was being a carer, but that wasn't being recognised."

Of significant concern is the role that the state is playing to enhance these issues during austerity. While these inequalities are part of a historical lineage of gender-based inequality and the localised consequences of the economic decline of the region in recent decades, they are seen to be getting worse due to welfare reforms. As Tara put it, seen through her work at a charity in Stockton-on-Tees:

"Austerity has had a huge impact on people. People have always struggled, but now you don't have enough income to pay for food, gas, electric. And now households are paying council tax, they might be paying a top-up on rent, bedroom tax, it's all had a massive impact on a limited budget that they already had."

As this quote illustrates, there is a clear emergence of newly intensified inequalities widening due to austerity measures.

Conclusion

This chapter has examined the effects of austerity on geographical inequalities in health using case studies of the North–South health divide in England and inequalities in health between local neighbourhoods. The chapter has shown how and why geography matters for health, arguing particularly that the relationship between health and place is a political one. It has taken austerity as an example of the latter and outlined its effects on socio-economic and spatial inequalities in health in England since 2010. Drawing on both quantitative and qualitative data, the chapter has shown that it is very clear that austerity is having uneven implications for health across localities and regions, and between different socio-demographic groups, further increasing existing health inequalities. This is in stark contrast to the claims of the government and austerity advocates that 'we are all in it together'.

Acknowledgements

With permission of the relevant publishers, this chapter is based on Bambra (2016), Garthwaite (2016) and Greer Murphy (2016).

References

Bambra, C. (2016) *Health divides: Where you live can kill you*, Bristol: Policy Press.

Bambra, C., Fox, D. and Scott-Samuel, A. (2005) 'Towards a politics of health', *Health Promotion International*, 20(2): 187–93.

Bambra, C., Barr, B. and Milne, E. (2014) 'North and South: addressing the English health divide', *Journal of Public Health*, 36: 183–6.

Barnes, M., Gunnell, C., Davies, D., Hawton, R., Kapur, K., Potokar, N. and Donovan, J.L. (2016) 'Understanding vulnerability to self-harm in times of economic hardship and austerity: a qualitative study', *British Medical Journal*, 6(2), doi: 10.1136/bmjopen-2015-010131

Barr, B., Taylor-Robinson, D., Stuckler, D., Loopstra, R., Reeves, A. and Whitehead, M. (2015) 'First, do no harm: are disability assessments associated with adverse trends in mental health? A longitudinal ecological study', *Journal of Epidemiology and Community Health*, 70(4): 339–45.

Beatty, C. and Fothergill, S. (2016) 'The uneven impact of welfare reform. The financial losses to places and people', Centre for Regional Economic and Social Research, Sheffield Hallam University, Sheffield.

Davis, L.B., Sengul, I., Ivy, J. and Brock, L. (2014) 'Scheduling food bank collections and deliveries to ensure food safety and improve access', *Socio-Economic Planning Sciences*, 48(3): 175–88.

DCLG (Department for Communities and Local Government) (2011) *English indices of deprivation 2010*, London: Department for Communities and Local Government.

De Agostini, P., Hills, J. and Sutherland, H. (2014) 'Were we really all in it together? The distributional effects of the UK Coalition government's tax-benefit policy changes', Social Policy in a Cold Climate, Working Paper 10, CASE, London.

Dorling, D. (2010) 'Persistent North–South divides', in N.M. Coe and A. Jones (eds) *The economic geography of the UK*, London: Sage Publications, pp 12–24.

Dorling, D. (2013) *Unequal health: The scandal of our times*, Bristol: Policy Press.

Dorling, D. and Thomas, B. (2009) 'Geographical inequalities in health over the last century', in H. Graham (ed) *Understanding health inequalities*, Maidenhead: Open University Press, pp 66–83.

Dwyer, P. and Wright, S. (2014) 'Universal Credit, ubiquitous conditionality and its implications for social citizenship', *Journal of Poverty and Social Justice*, 22: 27–35.

Elliott, E., Popay, J. and Williams, G. (2015) 'Knowledge of the everyday: confronting the causes of health inequalities', in K. Smith, S. Hill and C. Bambra (eds) *Health inequalities: Critical perspectives*, Oxford: Oxford University Press, pp 222–37.

Fawcett Society (2014) *The changing labour market 2: Women, low pay and gender equality in the emerging recovery*, London: Fawcett Society.

Garthwaite, K. (2016) *Hunger pains: Life inside foodbank Britain*, Bristol: Policy Press.

Garthwaite, K., Collins, P. and Bambra, C. (2015) 'Food for thought: an ethnographic study of negotiating ill health and food insecurity in a UK foodbank', *Social Science & Medicine*, 132: 38–44.

Greer Murphy, A. (2016) 'Austerity in the United Kingdom: the intersections of spatial and gendered inequalities', *Area*, 49(1): 122–24.

Hacking, J.M., Muller, S. and Buchan, I.E. (2011) 'Trends in mortality from 1965 to 2008 across the English North–South divide: comparative observational study', *British Medical Journal*, 342: d508.

Konzelmann, S. (2014) 'The political economics of austerity', *Cambridge Journal of Economics*, 38: 701–41.

Krieger, N., Rehkopf, D.H., Chen, J.T., Waterman, P.D., Marcelli, E. and Kennedy, M. (2008) 'The fall and rise of US inequities in premature mortality: 1960–2002', *Plos Medicine*, 5(2): 227–41.

Loopstra, R., Reeves, A., Taylor-Robinson, D., Barr, B., McKee, M. and Stuckler, D. (2015) 'Austerity, sanctions, and the rise of food banks in the UK', *British Medical Journal*, 350, p.h1775.

Loopstra, R., McKee, M., Katikireddi, S.V., Taylor-Robinson, D., Barr, B. and Stuckler, D. (2016) 'Austerity and old-age mortality in England: a longitudinal cross-local area analysis, 2007–2013', *Journal of the Royal Society of Medicine*, 109(3): 109–16.

Macintyre, S., Ellaway, A. and Cummins, S. (2002) 'Place effects on health: how can we conceptualise, operationalise and measure them?', *Social Science & Medicine*, 55(1): 125–39.

Moffatt, S., Lawson, S. and Patterson, R. (2015) 'A qualitative study of the impact of the UK "bedroom tax"', *Journal of Public Health*, 38(2): 197–205.

Niedzwiedz, C.L., Mitchell, R.J., Shortt, N.K. and Pearce, J.R. (2016) 'Social protection spending and inequalities in depressive symptoms across Europe', *Social Psychiatry and Psychiatric Epidemiology*, 51(7): 1005–1014.

ONS (Office for National Statistics) (2014) *Statistical bulletin adult health in Great Britain*, London: Office for National Statistics.

ONS (2015) *Inequality in healthy life expectancy at birth by national deciles of area deprivation: England, 2011 to 2013*, London: Office for National Statistics.

Pearce, J. and Dorling, D. (2006) 'Increasing geographical inequalities in health in New Zealand, 1980–2001', *International Journal of Epidemiology*, 35: 597–603.

Pearce, J., Dorling, D., Wheeler, B., Barnett, R. and Rigby, J. (2006) 'Geographical inequalities in health in New Zealand, 1980–2001: the gap widens', *Australian and New Zealand Journal of Public Health*, 30: 461–6.

Perry, J., Williams, M., Sefton, T. and Haddad, M. (2014) 'Emergency use only: understanding and reducing the use of food banks in the UK', CPAG, Church of England, Oxfam GB and the Trussell Trust.

Public Health England (2015) 'Stockton-on-Tees health profile 2015', APHO.

Schrecker, T. and Bambra, C. (2015) *How politics makes us sick: Neoliberal epidemics*, London: Palgrave Macmillan.

Scott-Samuel, A., Bambra, C., Collins, C., Hunter, D.J., McCartney, G. and Smith, K. (2014) 'The impact of Thatcherism on health and wellbeing in Britain', *International Journal of Health Services*, 44: 53–72.

Taylor-Robinson, D., Rougeaux, E., Dominic, H., Whitehead, M., Barr, B. and Pearce, A. (2013) 'The rise of food poverty in the UK', *BMJ*, 347: p.f7157.

Walby, S. (1997) *Gender transformations*, London: Routledge.

Whitehead, M. and Doran, T. (2011) 'The north–south health divide', *BMJ*, 342: d584

Whitehead, M., Bambra, C., Barr, B,. Bowles, J.R., Caulfield, R., Doran, T., Harrison, D., Lynch, A., Pleasant, S. and Weldon, J. (2014) *Due North: Report of the inquiry on health equity for the North*, Liverpool and Manchester: University of Liverpool and Centre for Local Economic Strategies.

TWENTY-ONE

Health and well-being of refugees and migrants within a politically contested environment

Gayle Munro

Introduction

The chapters in this volume have demonstrated how health and well-being can be impacted by a number of wider societal contexts affecting the daily lives of individuals, families and communities. Those arriving as newcomers to the UK are likely to have differing experiences of what has been described as the context of reception (Portes and Rumbaut, 2006) as they make lives for themselves in a new country. The heterogeneity of such experiences is likely to reflect the diversity of the demographic make-up of those who seek to make the UK their home, whether that is on a temporary or a permanent basis. Both the contexts of departure and the contexts of reception will have an influence over an individual migrant's experience of migration and will impact upon the daily life of a migrant in the country of destination.

Contexts of departure are likely to be affected by: the circumstances leading up to the decision to migrate; motivations for making the decision to leave; the year of departure; the country of origin; age and place on the life cycle on departure; socio-economic background; education; and the degree to which the decision to leave was 'forced' or 'voluntary' (or somewhere on a continuum). The context of reception into which the newly arrived migrant will find him/herself will similarly depend on: gender; age and place on the life cycle; the experience of the immigration system; experience in the local area of 'settlement' (urban, rural, extent to which the area is welcoming to newcomers); wider discourse (eg media) around (im)migration and/or coverage of events in the country of origin; experience in the labour market; extent to which the newcomer is familiar with the local language; and sociocultural-political circumstances in the country of destination.

All the factors just cited can have an impact upon the health and well-being of a migrant.[1] Due to the nature of his/her experience in the country of origin and an immigration status that is likely to dominate so many aspects of his/her life, refugees and migrants will frequently be 'fine-tuned' to the socio-political-cultural context in the country of destination in a way that those whose place of birth grants them a secure, unquestionable right to reside in the country have the luxury of ignoring. This wider context came to the fore in public debate in two main ways in 2015/16: the first through the rise in the numbers of those seeking refuge in and across Europe; and the second through the referendum result of the UK vote to leave the European Union (EU).

This chapter therefore discusses how the health and well-being of refugees and migrants can be socially (or politically) determined in three main and interconnected ways: the control of access to health care; the individual response to pre-migration factors; and the effects of a general political 'shift' (in this case, the societal aftermath of the EU referendum result).

Health and migration: general context

There is evidence that many migrants have reported good health on arrival in the UK but that this can often deteriorate over time, possibly because of a combination of post-migration stressors (Li et al, 2016) and issues with accessing appropriate health care (Rechel et al, 2013; Jayaweera, 2014). Much of the literature on health and migration will focus on the needs of specific groups of migrants, often defined by either their lived experience of migration or linked to their immigration status. Work has been carried out, for example, on the health needs of trafficked people (Westwood et al, 2016), migrants in detention (Medical Justice, 2013), asylum seekers and refugees (Bogić et al, 2012), and undocumented migrants (Woodward et al, 2014), or has focused on the health needs of particular ethnic groups.

The purpose of this chapter is not to provide a comprehensive review of the health-care needs of migrants, which can be read *inter alia* in the literature referenced earlier. When considering the socio-political contexts of health and migration, certain key and ongoing events occurred during 2015 and 2016 that could potentially have a profound effect on the health of migrants, both now and years into the future. Ongoing conflict and unrest in many countries of the Middle East (particularly Syria) and across the African continent has led to a significant increase in the numbers of those seeking asylum across Europe in 2015 and 2016. The number of asylum seekers across the

28 member states[2] of the EU more than doubled from 627,000 in 2014 to 1.3 million in 2015 (compared with an increase of less than 200,000 between 2013 and 2014).[3] The physical conditions for those seeking refuge across Europe are dire. For many of those who do survive the journey by sea, what awaits them is a long wait languishing in a refugee camp, fraught with difficult living conditions.

Dhesi et al (2015), for example, reported on conditions within the camp at Calais (often referred to as the 'Jungle') as 'diabolical', likely to have lifelong health repercussions for camp residents and not meeting standards recommended by the United Nations High Commissioner for Refugees (UNHCR) or World Health Organization (WHO). Not surprisingly, reports of physical and especially mental ill health are high within the populations, with many camp residents reporting symptoms associated with post-traumatic stress disorder (PTSD). At the time of writing, the 'Jungle' had been closed by the French authorities. However, there is evidence of the displaced former residents of the camp sleeping rough on the streets of Paris and other cities. Conditions in other camps, for example, in Greece, especially during the cold winter of 2016/17, have also come under heavy criticism from the European Commission and a number of media outlets.

Contexts of support

It would be natural to assume that for an individual fleeing persecution and/or a conflict situation, the place of refuge should represent a place of safety, a space where recovery and healing can begin, whether from physical or psychological wounds. In some cases, however, the migration experience itself is dominated by such exploitative conditions – either as part of the journey or continuing at the country of destination – that what should represent a safe space, a refuge, is anything but. In such cases where the pre-departure experience, journey itself and life in the country of destination forms one continuum of trauma, the amount of time necessary for eventual recovery can be lengthy and punctuated with setbacks.

Trafficked people, for instance, are often considered by service providers and policymakers as a distinct category from refugees, other vulnerable migrants or migrants in general. While it is the case that many individuals who have experienced a trafficking situation may present with different health needs than those migrants who have not been trafficked (Munro and Pritchard, 2013), it is also increasingly the case, in the UK, that trafficked individuals who are also eligible to claim asylum are being encouraged to do so. At the time of writing, victims of trafficking in the UK are identified as such via a process known as the National Referral Mechanism (NRM). Under the NRM, there is a two-stage decision-making process as to whether an individual has, indeed, been trafficked or not. One of the UK's 'competent authorities' makes a decision, based on a completed NRM referral, on whether there are 'reasonable grounds' (RG) or 'conclusive grounds' (CG) to determine that an individual has been trafficked or not. If there is a positive CG decision made in an individual's case, then that person is entitled to 45 days of support under the Council of Europe Convention on Action against Trafficking in Human Beings (ECAT).[4] However, once that 45-day period of support has come to an end, that positive CG decision entitles the trafficked individual to very little in terms of statutory support within the UK. Those non-European nationals who are eligible to claim asylum are often encouraged by their solicitor to do so for two reasons: first, the asylum process will usually take considerably longer than 45 days, and while the process is ongoing, the claimant is often entitled to support; and, second, if the claim results in a positive outcome, then the individual will be granted leave to stay in the UK, a conclusion that a positive CG decision does not guarantee.

Segregation of services

For reasons often connected to immigration status and a right to remain, (non-European) trafficked individuals will often enter the asylum process at some stage. Discourse exists on the nexus between trafficking and asylum but is often based on legal definitions. Less frequently considered within the literature is how the relationship between trafficking and asylum plays out within a support provider context, especially in the field of health and well-being. Services are frequently siloed, for instance, with many providers working with 'single-issue' clients. There are agencies, often non-governmental organisations (NGOs), which work with homeless populations, for instance, or with refugees, or with migrants, or in mental health, or with trafficking victims or victims of torture, or with individuals in or leaving immigration detention centres. The very nature of the support sector is piecemeal and does little to encourage the provision of holistic services which consider that one individual could potentially encompass all these categories simultaneously. Voluntary support services are frequently funded through commissioned contracts via local or central government departments, which, in turn, operate separate budget streams. One somewhat inevitable outcome of this financial segregation of services throughout the support sector via commissioning routes is that on the sharp end of the process, the individual in need of assistance can be in receipt of different kinds of services from a multitude of providers, depending on which organisation is awarded which contract, and which migration 'box' the individual fits into at the time.

This segregation of support is reinforced by the common practice of defining an individual who has moved from one country to another via a label designed to categorise by migration 'type', usually based on motivation for migrating. However, highlighted by many (eg Turton, 2003) is the way in which the migration experience is rarely so straightforward and so easily defined by one (set of) motivation(s). A response such as 'That's not really migration is it? That's trafficking'[5] before packaging that individual and any support needs that he/she may have into the 'trafficking box' may therefore suit the contract culture as a whole, the service commissioners and the contract deliverers but may not ultimately be the best response for the human being in need of help – help that is not necessarily defined by the trafficking experience, or even by the experience of migration at all.

Contexts of politics

The British government, as part of the creation of its hostile environment strategy, passed an Immigration Act in 2016 that embeds immigration control into everyday life in a way hitherto not experienced in the UK.[6] The rules and regulations around access to health care are governed by who and, more importantly, who does not have the right to different types of treatment. The Department of Health (DH) led a consultation in 2015/16 around the charging process for overseas visitors.[7] The consultation process revealed a level of confusion and misunderstanding on the 'front line' of service delivery, especially in general practitioner surgeries, around entitlements to health care. NGOs within the sector, for instance, have long reported their concerns around the (often erroneous) 'policing' of access to services by practice managers and overzealous GP receptionists.[8]

Health and the experience of (forced) migration

The politicisation of health care in terms of accessing services and the gatekeeping of treatment based on immigration status is one clear, overt way that politics and health are wedded together in an unhappy marriage. The psychosocial model within migration studies emphasises the way in which interventions within the 'social space' can have positive benefits on the health and well-being of individuals and communities. In the case of those forced to flee conflict within the country of origin, the social, political and cultural circumstances related to their original flight can have an impact on the physical and mental well-being of refugees for years following the original departure. Unrelated to the field of migration, observers have highlighted how the emotional stress brought about by the experience of 'trauma', however that may be defined, can have an impact upon physical and mental health. An individual response to a traumatic event will obviously vary depending on a whole host of factors. There is anecdotal but thus far under-studied evidence specifically on how the experience of *injustice* and its associated stressors impacts upon physical and psychological health. In the case of the Hillsborough[9] tragedy, for example, there has been much discussion around how the physical and, in particular, the mental health of survivors and the families of those killed have been affected since 15 April 1989. Of course, it is not possible to isolate the extent to which any existing mental health problems experienced by survivors could be attributed to the events of the day itself or to the ongoing struggle for justice for more than 25 years since. Similarly, it is possible to speculate but not to 'prove' that any health issues experienced by the families of those killed at Hillsborough were 'caused' or exacerbated by either the tragedy or by the experience of the stress of injustice for so many years following.

The link between stress and health problems has, however, been well established (Schneiderman et al, 2005). Endured by those who have experienced trauma, some for many years, is the feeling of constantly being denied a sense of control over unsolicited life events. When the original trauma is combined with a lack of reckoning concerning the experience, this combination of the trauma and a constant feeling of having been severely 'wronged' can lead to a toxicity that may have a dramatic result on the health of the individual. Concerning the often-cited mental health issues related to refugees, for example, particular references have been made to the health impacts of not only the circumstances leading up to and surrounding the act of migration itself, but also the ongoing corrosive effect of *injustice* upon the mental health of a forced migrant.

The health and well-being of a refugee sometimes have to withstand the accumulative effect of persecution and/or acts of or threats of violence associated with conflict in the country of origin, accompanied by: the loss of family members and friends; the unsolicited experience of having to 'abandon' their home and life in the country of origin; and stressors associated with the journey itself. This is all before arrival in the country of 'refuge', where the 'post-migration' stage can be characterised by: a difficult and sometimes protracted negotiation of the immigration system, with months or years being in a state of 'limbo'; an inability to travel while the authorities make a decision about immigration status; feelings of being 'unwanted' in an area that may not be welcoming to newcomers; and difficulties adapting to daily life in a new country. The post-migration stage can also frequently be underpinned by a heavy dose of survivor guilt or guilt at leaving the country of origin, as well as family and friends in the country of origin (Munro, 2017). The accumulative effect of such post-migration stressors occurring after the experience of forced migration would be a significant burden for the mental health of any individual. However, some refugees have to cope with additional challenges to their health and well-being: the knowledge that some of those responsible for their forced departure from the country of origin have not only escaped justice, but may be thriving in positions of responsibility; being confronted with denial from some about the circumstances surrounding the flight from the country of origin; an ongoing fight to raise awareness of events within the country of origin; and a fight to gain an acceptance of responsibility from those who have caused such pain.[10]

Health and public/political discourses

The political discourse surrounding migration is such that, in some contexts, this can easily contribute to the toxicity that can have such a destructive effect on the health and well-being of a migrant. Observers of the presentation of migrants and migration within certain British mainstream media have long highlighted how the discourse around migration has been conflated by inflammatory headlines and provocative statements, implying or sometimes outright claiming that the UK is being beset by large numbers of migrants, sometimes with the accompanying suggestion that these migrants are 'illegal' or 'bogus', or that they are intent on 'taking our jobs' and/or 'destroying our culture'.[11] Some directly imply that the phenomenon of 'health tourism' has led to some capitalising on their immigration status by seeking to 'exploit' the NHS.

The result of the referendum held on 23 June 2016 around the UK's membership of the EU has led some to interrogate the extent to which such media coverage, some of which dates back years, contributed to a public fear of uncontrolled (im)migration. The UK consistently features among those European countries that have the lowest numbers of asylum claims[12] and it is certainly not EU member states that have had the responsibility of absorbing the largest numbers of those seeking asylum during 2015/16. However, headlines such as those propounded by much of the British tabloid media would suggest otherwise. It is not possible to 'prove' the extent to which such headlines, drip-fed over months and years and intensifying in the run-up to the referendum, contributed to the results of the vote. Yet, statements issued by those who voted and campaigned to leave the EU would suggest that immigration played a significant role in both the campaign itself and in the decision-making of leave voters.

The result of the vote to leave the EU will have potentially far-reaching implications for the health of migrants in the UK in a number of different areas. At the time of writing, as the UK grapples with the overall implications of the 'leave' vote, the wider repercussions of the vote result, as well as those specifically related to health and/or migration, are still unknown. However, it is possible to determine a number of areas in which the UK leaving the EU is likely to have an impact upon health outcomes for migrants (and for those of the wider non-migrant population). These can be broadly defined by the following:

- *Research*: as with so many 'Brexit' outcomes, the eventual wider impact is still unknown. However, there have been a number of anecdotes of UK-based university researchers being asked to remove their names from grant applications involving EU funds. There is also an indication that some research centres are considering moving their work from the UK to a EU-based university (Boffey, 2016).
- *Staffing*: the reliance of the NHS on staff from overseas is well documented. The NHS benefits from the services of overseas workers from both within and outside the EU. It remains to be seen how a UK exit from the EU is going to impact the UK's attraction to health workers from outside the EU.
- *Entitlement to services*: entitlement to health care and treatment in the UK is complex, often misunderstood even by those responsible for implementing such a system. An already-complicated system is likely to be made even more so when the, as yet undefined, entitlements to reciprocal health care are negotiated between the UK and the EU. This is also likely to impact upon victims of trafficking from EU member states, most of whom currently have the right to reside in the UK after leaving a support service.
- *Rise in racism and increased hostility*: since 23 June 2016, there has been a reported increase in racist incidents across the UK. Migrants from both EU and non-EU member states have described how

this increase, even if they have not personally experienced any such incidents, has increased anxiety levels, which in the case of those migrants living with PTSD, may not have been far below the surface. In many ways, governmental efforts to create a 'hostile environment' are reflected in the general public discourse. Again, the corresponding increase in demand on health services (particularly in the field of mental health) is yet to be felt.

Conclusion

The link between housing and health has been well established (World Health Organization, 2011). It could be argued that the living conditions experienced by many migrants both in the UK and across Europe, whether through an existence in a refugee camp, in poor-quality accommodation for asylum seekers or for those migrants whose immigration status leaves them with no recourse to public funds in the UK and who are struggling to make a life for themselves and their families, represent a health-care crisis in waiting. It is important to note that for many migrants, the journey to the UK is uncomplicated and is followed by a positive experience of the immigration system and a relatively straightforward transition to life in the UK. At the other end of the spectrum, however, poor living conditions, combined with limited access to health care and the still-to-be-realised effects on the individual migrant's health of the pre- and post-migration process, together with the effects of the journey itself, represent a toxic cauldron of physical and mental health problems in waiting. The median age of the international migrant within the EU is 28 years.[13] This means that any health issues associated with the migration experience in need of treatment could potentially last many years. There is a need for more research – especially longitudinal in nature – into the impact of socio-political discourses surrounding the migration experience upon the mental and physical health of the individual migrant; unfortunately, the current political climate affords an ideal 'laboratory' for such reflections.

This chapter has briefly outlined how services for refugees and migrants are frequently siloed by migration 'type'. It is individual migrants, their future families and health support services that will reap the results of poorly designed immigration policy and practice. Given the likely future demand on health services as a result of hostile migration policies, service commissioners and policymakers around immigration marginalise health services at their peril.

Notes

1 Much has been made in recent public discourse around the use of the terms 'migrants'/'refugees' (for a wider discussion around the lexicon associated with migration, see Munro, 2017: ch 3). In this chapter, I use the term 'migrant' simply to describe the condition of someone who has moved from one place to another, and in using the term, I am making no qualitative stance on the reasons for that migration or legal status. At relevant points, I also refer specifically to 'refugees' but that is more reflective of the forced nature of the migration rather than the (relatively narrow) definition of how a 'refugee' is understood by the immigration authorities.

2 At the time of writing.

3 Data from Eurostat's asylum statistics, available at: http://ec.europa.eu/eurostat/statistics-explained/index.php/Asylum_statistics#Further_Eurostat_information

4 Again, this 45-day period can be (and often is) extended in cases where the individual has ongoing support needs or is assisting with an ongoing police investigation against the trafficker(s).

5 Comments frequently heard to be made by staff.

6 A process that has been described as 'everyday bordering' (Yuval-Davis, 2013).

7 See the consultation website, available at: https://www.gov.uk/government/consultations/overseas-visitors-and-migrants-extending-charges-for-nhs-services

8 Researcher attendance at consultation meetings (see also Doctors of the World, 2015).

9 The tragedy at Hillsborough football stadium where 96 Liverpool fans were crushed to death. The behaviour of fans was initially erroneously blamed, by the authorities, the police and some media, for contributing to the crushing inside the stadium. After 25 years, a number of official inquiries and the publication of the report of the Hillsborough Independent Panel, an inquest reported in April 2016 that the 96 Liverpool fans had been unlawfully killed and that those surviving fans attending the game were exonerated from blame. Practice around initial investigations into the disaster in 1989, which included the doctoring of police statements, has been described by MP Andy Burnham as the *"greatest miscarriage of justice of our times"*.

10 Summerfield (2003) and Halilovich (2013) discuss of the dangers of 'over-pathologising' the experience of refugees whose mental health, they hypothesise, is a 'normal' reaction to their experiences that would ameliorate steps towards justice against their tormentors in the country of origin.

11 Examples of such headlines, far too numerous to list here, permeate the British print media.

12 In 2015, for example, the UK received 3% of the EU's total asylum claims, see: http://www.migrationobservatory.ox.ac.uk/resources/briefings/migration-to-the-uk-asylum/

13 Data from Eurostat, available at: http://ec.europa.eu/eurostat/statistics-explained/index.php/Migration_and_migrant_population_statistics

References

Boffey, D. (2016) 'EU countries in scramble to "steal" UK-based research centres', *The Guardian*, 18 September.

Bogić, M., Ajduković, D., Bremner, S., Franciskovič, T., Galeazzi, G.M., Kučukalić, A., Lečić-Toševski, D., Morina, N., Popovski, M., Schützwohl, M., Wang, D. and Priebe, S. (2012) 'Factors associated with mental disorders in long-settled war refugees: refugees from the former Yugoslavia in Germany, Italy and the UK', *The British Journal of Psychiatry*, 200: 216–23.

Dhesi, S., Isakjee, A. and Davies, T. (2015) 'An environmental health assessment of the new migrant camp at Calais', University of Birmingham and Doctors of the World.

Doctors of the World (2015) *Registration refused: A study on access to GP registration in England*, London: Doctors of the World.

Halilovich, H. (2013) *Places of pain: Forced displacement, popular memory and trans-local identities in Bosnian war-torn communities*, New York, NY, and Oxford: Berghahn.

Jayaweera, H. (2014) 'Health of migrants in the UK: what do we know?', briefing paper from the Migration Observatory, University of Oxford.

Li, S., Lidell, B. and Nickerson, A. (2016) 'The relationship between post-migration stress and psychological disorders in refugees and asylum seekers', *Current Psychiatry Reports*, 18(9): 82.

Medical Justice (2013) *Mental Health in Immigration Detention Action Group: Initial report 2013*, London: Medical Justice.

Munro, G. (2017) *Transnationalism, diaspora and migrants from the former Yugoslavia in Britain*, London and New York, NY: Routledge.

Munro, G. and Pritchard, C. (2013) 'Support needs of male victims of human trafficking: research findings', The Salvation Army.

Portes, A. and Rumbaut, R.G. (2006) *Immigrant America: A portrait* (3rd edn), Berkeley, CA: University of California Press.

Rechel, B., Mladowsky, P., Ingleby, D., Mackenbach, J.P. and McKee, M. (2013) 'Migration and health in an increasingly diverse Europe', *Lancet*, 381: 1235–45.

Schneiderman, N., Ironson, G. and Siegel, S. (2005) 'Stress and health: psychological, behavioural and biological determinants', *Annual Review of Clinical Psychology*, 1: 607–28.

Siddique, H. (2014) 'Figures show extent of NHS reliance on foreign nationals', *The Guardian*, 26 January.

Summerfield, D. (2003) 'War, exile, moral knowledge and the limits of psychiatric understanding: a clinical case study of a Bosnian refugees in London', *International Journal of Social Psychiatry*, 49: 264–8.

Turton, D. (2003) 'Conceptualising forced migration', RSC Working Paper No. 12, Queen Elizabeth House, University of Oxford.

Westwood, J., Howard, L.M., Stanley, N., Zimmerman, C., Gerada, C. and Oram, S. (2016) 'Access to and experiences of healthcare services by trafficked people: findings from a mixed methods study in England', *British Journal of General Practice*, 66(652): e794–e801.

Woodward, A., Howard, N. and Wolffers, I. (2014) 'Health and access to care for undocumented migrants living in the European Union: a scoping review', *Health Policy and Planning*, 29(7): 818–30.

World Health Organization (2011) *Environmental burden of disease associated with inadequate housing*, Geneva: World Health Organization.

Yuval-Davis, N. (2013) 'EUBorderscapes: a situated intersectional approach to the study of bordering', EUBorderscapes Working Paper No. 2.

TWENTY-TWO

The Care Act 2014

Paul Burstow

The Elizabethan Poor Law punished the homeless vagrant in the most savage manner. I have been looking up the Elizabethan statute. This is what it says: And every such person, upon his apprehension, shall, by order of a justice or constable assisted by advice of the Minister and one other of the parish, be stripped naked from the middle upwards and be openly whipped until his body be bloody. (*Hansard*, 1947)

From the Poor Law to well-being

To understand the significance of the Care Act, it is first necessary to understand its antecedents. The Care Act is both a break with the past and a continuation of some long-established approaches to administering state social policy.

For 60 years, the legal framework governing adult social care in England and Wales was the National Assistance Act 1948. It marked the end of the Poor Law in this country. The Poor Law lasted – albeit with reforms – for 350 years. The first Poor Law legislation was enacted during the reign of Elizabeth I. It made provision for the relief of the 'impotent poor'. Feudal in character and inconsistently applied, the focus was on 'setting the poor on work', not on confining people to the workhouse, which would come later. The system remained in place with minor amendment until the Poor Law Amendment Act 1834.

The 1834 New Poor Law was born out of the Industrial Revolution, rapid population growth and the shift from the country to the towns and cities. It was based on two principles: first, less eligibility – the poor were to be treated less favourably than an 'independent labourer'; and, second, the workhouse test meant that there would be no relief outside of the workhouse. A Poor Law Commission was established to provide national oversight of the system.

Punitive in character and often appalling in its execution, the workhouse system was intended to act as a deterrent, stigmatising the poor. Despite much debate in the early 20th century, a Royal Commission in 1909 left the essentials of the Poor Law unchanged. However, while Beatrice Webb's minority report (HMG, 1909), which made the case for a 'national minimum of civilised life', was rejected at the time, it was influential on the thinking of the 1942 Beveridge Report.

Responsibility for the Poor Law was transferred to local authorities by the Local Government Act 1929, which abolished the Poor Law Boards of Guardians and public hospitals. This did not mark the end of the workhouses; instead, they were given a new name, Public Assistance Institutions. It was not until the National Assistance Act 1948 that the Poor Law was finally removed from the statute book, sweeping away over 20 Poor Law Acts.

The Poor Law had been punitive in character, offering a residual safety net. Condemned in the Beveridge Report, post-war reform sought to break the pattern. The National Assistance Act was one of the sets of laws enacted by the Attlee government to implement the Beveridge Report. However, investigations across Britain at the end of the 1950s found that despite the National Assistance Act, 'poor law attitudes and practices still lingered in institutions' (Townsend, 2008). The Victorian idea of 'less eligibility' persisted.

Part III of the National Assistance Act remained the foundational law for social services in England and Wales until the Care Act came into effect in April 2015. Over the course of 60 years, the provisions of Part III were much amended. The Law Commission (2011) described the law relating to adult social care as 'a confusing patchwork of conflicting statutes'. Between 2008 and 2011, the Law Commission undertook a major project to reform the law on adult social care in England and Wales. This culminated in its report, published in May 2011 (Law Commission, 2011).

The government responded to the report, publishing a draft Bill in July 2012 (HMG, 2012a) alongside a White Paper (HMG, 2012b). This was subject to a period of pre-legislative scrutiny by a Joint Committee of Commons and Lords, which took evidence and made a series of recommendations (Joint Committee on the Draft Care and Support Bill, 2013), the majority of which were accepted by the government (HMG, 2013b). In its response to the Joint Committee, the government summarised the main features of the legislation (see Box 22.1).

Box 22.1: Main features of the Care Act

- Modernises over 60 years of care and support law into a single, clear statute, which is built around people's needs and what they want to achieve in their lives.
- Clarifies entitlements to care and support to give people a better understanding of what is on offer, help them plan for the future and ensure they know where to go for help when they need it.
- Provides for the development of national eligibility criteria, bringing people greater transparency and consistency across the country.
- Treats carers as equal to the person they care for – putting them at the centre of the law and on the same legal footing.
- Reforms how care and support is funded to create a cap on care costs that people will pay, and give everyone peace of mind in protecting them from catastrophic costs.
- Supports our aim to rebalance the focus of care and support on promoting well-being and preventing or delaying needs in order to reduce dependency, rather than only intervening at crisis point.
- Provides new guarantees and reassurance to people needing care in order to support them to move between areas or to manage if their provider fails, without the fear that they will go without the care they need.
- Simplifies the care and support system and processes to provide the freedom and flexibility needed by local authorities and care professionals to integrate with other local services, innovate and achieve better results for people

Source: HMG, 2012b.

At the time of writing, the Care Act is a little more than a year into implementation, the provisions for capping care costs have been put on hold (at least until 2020) and budget pressures and cuts are the main preoccupation of local authorities. The Act repealed in whole or in part 12 Acts of Parliament and pages of secondary legislation consolidating and simplifying the decision-making part of the legal framework. However, just because the law changes does not mean that practice follows. It took time for the National Assistance Act to bed in. The Poor Law may have been repealed in 1948 but it took a decade or more for it to be repealed in the hearts and minds of those who administered the system. The Care Act is likely to suffer the same fate.

A monumental reform? Shifting the focus from deficits to assets

The Care Act marks a break with the Poor Law principle of less eligibility, which persisted in the National Assistance Act. Rather than taking a punitive or judgemental view in assessing need, it requires social workers to use a different lens.

The 2012 Care and Support White Paper (HMG, 2012b) championed an asset-based approach to stem the tide of need and harness the strengths of the individual and their community. However, will it prove to be a milestone on the road to real change or a gravestone marking the end of a brief period of optimism? One of the premises of this White Paper is that independence, at its best, is achieved within a community of interdependence. The strength of communities is their capacity to mobilise individual and collective responses to adversity.

Community is more than a simple matter of geography. It is about how people connect with each other and the power of relationships and reciprocity, whether based on common interests, friendship or the giving and receiving of support. These networks of informal ties are what make up the many and diverse communities that each of us benefit from. Without community, independence can become miserable isolation.

Yet, these networks are not a given. The White Paper was clear that practice needs to be much more focused on recognising and building links between the strengths of individuals and communities, not only on waiting to come to the rescue of casualties when networks fail. This approach suggests that if the care plan for an older person just looks at the two hours a day when they need formal help and ignores the other 22, it has missed the point.

The most important links in that person's network may be their neighbours who pop round for a chat, their children who deal with the bills while they watch their grandchildren or the weekly scrabble tournament with an old friend. Mapping these networks, whether they consist of five people or 50, whether they are local or more distant, should be the starting point for care planning, not an optional extra. This is the only way to achieve the White Paper's aspiration of putting prevention and well-being at the heart of social care.

Community-based approaches

These ideas are not new. For example, Leeds' Neighbourhood Networks have evolved over the past 20 years and have changed the way in which care and support are organised and delivered in that city. More recently, Derby, Shropshire and North Tyneside have adopted asset-based approaches.

As part of work led by the Local Government Association, Shropshire and North Tyneside have redesigned the front end of their services to make sure that every contact they have with their public counts. In Shropshire, the council has established a community interest company, called People2People, to deliver the front end of its adult social care service. Staff and service users are involved in running the company at all levels. People2People provides a bespoke response to people who are referred to social care services, offering information and advice and booking people into community contact sessions in their neighbourhood.

All staff are trained in person-centred approaches, and social workers carrying out assessments are encouraged to have different conversations to capture information about what really matters to the person and their family, with much shorter recording and form-filling processes. Peer support volunteers, who have experience of using social care, work alongside practitioners and offer support, guidance and information.

Traditional services are only considered once community-based solutions have been exhausted. A key measure of the success of this approach is what proportion of these initial discussions identifies workable answers without the need for formal assessments and care packages. In 2014, three quarters of enquiries were dealt with during the first discussion.

North Tyneside has also redesigned its front end. It means that while the overall number of people contacting the service for help is increasing, fewer go on to receive formal care packages. Over a three-year period, the council has increased the number of contacts dealt with at or near the first contact from 46% to 66%; they are aiming for 75%. They have achieved this by using a robust triage system for when people first make contact. For those who receive low-level services, such as meals or simple equipment, the council directly provides and charges for services. Low-level occupational therapy screening for equipment takes place over the phone as part of the initial contact.

A new, free community-based service called Care and Connect is helping to bring local community services and people who need them together. The service also works with communities to set up groups and activities. North Tyneside is also tracking the effectiveness of its reablement service, which provides short-term rehabilitative support. The national target is for the person to still be at home 91 days after being discharged from hospital, but the council are measuring more than this. They follow up with the patient after three months and sixth months to see if reablement is still working, and to identity anyone who may be on the verge of readmission.

In both Shropshire and North Tyneside, the approach has been to widen the information and advice that they provide to see it as an intervention in itself. The focus has been on maintaining independence and social connectedness. The results from both councils are encouraging as they reveal that large numbers of people can be supported without recourse to formal services.

Derby City Council has taken a different model but with similar goals, having introduced Local Area Coordination in 2012, starting in two wards in the city. The aim of Local Area Coordination is to support people in the local community to 'get a life, not a service', empowering individuals to find community-based solutions instead of relying on services. According to the Centre for Welfare Reform (2015), Local Area Coordination puts a 'focus on people and places, and so generates new possibilities for positive change.... It looks for solutions that help people sustain themselves in full community life from the very beginning – even before people come into contact with services'.

A Social Return on Investment Analysis (SROI) (TLAP, 2016) found that over a three-year forecast period with 10 Local Area Coordinators, Local Area Coordination would deliver significant social value, with up to £4 of value for every £1 invested.

Well-being: a new organising principle

Over 50 years ago, the Seebohm Report (HMSO, 1968) recognised the need to break the vicious circle of crisis care and argued against a 'symptom-based approach'. This vision of well-being and community involvement was restated in the 1982 Barclay Report (Barclay, 1982), which argued that social work should be a balance between casework and community work. Neither Seebohm nor Barclay prevailed. So, will it be different this time?

One of the reasons that past attempts at shifting the focus onto well-being and community have failed is that when resources are under pressure, practice defaults to the minimum requirements of the National Assistance Act 1948. That is where the Care Act comes in. It establishes a new mission for social care: the promotion of individual well-being.

Some have described the Care Act as 'monumental', pointing to the inclusion of what the Law Commission (2011) described as a 'single overarching principle that adult social care must promote or contribute to the well-being of the individual'. The well-being principle set out in Section 1 of the Care Act are outlined in Box 22.2.

Box 22.2: Section 1, Care Act 2014

Promoting individual well-being

(1) The general duty of a local authority, in exercising a function under this Part in the case of an individual, is to promote that individual's well-being.

(2) 'Well-being', in relation to an individual, means that individual's well-being so far as relating to any of the following –

(a) personal dignity (including treatment of the individual with respect);

(b) physical and mental health and emotional well-being;

(c) protection from abuse and neglect;

(d) control by the individual over day-to-day life (including over care and support, or support, provided to the individual and the way in which it is provided);

(e) participation in work, education, training or recreation;

(f) social and economic well-being;

(g) domestic, family and personal relationships;

(h) suitability of living accommodation;

(i) the individual's contribution to society.

(3) In exercising a function under this Part in the case of an individual, a local authority must have regard to the following matters in particular –

(a) the importance of beginning with the assumption that the individual is best-placed to judge the individual's well-being;

(b) the individual's views, wishes, feelings and beliefs;

(c) the importance of preventing or delaying the development of needs for care and support or needs for support and the importance of reducing needs of either kind that already exist;

(d) the need to ensure that decisions about the individual are made having regard to all the individual's circumstances (and are not based only on the individual's age or appearance or any condition of the individual's or aspect of the individual's behaviour which might lead others to make unjustified assumptions about the individual's well-being);

(e) the importance of the individual participating as fully as possible in decisions relating to the exercise of the function concerned and being provided with the information and support necessary to enable the individual to participate;

(f) the importance of achieving a balance between the individual's well-being and that of any friends or relatives who are involved in caring for the individual;

(g) the need to protect people from abuse and neglect;

(h) the need to ensure that any restriction on the individual's rights or freedom of action that is involved in the exercise of the function is kept to the minimum necessary for achieving the purpose for which the function is being exercised.

Everything else in Part 1 of the Care Act is governed by this organising principle. It should have a profound effect on the way in which adult social care is organised, placing the individual and the outcomes that matter to them at the heart of decision-making. The radical idea is that instead of building the state's response to need around people's 'deficits' to be met by the provision of services, the focus should be on people's strengths, their networks, social capital to promote resilience and reciprocity (RSA, 2013).

However, is it not just the well-being principle that the Care Act brings into law; the Act also places informal carers on a par with those who need care and support. This legal parity – the recognition that the well-being of the informal carer matters too – represents a fundamental shift. Not every social worker has understood that yet, and most carers are blissfully unaware of the potential revolution that this could unleash.

Along with well-being and parity of esteem for informal carers, the Care Act places a duty on local authorities to prevent and postpone the need for care – just 50 years after Seebhom had set out a well-argued case for prevention to be at the heart of social services departments. Some will argue that all these changes are simply the law catching up with the personalisation agenda and ideas in social work practice of self-determination that date back decades. However, the statutory status it now has can be transformative – but we are not there yet.

The elephant in the room

To say that social care is facing tough times barely describes the magnitude of the challenge. Even before the Care Act, social workers found themselves deployed principally as border patrol, policing access to increasingly insufficient resources against a seemingly limitless need. It is a deficit model that has dominated practice and policy for decades. Yet, it is now clearer than ever that it is unsustainable. Social care is consuming an ever-greater share of falling council resources while the number whose needs it meets is paradoxically diminishing, shunting costs onto the National Health Service (NHS) and leaving increasing numbers of people struggling to cope.

According to the National Audit Office, local authorities have 'reduced the total amount of State-funded care provided through individual packages of care every year since 2008–09' (NAO, 2014). Public spending on social care as a proportion of gross domestic product (GDP) will fall back to around 0.9% by 2019/20, despite the ageing population and rising demand for services (King's Fund, 2015).

In the end, it is informal carers who will be left to pick up the pieces – family and friends who, out of love, solidarity, circumstance or duty, find themselves taking on a caring role. This can include anything from practical tasks, such as cooking, housework and shopping, to managing the family budget and collecting benefits and prescriptions. There is also emotional support, or physical care, such as lifting, as well as personal care, such as dressing, washing and helping with toilet needs. It can be exhausting, it can be rewarding; either way, it takes a toll.

The evidence of the negative health and wealth impacts (Carers UK, 2015) of caring is well documented. The impact on the labour market and the wider economy (HMG, 2013a) is just beginning to be understood.

To integrate or not to integrate?

In its report on 'Adult social care', the National Audit Office (2014) observes that how 'well adults' needs are met depends on all parts interacting effectively', and provides a graphic representation of the interactions, reproduced in Figure 22.1. The graphic sums up perfectly the independencies that go to make up a person's experience of 'the system' and why integration is so hard to define and deliver in practice.

Just as it is necessary to take the long view to understand the significance of the Care Act, the same can be said for the long-running debates about integrating health and social care. So much of the present debate and preoccupation with integration is shaped by decisions taken over 70 years ago, taking the Beveridge Report as the starting point, although some would argue that the question was a live one much earlier with Beatrice Webb's minority report on the Poor Law, arguing for health and social services to be unified within local government.

Beveridge, and the enacting into law of his report, treated health and social services as separate things, reflecting professional preferences and a difference in status and power of the medical and social work professions. The NHS Act 1946 and the National Assistance Act 1948 institutionalised this divide.

In 1962, the first 10-year Hospital Plan for the NHS was described as complimentary to the preventive and community care services, which local authorities were meant to develop over the same period. When the impact of the Hospital Plan was evaluated, it was found that there was a lack of whole-system planning, cost shunting, underfunding, disputes over responsibilities and a focus on structure over purpose – sounds familiar.

Figure 22.1: Adult care services and other services

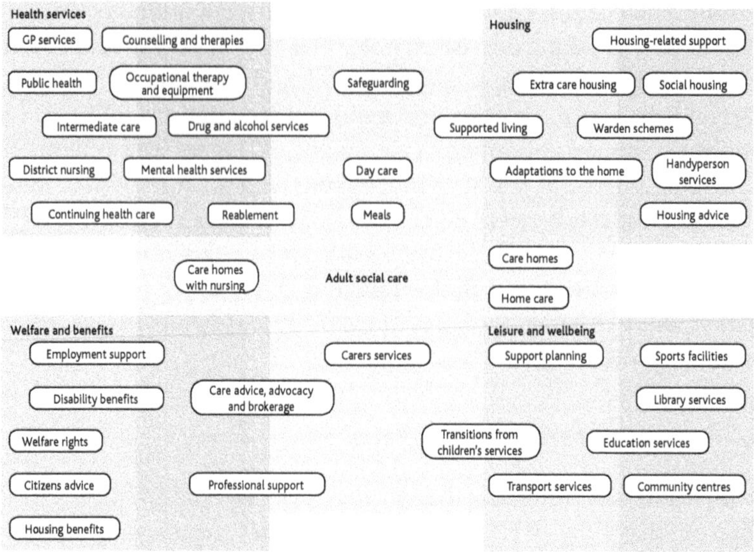

Source: NAO (2014)

A decade later saw the formation of joint committees and a duty to cooperate. In the 1970s, the Seebohm Report, Redcliffe-Maud Royal Commission on Local Government Reform and NHS Reorganisation all took as their principle that services should be organised around the skills of the provider. The result was further entrenchment of different institutional objectives, cultures, systems and professional views; put simply, one, the NHS, looking up to Whitehall, the other, local government, looking out to the community.

The 1980s saw further tinkering to try and make joint planning work. There was talk of shifting the focus from process to outcomes. However, the institutional divide was still taken as read. In the 1990s, New Labour introduced pooled budgets, lead commissioning and other 'flexibilities' aimed at promoting integration. A new century saw a new 10-year plan; this time, the Secretary of State even threatened to impose Care Trusts to end the divide – a few were set up but, in practice, this was an experiment that never escaped the laboratory. This was followed by integrated care pilots.

Joint commissioning and aligning NHS and local government planning cycles were the order of the day. The Coalition government revisited the joint committee idea, legislating for Health and Wellbeing Boards, but resisted calls for them to be given a power of veto. A new programme of integration pioneers was launched and the NHS Five

Year Forward View saw the launched an NHS-led process of system redesign around new models of care, called the Vanguard programme. A series of devolution deals were negotiated, with health and care integration as one of the goals. However, while the governance of the devolution deals appears to put more power in local hands, it remains to be seen whether NHS budgets will come without strings attached.

Over the past 70 years, successive attempts to 'integrate' have foundered because of: the tendency to focus on institutions rather than people and place; performance being judged by institution and process rather than outcomes; payment and contracting reinforcing the status quo; and a lack of clear definition or clarity of responsibilities. Put simply, there are two institutions with different accountabilities and core business. The last 70 years have seen countless efforts to bridge the gap between the two silos. Einstein is credited with saying that the definition of insanity is 'doing the same thing over and over again and expecting a different result'. The Department of Health should have a resident historian, the corporate memory. A meeting with the departmental historian should be a must-do for every minister who turns up at the Department of Health.

Conclusions: two systems, one purpose?

In 2012, NHS England commissioned National Voices to co-develop a definition of integration. After an extensive process of research on what matters most to people, a definition emerged. It boiled down to the following proposition: 'I can plan my care with people who work together to understand me and my carer(s), allow me control, and bring together services to achieve the outcomes important to me' (National Voices, 2013).

Rather than getting bogged down in yet more attempts to break down institutional barriers, National Voices' definition of integration and the Care Act's promotion of individual well-being offer a new way forward. The promotion of well-being and wellness should become the common purpose of health and social care. It puts the people rather than institutions at the heart of designing and delivering solutions which recognise that relationships are critical to a good life; maintaining social connections and looking to the strengths and resources that we can draw on help people to have a life, providing a service is just the enabler.

Time for dialogue without preconditions?

The Care Act's well-being principle offers a blueprint for reshaping health and social care. However, the outcome will hinge on three things: funding, eligibility and workforce. At the time of writing, the social care system in England is under huge strain. The scale of the challenge has been documented by leading health think tanks and the prime minister has acknowledged the need for a long-term solution.

A cross-party–civil society dialogue about the cost of care and how we pay and share the responsibility for it is long overdue. It will only succeed if the survival of sacred cows is not made preconditions of dialogue. Gatekeeping has always been part of the system. Eligibility and the rules that govern it have remained firmly wedded to Poor Law principles despite the best intentions of the Care Act. Getting a more accurate fix on the numbers who are shut out is essential to the dialogue too.

Even before the 'Brexit' vote, there were serious concerns about the difficulties in retaining and recruiting care workers. Developing new career paths and opportunities and significantly improving the pay, conditions and status of care work should also be part of the dialogue. As John Maynard Keynes said: 'The difficulty lies not so much in developing new ideas as in escaping old ones'. This is certainly true with the NHS and social care. Yet, the forces driving the need for change are overwhelming.

References

Barclay, P. (1982) *Social workers: their role and tasks (the Barclay Report)*, London: Bedford Square Press.

Carers UK (2015) 'State of care'. Available at: http://socialwelfare. bl.uk/subject-areas/services-activity/social-work-care-services/ carersuk/175462carers-uk-state-of-caring-2015-report-final-web.pdf

Centre for Welfare Reform (2015) 'People, places, possibilities, progress on local area coordination in England and Wales', Ralph Broad, August.

Hansard (1947) 'National Assistance Bill', HC Deb, 24 November, vol 444, cc1603–716.

HMG (Her Majesty's Government) (1909) 'Royal Commission on the Poor Laws and the Relief of Distress', Cd 4499, minority report, vol III.

HMG (2012a) 'Draft Care and Support Bill', July, Cmnd 8386, Department of Health. Available at: https://www.gov.uk/government/uploads/system/uploads/attachment_data/file/137709/dh_134740.pdf

HMG (2012b) 'Caring for our future: reforming care and support', July, Cmnd 8378. Available at: https://www.gov.uk/government/uploads/system/uploads/attachment_data/file/136422/White-Paper-Caring-for-our-future-reforming-care-and-support-PDF-1580K.pdf

HMG (2013a) 'Supporting working carers: the benefits to families, business and the economy', August. Available at: www.carersuk.org/for-professionals/policy/policy-library/supporting-working-carers

HMG (2013b) 'The Care Bill explained including a response to consultation and pre-legislative scrutiny on the Draft Care and Support Bill', May, Cmnd 8627. Available at: https://www.gov.uk/government/uploads/system/uploads/attachment_data/file/228864/8627.pdf

HMSO (Her Majesty's Stationery Office) (1968) 'Report of the Committee on Local Authority and Allied Personal Services', July, Cmnd 3703.

Joint Committee on the Draft Care and Support Bill (2013) 'HL Paper 143', HC 822, March. Available at: www.publications.parliament.uk/pa/jt201213/jtselect/jtcare/143/143.pdf

King's Fund (2015) 'The Spending Review: what does it mean for health and social care?', December. Available at: www.health.org.uk/sites/default/files/Spending-Review-Nuffield-Health-Kings-Fund-December-2015_spending_review_what_does_it_mean_for_health_and_social_care.pdf

Law Commission (2011) 'Adult social care', Law Com No 236, May. Available at: www.lawcom.gov.uk/app/uploads/2015/03/lc326_adult_social_care.pdf

NAO (National Audit Office) (2014) 'Adult social care: an overview', March. Available at: https://www.nao.org.uk/wp-content/uploads/2015/03/Adult-social-care-in-England-overview.pdf

National Voices (2013) 'A narrative for person-centred coordinated care', TLAP. Available at: www.nationalvoices.org.uk/sites/default/files/public/publications/narrative-for-person-centred-coordinated-care.pdf

RSA (Royal Society for the Encouragement of Arts, Manufactures and Commerce) (2013) 'The new social care: strength based approaches', May. Available at: https://www.thersa.org/discover/publications-and-articles/reports/new-social-care-strength-based-approaches/

TLAP (Think Local Act Personal) (2016) 'Social value of local area coordination in Derby', March. Available at: www.thinklocalactpersonal. org.uk/_library/BCC/Assured_SROI_Report_for_Local_Area_ Coordination_in_Derby_March_2016.pdf

Townsend, P. (2008) '1909–2009: Beatrice Webb and the future of the welfare state', Lecture, 20 May, Fabian Society.

TWENTY-THREE

Health and social care in an age of austerity

Charles West

Introduction

One of the first lessons I was taught at medical school was that the career we were being trained for was by no means the most important factor in promoting good health or a long life. Clean water, sanitation, nutrition, housing, employment and money are all more important than medical care as factors in the improvement in life expectancy. One might now add to the list social networks (Wilkinson and Marmot, 2003) and equality (Wilkinson and Pickett, 2009).

It remains true, however, that medical care does contribute to improvements in both the quality and duration of life. It is also true that societies generally place a high value on the provision of such care; when we are ill we all want someone to look after us, and, if possible, to make us better. In this chapter, therefore, I shall concentrate on the health care that is provided by health services such as the National Health Service (NHS). In the same way, I shall focus on the social care that is normally paid for, rather than the wider social support provided by family, friends, neighbours or colleagues.

The second point of clarification that I need to make is that austerity is a conscious act of policy. It is not an 'act of God'. Total government spending is a choice, and I would argue that the policy of austerity as exhibited by the UK government, among others, has deepened and prolonged the economic downturn since 2007:

> The austerity arguments focused on deep cutbacks to public policies and shrinking the state as a main way to fix the deficit, calm the markets and revitalize the economy; following this logic, the social welfare state was depicted as unaffordable and burdensome, which ultimately reduced competitiveness and discouraged growth.

Numerous studies have highlighted the fallacious basis of austerity programs. In the short term austerity depresses incomes and jobs, hinders domestic demand and ultimately recovery efforts. Austerity also has negative impacts on employment, economic activity and development over the long term. (Ortiz and Cummins, 2013: 11; see also Chu, 2015; Krugman, 2015; Crescenzi et al, 2016)

The economic case for spending on health and social care

It does nevertheless fall to governments at a time of reduced government revenue to consider carefully what their priorities for spending should be. In pure economic terms, there is logic in pursuing spending policies that carry a high economic multiplier.

The economic multiplier favours giving more money (through earnings, welfare or tax regimes) to the poor and less to the rich (Lysy, 2013; Elliot, 2015; Kenny, 2015). Spend on health care has a high economic multiplier (Ku, 2010; Reeves et al, 2013). This is perhaps not surprising when one considers that about three quarters of health spending is salaries, and that those earning the salaries will spend most of their earnings in the local economy. Better access to health care also, unsurprisingly, improves physical and mental health status, including the health status of working people. This, in itself, carries economic benefits. It is perhaps fortunate that, in this regard, hard economic facts point in the same direction as the softer motives such as compassion and social justice: governments' spending should favour spending on health care.

There might, of course, be an argument for limiting or reducing government expenditure on health care if the UK were spending greatly more than similar countries. However, we are not. Whether we look at ranking within the European Union (EU) or Organisation for Economic Co-operation and Development (OECD), the UK spends significantly less on health care than other countries, and has done so for many years (Appleby, 2016). Between 2000 and 2009, the gap between the UK and other EU countries was narrowing, but since then, the gap has widened and the UK has reduced its spending on health care. Current government plans are to reduce that even further.

Getting better value from the money spent

There is, therefore, a strong case for the UK to spend more on health care. There still remains, though, a powerful duty on governments and those working in health care to achieve good value for the money spent. International comparisons would suggest that, in the past, the UK NHS has provided excellent value for money. From 1998 to 2014, the Commonwealth Fund has published international comparisons of health-care systems. The NHS has repeatedly come top, not only in terms of value for money, but also, by many parameters, in terms of the quality of service provided as well (Davis et al, 2014).

Unfortunately, for 25 years, all governments have been pursuing a misguided policy of increasing competition within the provision of health care. What might at one time have been a reasonable assumption that competition would drive up efficiency and drive down costs has long since been discredited. For a competitive market to work, there must be numerous providers and numerous consumers. There are five principles underlying a competitive market:

- *Profit*: the providers must see a profit to be derived from delivering the goods or services in question.
- *Limited supply*: as the supply of a given product or service becomes more scarce, its price will rise.
- *Rivalry*: consumers also need to compete for the item being sold. We cannot all sit in the best seat of the centre court at Wimbledon.
- *Excludability*: the provider can refuse to serve or sell to a consumer if, for example, they are not willing to pay the price being asked.
- *Rejectability*: the consumer has the right to reject a product or service if they believe that the price is too high, or the quality too low.

It will immediately become apparent that the delivery of health care in the NHS is not, and cannot be, a true market. For a start, the consumer is not buying the service directly; it is being bought for them. Looking further at the five principles just outlined, we can see that with the exception of the consumer having the right to reject treatment, the others all generate ethical or practical problems for a civilised caring society. It would not be acceptable for patients to be excluded from treatment that they need simply because they cannot afford to pay, because someone else is prepared to pay more or because providers have decided to stop delivering that service.

Even if one attempts to run a pseudo-market in health care, the practical difficulties are legion. Health care is complex. Let us think briefly about the necessary links between services. Consultant obstetricians also perform gynaecological operations, so it makes sense for an obstetric unit to be attached to a gynaecological one. The outcome of a successful obstetric procedure is a baby, so we need paediatricians. Children are common users of head and neck services, so it makes sense to have those close at hand. The other main users of head and neck specialists are cancers and major trauma. So, our hospital should have radiotherapy and accident and emergency departments. All these services will need anaesthetics, X-rays, blood tests and good links to community services. There are many more essential links between departments. There are also important issues about the mix of workload within a department. An orthopaedic department may perform many routine hip replacements but only occasionally be faced with a complex one where complications arise. However, you cannot run a unit that only caters for the rare case: the staff would become deskilled and it becomes impossible to train the next generation of clinicians. There have been several examples in recent years of NHS hospital departments becoming non-viable because an alternative provider has creamed off the easy and profitable work.

It is apparent that the provision of any health-care service needs to have a certain critical mass. If we are to have multiple providers competing and each provider needs to be large enough to offer a sufficient range and mix of services, such provision would only be possible in the very largest centres of population. This would deprive most of the country of any reasonable access to health care.

There are other losses of efficiency inherent in running even a pseudo-market. If you want to get your bedroom decorated and decide to get six decorators to quote for the job, you have to show round six different decorators. They all need to measure up, find out prices for paint and wallpaper, calculate how long the job will take them, and send you a quotation. Only one will get the job, but they all need to cover the costs of tendering for the work, so they need to price in enough time to quote for all the jobs they do not win. You have also spent six times as long explaining the work you want done.

In 1990, the government introduced what they called an internal market in the NHS. The services were still provided by NHS providers but each provider produced theoretical bills for work and the purchasers had to check them and pay with theoretical money. Since then, successive Conservative, Labour and Coalition governments have administered larger and larger doses of the same medicine to the NHS, ostensibly in the pursuit of increased efficiency. The Health and Social Care Act 2012 was the culmination of this process. Purchasers are required to put work out to tender. Private providers are encouraged to take on work and apart from the necessary routine administration and accounting work that this has generated, the inevitable disputes and contested decisions are diverting large sums of much needed money from health care.

Both international comparisons and trends in the UK show that the march of the market is correlated with increased and increasing administrative and management costs, and is therefore making the whole system *less* efficient. The recent promotion of private health-care provision has greatly exacerbated this trend. Let us look, then, at the actual experience of the NHS with regard to administration and management costs and attempt to project forward the likely effect of the changes that the service is currently undergoing.

The 1979 Royal Commission said that the NHS provided good value for money and high levels of satisfaction, and that it did not need 'major surgery'. This view did not suit Prime Minister Margaret Thatcher, who commissioned a further report from businessman Roy Griffiths. His report took the form of a letter to the prime minister written in 1983 and signalled the onset of a series of changes, starting with general management and followed by the introduction of the internal market in 1990. Until the 1980s, the NHS spent 5% of its total expenditure on administration (House of Commons Health Committee, 2010). After the introduction of the internal market, administrative costs soared; in 1997, they stood at about 12%, and by 2010, costs had risen to 14%. Between 2000 and 2010, as the Labour government placed more and more contracts with external providers, the number of NHS managers increased twice as fast as the number of doctors (Smith, 2010) and five times as fast as the number of nurses (Ramesh, 2010). We have seen, therefore, over a period of 20 years or so, an increase in the costs of management and administration from 5% of the budget to 14% of the budget. Over the same period, the total NHS budget more than doubled, even after allowing for inflation. In effect, not only had management consumed a much larger share of the cake, but the cake had grown. These increases coincided with the development of the market in health care, at first an internal market and then, increasingly over time, a mixed internal and external market. This amounts to an increased cost of at least £9 billion per year (Paton, 2014).

International comparisons tell a similar story, and suggest that with increasing fragmentation of the supply of health care and the mix of state and private providers, management costs will continue to rise. Administrative costs in countries with a purchaser–provider split and a mix of state and private insurance tend to be higher still, purchaser costs alone typically amounting to around 20% (Nicolle and Mathauer, 2010). In the US in 1999, administrative spending consumed at least 31.0% of health spending (Woolhandler et al, 2003; Himmelstein et al,

2004). Billing alone costs up to 13%. It is worth noting that the billing costs of health-care providers are 10 times the average of all businesses in the US (Yong et al, 2010). There is an inherent complexity to the business of delivering health care.

Combining the experience of the NHS so far and international studies suggests that in the near future, running a pseudo-market in health care could be costing the NHS around £20 billion per year. In addition to these powerful economic factors, running a competitive market in health care has other damaging effects. It reduces cooperation and trust between providers and thereby impedes the flow of information, patients and test results between providers. It also militates against effective training and manpower planning. It also reduces equity (Bambra et al, 2014; Footman et al, 2014). It is little wonder that the Health Committee reported in March 2010 that 'the purchaser/provider split may need to be abolished' (House of Commons Health Committee, 2010: 60).

The second large and unnecessary financial burden faced by the NHS is the Private Finance Initiative (PFI). This is a form of financial manipulation whereby public infrastructure projects are financed by a consortium typically involving a source of finance, a developer and an operating company. It was first used in 1992 by John Major's Conservative government and though initially criticised by the Labour opposition, PFI was enthusiastically espoused by the New Labour governments of Blair and Brown.

The apparent advantage for governments was that they thought that PFI was a way of financing infrastructure projects without the cost appearing as government debt. Even this 'advantage' turned out to be illusory. The immediately obvious disadvantages were the cost and the fact that users were locked into an agreement to buy certain support services that might, in time, become outdated, unnecessary or wasteful. The charges on PFI schemes amounted to an effective interest rate of 16% at a time when governments could have borrowed for 6%. The NHS is now paying over £2 billion per year on PFI schemes. If one considers that interest rates since 2010 have been close to 0%, one might argue that there has never been a better time for the government to invest in infrastructure. This has been a tragic missed opportunity. Even now, it is not too late to refinance the debts incurred under PFI schemes. The burden of PFI has already led directly to highly unpopular closure proposals (Campbell, 2013; Shepherd, 2014). Other hospitals throughout the country are struggling with the costs imposed by their PFI contracts (Kingman, 2013; Pollock and Price, 2013; Mendick et al, 2015; Campbell, 2016). If these debts are not refinanced, or rescheduled in some way, they will threaten the very viability of large parts of the NHS.

Social care

Social care contributes directly to good health (Clark, 2005) and has synergies with health care. Good social care may prevent the need for hospital admission, and, conversely, lack of adequate social care is a major reason for the delayed discharge of patients from hospital. As a result, many patients who do not otherwise need to be in hospital are being cared for in an inappropriate and unnecessarily expensive environment, and other patients who are in more urgent need of hospital facilities are denied access to them.

The onslaught by governments on social care spending preceded that on health by about 10 years. It was marked by the outsourcing of most residential and nursing home care and has been affected by years of downward pressure on local authority budgets. When budgets are under pressure, the artificial boundaries between health care, social care and housing provision encourage cost-shifting and buck-passing. As a result, some have advocated the merging of health and social care. Closer working between health and social care teams is vital, but the merging of budgets presents significant risks.

The UK has a long tradition of delivering health care free at the point of use. Social care has traditionally been paid for by the individual with or without means-tested support from the state. Health care has a long tradition of trust in the health-care professionals who determine whether a patient 'needs' (would benefit from) a given medical intervention. Social care needs are much less clearly defined. The current political climate, dominated as it is by neoliberal thinking, would be more likely to see the merging of health and social care budgets as an opportunity to stop free health care than to remove charges for social care. The full implementation of the report of the Dilnot Commission (Dilnot, 2010) would go a long way to reducing the risk of extreme social care costs. The Care Act 2014 had intended to set a cap on the costs of social care met by individuals, albeit at a less generous level than Dilnot, but we have seen in Chapter Twenty-two that even these proposals have been shelved. The problem of who defines social care needs would still remain. How, then, are we to minimise cost-shifting and gaming between departments if budgets for health care, social care, housing and welfare all remain separate and continue to be under pressure?

One tool much used by governments in managing public services is the imposition of targets. Targets may be argued to concentrate the mind and it has been argued that the imposition of targets has led to raised standards, particularly in the specific measure to which the target applies. However, if ever there was a time for targets, it is now clear that governments' reliance on multiple targets is counterproductive. It has been claimed that the imposition of targets was responsible for improvements in delivering health care, for example, as in the reduction of waiting times. We should note, however, that this improvement occurred at a time when there was an effective doubling in resources available to the NHS – an unprecedented increase. We hear of services that concentrate so hard on delivering the targets that they forget or ignore the needs of the patient, client or customer. This was part of the problem at Mid Staffordshire NHS Trust, where management were so focussed on delivering the financial targets required to become a foundation trust that they forgot many of the basic requirements of humane clinical care. We hear of accident and emergency departments where patients are admitted to a ward within the four-hour target time, even if that means sending them to an inappropriate ward. We hear of the scandalous treatment of young people in privately run secure training centres, partly because of a powerful incentive to deliver targets defined in their contract. Using targets and contracts in the pursuit of efficiency takes the focus off the needs of the patient. In effect, the system may become more efficient at delivering something that is not what the patient wants or needs. This creates a great increase in activity, but it is non-productive activity. It is what John Seddon (2008) describes as 'failure demand'. A service provider may achieve a target for answering the telephone within 30 seconds by employing a call centre that answers the phone but actually cannot answer any of the enquirers' questions. People accessing our public services want their particular need fulfilled at a time convenient to them. They do not want to be handed off from person to person and agency to agency, and they do not wish to be fitted into an arbitrary category. Much unproductive work can be eliminated if we 'get it right first time'.

Health care and social care can be made to work more effectively together. For this to happen, there needs to be much more contact between the professionals of both services. There also needs to be more clarity around what can be expected of social care services, and the resources that they can expect. Whereas there are known expectations of what the health-care system should provide, there are not similar expectations of social care. Indeed, the health-care sector is almost certainly too 'micromanaged' from the centre, whereas social care is pretty well ignored by the centre unless a child is killed, in which case, there is a witch-hunt as everyone looks for someone to blame.

Summary

In summary, it is clear that the policy of austerity has had an adverse effect on the health and well-being of the people of the UK, not least through the damage it has inflicted and continues to inflict on the health and social care services. There are things that could be done to reverse many of these damaging effects. Some of these recommendations are listed as follows:

- Abolish the market in health care, both internal and external.
- Restore direct provision as the norm for NHS health-care services.
- Establish clear expectations in a broad sense of what social care should be provided.
- Define social care budgets in relation to those expectations and the needs of the community concerned.
- Encourage health-care and social care staff to meet and cooperate.
- End central government's micromanagement of services by the use of multiple targets.
- Define instead the high-level purpose of each service.
- Promote a new culture where performance measurement is used as a tool for learning rather than a stick with which to beat those delivering services.
- Refinance PFI debts.
- Increase the total budget for the NHS.

We read in Chapter One that compassion for the weak and sick was not a feature of the society of ancient Rome. Modern society is rather different. Every major world religion and civilised nation sees the value in caring for the needy. The UK was among the first nations in the world to offer a health service that was universal, comprehensive and free. By pooling the risk and delivering a universal service, the NHS achieved levels of efficiency and effectiveness that were admired throughout the world, and the NHS has been a model for the development of health-care systems in many other countries.

In recent years, governments and individuals alike have been faced with economic pressures. This has presented governments with a challenge but also an opportunity to invest in health care, social care, housing and education in a way that will bring real benefits to the whole country and at a time when interest rates have been near zero.

Looking forward, we can see two possibilities. We could see governments continuing to impose spending restrictions on health and social care, with the inevitable collapse of the publicly provided service. Private providers of both health and social care will be encouraged to take over any services that are profitable, and individuals who can afford to do so will be urged to take out private insurance. The result would be a deterioration in health and quality of life for everyone, but it would most severely impact the poor and vulnerable. The alternative would be for governments to grasp the opportunity to invest in universal public services in a way that makes a reality of the compassionate and caring society to which we all aspire.

References

Appleby, J. (2016) 'How does NHS spending compare with health spending internationally?', The King's Fund. Available at: www.kingsfund.org.uk/blog/2016/01/how-does-nhs-spending-compare-health-spending-internationally

Bambra, C., Garthwaite, K. and Hunter, D. (2014) 'All things being equal: does it matter for equity how you organize and pay for health care? A review of the international evidence', *Int J Health Serv*, 44(3): 457–77.

Campbell, D. (2013) 'Lewisham hospital's fury at £195m bill for A&E closure', *The Guardian*, 21 January.

Campbell, D. (2016) 'London hospital trust heading for biggest overspend in NHS history', *The Guardian*, 7 February.

Chu, B. (2015) 'Two thirds of economists say Coalition austerity harmed the economy', *The Independent*, 1 April.

Clark, C. (2005) *Relations between social support and physical health*, Evanston, IL: Northwestern University.

Crescenzi, R., Luca, D. and Millio, S. (2016) *Austerity has slowed regional recovery during the post-2008 recession*, London: LSE.

Davis, K., Stremikis, K., Schoen, C. and Squires, D. (2014) *Mirror, mirror on the wall: How the performance of the US health care system compares internationally, 2014 update*, New York, NY: The Commonwealth Fund.

Dilnot, A. (ed) (2010) *Fairer care funding: The report of the Commission on Funding of Care and Support*, London: UK Government.

Elliot, L. (2015) 'Pay low-income families more to boost economic growth, says IMF', *The Guardian*, 15 June.

Footman, K., Garthwaite, K., Bambra, C. and McKee, M. (2014) 'Quality check: does it matter for quality how you organize and pay for health care? A review of the international evidence', *Int J Health Serv*, 44(3): 479–505.

Himmelstein, D.U., Woolhandler, S. and Wolfe, S.M. (2004) 'Administrative waste in the US health care system in 2003', *International Journal of Health Services*, 34(1): 79–86.

House of Commons Health Committee (2010) *Commissioning*, HC268, 30 March, London: The Stationery Office.

Kenny, C. (2015) 'Give poor people cash', *The Atlantic*. Available at: www.theatlantic.com/international/archive/2015/09/welfare-reform-direct-cash-poor/407236/

Kingman, D. (2013) 'New figures reveal weight of PFI burden on NHS trusts'. Available at: www.if.org.uk/archives/3453/new-figures-reveal-weight-of-pfi-burden-on-nhs-trusts

Krugman, P. (2015) 'The case for cuts was a lie. Why does Britain still believe it? The austerity delusion', *The Guardian*, 29 April.

Ku, L. (2010) 'Can health care investments stimulate the economy?', *Health Affairs*. Available at: http://healthaffairs.org/blog/2010/03/16/can-health-care-investments-stimulate-the-economy/

Lysy, F. (2013) 'The fiscal multiplier', *AnEconomicSense*. Available at: https://aneconomicsense.org/about-3/

Mendick, R., Donnelly, L. and Kirk, A. (2015) 'The PFI hospitals costing NHS £2bn every year', *The Telegraph*, 18 July.

Nicolle, E. and Mathauer, I. (2010) *Administrative costs of health insurance schemes: Exploring the reasons for their variability*, Geneva: World Health Organization.

Ortiz, I. and Cummins, M (2013) *The age of austerity: A review of public expenditures and adjustment measures in 181 countries*, New York, NY, and Geneva: Initiative for Policy Dialogue and The South Centre.

Paton, C. (2014) *At what cost? Paying the price for the market in the English NHS*, London: The Centre for Health and the Public Interest.

Pollock, A. and Price, D. (2013) 'PFI and the National Health Service in England'. Available at: www.allysonpollock.com/wp-content/uploads/2013/09/AP_2013_Pollock_PFILewisham.pdf

Ramesh, R. (2010) 'NHS management increasing five times faster than number of nurses', *The Guardian*, 25 March.

Reeves, A., Basu, S., McKee, M., Meissner, C. and Stuckler, D. (2013) 'Does investment in the health sector promote or inhibit economic growth?', *Globalization and Health*, 9: 43. Available at: http://doi.org/10.1186/1744-8603-9-43

Seddon, J. (2008) *Systems thinking in the public sector*, Axminster: Triarchy Press.

Shepherd, J. (2014) 'Some facts and figures about Calderdale Royal Hospital PFI debt repayments', 14 April. Available at: www.energyroyd.org.uk/archives/11434

Smith, R. (2010) 'NHS managers numbers rise at twice rate of doctors', *The Telegraph*, 12 February.

Wilkinson, R. and Marmott, M. (eds) (2003) *Social determinants of health: The solid facts* (2nd edn), Copenhagen: World Health Organization.

Wilkinson, R. and Pickett, K. (2009) *The spirit level: Why more equal societies almost always do better*, London: Allen Lane.

Woolhandler, S., Campbell, T. and Himmelstein, D. (2003) 'Costs of health care administration in the United States and Canada', *N Engl J Med*, 349: 768–75.

Yong, P.L., Saunders, R.S. and Olsen, L.A. (eds) (2010) *The healthcare imperative: Lowering costs and improving outcomes: Workshop series summary*, Washington, DC: National Academies Press.

Conclusion

Adrian Bonner

This interdisciplinary approach to social inequality and well-being began, in Part One, with a consideration of a person's early years' experience, involving a process of maturation and integration of physiological, psychological and social factors. Clearly relative poverty and a person's social capital will, to a greater or lesser extent, provide the resilience for that person to experience a sense of well-being and lead to successful ageing. Lifestyle choices and the support of a healthy community will reduce vulnerability to negative health behaviours. Upstream support from family, schools and community networks is important in promoting self-esteem and psychological health as the individual progresses into the working community. Not everyone has the capacity or opportunity to be employed; however, there are opportunities for meaningful activities beyond the traditional world of work, as noted in Chapters Nine and Thirteen of this book.

Personal well-being is related to the availability of personal, family and community resources. Clearly the economic status of a community will impact on individual health and the community resources to support the more vulnerable people in the community. There have been many references in this book highlighting the link between social gradient and health (Marmot, 2010), which is, to large extent, determined by political processes. The Children and Families Act 2014 gave greater protection to vulnerable children and better support for children affected by family breakdown and for children with special educational needs. The Care Act 2014 was aimed at promoting individual well-being (see Chapter Twenty-two). However, these and many other initiatives delivered by local authority and non-statutory providers have been decimated by reductions in public spending, unprecedented since the Second World War, due to austerity budgets initiated after the collapse of the world economy in 2008. Cuts in the welfare and social care budgets, and more recently, significant reductions in school budgets in real terms are increasing the gap between the rich and the poor (Beatty and Fothergill, 2014). More specifically, the health inequality gap in England 'is still growing', with life expectancy, vulnerability to disability and disease worsening in deprived areas of England (Bambra, 2016; Buck, 2017). Continued erosion in household incomes and a rising cost of living are already having an impact on the most vulnerable at the bottom end of the social gradient (Bambra, 2016). These regressive polices are being reinforced by a major economic impact on the UK economy from policies related to the process of the UK leaving the European Union (Brexit), resulting from a referendum in June 2016 in which 52% of the voting electorate voted to Leave the EU and 48% voted to Remain. The lower socioeconomic groups were over-represented in the Leave vote.

Currently, the Conservative Prime Minister, Theresa May, is in the initial stages of negotiating the terms of Brexit. To this end she called a snap General Election that was predicted to result in a 'landslide majority' which would strengthen her negotiating position in the Brexit process. The election result on 8 June 2017 resulted in a hung parliament, with significant implications for Brexit. Although the snap election was called to support May's Brexit campaign, the electorate was influenced by other issues, particularly ongoing austerity policies and other highly contentious policy intentions in the Conservative Party's manifesto.

From the perspective of this book, currently there is uncertainty about welfare proposals in relation to Universal Credit, social mobility, and free school meals. A key issue which was a turning point in the General Election was the Conservative manifesto policy on social care, the 'dementia tax'. The proposal related to the proportion of care costs to be paid by individuals (and their families) compared to the state. Four independent reviews, and a number of Green and White Papers on the funding of social care, including a Royal Commission and the Dilnot Commission (Dilnot, 2010), have not resolved this demographic crisis. The manifesto proposal appears to have been poorly considered and exposed May's 'strong and stable' government as being 'weak and wobbly', providing political capital for the other parties, with Labour as the main beneficiary (Campbell, 2017).

The minority government entered the Brexit process on 20 June 2017 in a weak negotiating position and, with the turmoil within the Conservative Party, might have a limited life. It appears that the UK will leave the EU but there are growing pressures for it to stay in the single market and the customs union. The predicted negative impact of Brexit on the UK economy and consequential costs of withdrawing from the EU, estimated to be in excess of £60 billion, plus the impact on employment and living standards is unknown at present. People who voted Leave in the EU Referendum in 2016 (disproportionately in the socially deprived areas) are those most likely to be adversely affected as the UK moves into a different position with regard to world trade and immigration, and with the unintended consequences on the social and welfare budgets and prospect of rising taxation to fund Brexit.

In the Marmot review (Marmot, 2010), there was a clear indication that the poor health status of those at the lower end of the social gradient was not solely the result of limited access to resources such as food and housing, but was associated with negative self-perceptions and lack of meaning and belonging. There is increasing concern for those who are powerless to live a life of freedom due to refugee status (see Chapter Twenty-one) and modern-day slavery (BBC News, 2017). One of the most important social determinants of health is inter-personal behavior, either through healthy relationships (note the salutogenesis model, described in Chapter Three), the development of supportive communities (Part Three) and the promotion of a tolerant, open and united society (Farron, 2016).

Considerations of a just and fair society, personal values and the role of faith-based communities are beyond the scope of this book. However, in advanced societies in which the treatment of non-communicable diseases (NCDs) is consuming increasing proportions of health-care budgets, consideration should be given to causative factors, such as stress-related anxieties, in this rapidly changing, interconnected, yet increasingly divided world (as expressed through emerging nationalism and 'popularism politics' [Shuster, 2015]). These psychosocial and political influences on the functioning of the nervous system, the immune system and homeostatic regulation of the body and mind are often related to isolation, marginalisation, loneliness and the search for meaning. It is hoped that this collection of chapters from the interconnected and interdependent domains of the 'Rainbow' model of social determinants of health (Dahlgren and Whitehead,1991) will stimulate a wholistic approach to inequality and well-being.

References

Bambra, C. (2016) *Health divides: Where you live can kill you*, Bristol: Policy Press.

BBC News (2017) 'Modern slavery and trafficking "in every UK town and city"'. Available at: www.bbc.co.uk/news/uk-40885353

Beatty, C. and Fothergill, S. (2014) 'The local and regional impact of the UK's welfare reforms', *Cambridge Journal of Regions, Economy and Society*, 7(1): 63-79.

Buck, D. (2017) 'Reducing inequalities in health: towards a brave old world', 13 August. Available at: https://www.kingsfund.org.uk/blog/2017/08/reducing-inequalities-health-towards-brave-old-world

Campbell, A. (2017) 'Weak and wobbly: Thanks to deluded Theresa we have no leadership', *The New European*, 10 June. Available at: http://www.theneweuropean.co.uk/top-stories/weak-and-wobbly-thanks-to-deluded-theresa-we-have-no-leadership-1-5056257

Dahlgren,G. and Whitehead, M. (1991) *Policies and strategies to promote social equity in health*, Stockholm: Institute for Futures Studies.

Dilnot, A. (2010) Commission on Funding of Care and Support, Documents available at: http://webarchive.nationalarchives.gov.uk/20130221130239/http://dilnotcommission.dh.gov.uk/

Farron, T. (2016) 'An open, tolerant and united Britain', speech made at IPPR: The Progressive Policy Think Tank, 31 August. Available at: https://www.ippr.org/event/tim-farron-an-open-tolerant-and-united-britain

Marmot, M. (2010) *Fair society, healthy lives: The Marmot Review. Strategic review of health inequalities in England post-2010*, London: UCL Institute of Health Equity.

Shuster, S. (2015) 'The populists: Europe is doomed – politically and financially', *Time*. Available at: http://time.com/time-person-of-the-year-populism/

Index

Page references for notes are followed by n

nutrition
  and alcohol use 62
  children 3, 4, 9, 42, 43, 46
  and homelessness 41–9

O

obesity 55, 88–9, 90
  and alcohol use 62
  and homelessness 44
  and physical activity 104
  and sedentary behaviour 105
Oddy, M. 258
offending
  and brain injury 257, 259–62
  and homelessness 196
Office for Civil Society 165
Office for National Statistics (ONS)
  31, 150–1, 181–2
Ohio State University Traumatic Brain
  Injury - Identification 257
Olson, C.M. 45
O'Mara-Eves, A. 153
opiate-using neural pathways 6
opioid replacement therapy 269
Orford, J. 73
Organisation for Economic Co-
  operation and Development
  (OECD) 139–40
Ortiz, I. 325–6

P

Paths for All 97
Pawson, R. 168, 169
Pay to Stay 218, 219
peer involvement 273
  community well-being 153
  educational inequalities 24
  Housing First 200–1, 203–4, 268–9,
    271
People2People 315
Percy-Smith, J. 247
pharmacological interventions 269–70
physical activity (PA) 88–9, 97
  guidelines 93–5
  health benefits 87, 88, 89–90
  international policy 90–3
  measuring 93
  public health and community
    interventions 87–8, 95–7
  see also exercise
physical inactivity (PIA) 29, 88, 89–90
  sedentary behaviour 94, 104–5,
    109–10

Pickett, K. 79
Pitman, I. 261
pleasure 34–5
Poland 140
Poor Law 311–12, 313, 322
Poor Law Amendment Act 1834 311
positive psychology 31
Post-Traumatic Stress Disorder (PTSD)
  xx, 12
poverty 9–10, 274
  and addiction 77–8
  and health outcomes 73
  and homelessness 195, 201–2
prefrontal cortex 6, 75
Private Finance Initiative (PFI)
  housing 215
  NHS 330–1, 333
private goods 121
private rented sector 213–14, 220–1
profound and multiple learning
  disability (PMLD) 136
proportionate universalism 80, 81, 272
prosocial behaviours xix, 7–8
protect-despair-detachment 8
public goods 121
Public Health England
  community well-being 152–4
  The eatwell guide 42
  Healthy Child Programme 26
  homelessness 204
  What Works centres 150
publication bias 157
Pupil Premium (PP) 21–2
Putnam, Robert 33, 123–4, 126

Q

quality of life xix, xxi
Queen's Nursing Institute (QNI) 42,
  44

R

racism 306–7
Raffo, C. 21
RAMESES Project 169
randomised controlled trials (RCTs)
  155–7, 158
realist evaluation and synthesis 119,
  165–75, 237
  added value 174–5
  living history 169–70
  Salvation Army community
    programme 170–5
  terminology 168–9

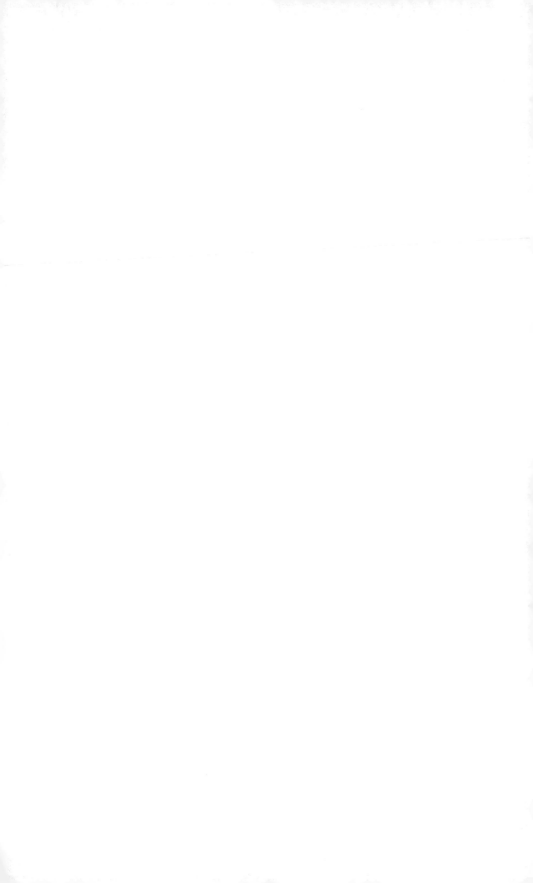

Lightning Source UK Ltd.
Milton Keynes UK
UKHW020654121021
392071UK00003B/169